Eating Disorders in Children and Adolescents

Eating Disorders in Children and Adolescents

Editor: Andrew Gibson

hayle medical

New York

Hayle Medical,
750 Third Avenue, 9th Floor,
New York, NY 10017, USA

Visit us on the World Wide Web at:
www.haylemedical.com

ISBN 978-1-64647-584-1 (Hardback)

Cataloging-in-Publication Data

Eating disorders in children and adolescents / edited by Andrew Gibson.
p. cm.
Includes bibliographical references and index.
ISBN 978-1-64647-584-1
1. Eating disorders in children. 2. Eating disorders in adolescence. 3. Eating disorders.
4. Child psychopathology. 5. Adolescent psychopathology. I. Gibson, Andrew.
RJ506.E18 E28 2023
618.928 526--dc23

Contents

Preface

Eating disorders are a range of psychological disorders related to abnormal eating behaviors that have a negative impact on health. There are several types of eating disorders including anorexia nervosa, bulimia nervosa, binge eating disorder, pica, rumination syndrome, and avoidant/restrictive food intake disorder (ARFID). Bulimia nervosa is a common type of eating disorder that occurs in children and adolescents. It is characterized by recurrent binge episodes of eating a large amount of food followed by purging behaviors such as self-induced vomiting, fasting, and excessive exercise for compensating for the binge behaviors. Doctors usually diagnose the eating disorders by first looking for the signs and symptoms of eating disorders and by evaluating the eating habits of the patient. Based on the preliminary examination, the doctor may perform physical examination, psychological evaluation, blood tests, and urine tests. Cognitive behavioral therapy (CBT) is the most common type of treatment for eating disorders. Antidepressants, hospitalization, and nutrition counseling are some other treatment options. This book unravels the recent studies on eating disorders among children and adolescents. It will serve as a valuable source of reference for graduate and postgraduate students.

After months of intensive research and writing, this book is the end result of all who devoted their time and efforts in the initiation and progress of this book. It will surely be a source of reference in enhancing the required knowledge of the new developments in the area. During the course of developing this book, certain measures such as accuracy, authenticity and research focused analytical studies were given preference in order to produce a comprehensive book in the area of study.

This book would not have been possible without the efforts of the authors and the publisher. I extend my sincere thanks to them. Secondly, I express my gratitude to my family and well-wishers. And most importantly, I thank my students for constantly expressing their willingness and curiosity in enhancing their knowledge in the field, which encourages me to take up further research projects for the advancement of the area.

Editor

1

Associations between symptoms of eating disturbance and frequency of physical activity in a non-clinical, population-based sample of adolescents

Ove Heradstveit[1,2*], Eva Holmelid[3], Helene Klundby[3], Birgitte Søreide[3], Børge Sivertsen[4,5,6] and Liv Sand[1]

Abstract

Background: Physical activity is an important factor related to eating disorders, but the relationship between symptoms of eating disorders and physical activity is multifaceted. The aims of this study were to investigate how symptoms of eating disturbance (ED) were associated with physical activity, and to explore potential sex differences and the potential moderating effects from body mass index (BMI) scores.

Methods: Data stem from a large population-based survey of 10,172 Norwegian adolescents aged 16 to 19 years, the youth@hordaland-survey. The main dependent variable was self-reported number of days with physical activity per week, while the main independent variable was self-reported symptoms of ED using the five-item Eating Disturbance Screening (EDS-5) questionnaire. Control variables included sex, age, socioeconomic status, and BMI.

Results: Girls reported substantially more symptoms of ED compared with boys ($M = 3.02$ versus 1.32, $d = 0.80$, $p < 0.001$), as well as fewer days with physical activity per week ($M = 2.88$ versus 3.46, $d = -0.28$, $p < 0.001$). For both sexes, symptoms of ED were negatively associated with physical activity (adjusted mean differences (adj. mean diff) ranging from −0.03 to −0.08, all $p < 0.05$). Interaction analyses showed, however, that associations between symptoms of ED and physical activity were significantly moderated by BMI scores for both girls ($p < 0.01$) and boys ($p < 0.05$). Specifically, ED symptoms were associated with lower physical activity levels among adolescents with higher BMI scores.

Conclusions: The present study indicates that symptoms of ED were overall negatively associated with physical activity for both sexes during adolescence. However, associations between ED symptoms and physical activity levels differed considerably across the weight spectrum.

Keywords: Eating disturbance, Disordered eating, EDS-5, Physical activity, Population-based study, Sex differences, Correlates, Heterogeneity

Plain english summary

Physical activity is related to eating disorders in multifaceted ways. This study aimed to disentangle how symptoms of eating disturbance (ED) relate to physical activity in a non-clinical, community-based sample. The study also investigated how these associations varied across sexes and across the weight-spectrum. A cross-sectional design was used, employing data from a large, Norwegian population-based study, the youth@hordaland-survey. The study included 10,172 adolescents that all reported symptoms of ED as well as physical activity levels per week. In addition, age, socioeconomic status, and body mass index were included in the analyses as covariates. The study revealed that symptoms of ED were negatively associated with physical activity for both sexes. However, body mass index (BMI) moderated these associations,

* Correspondence: ovhe@norceresearch.no
[1]Regional Centre for Child and Youth Mental Health and Child Welfare, Ove Heradstveit, NORCE Norwegian Research Centre, RKBU, Nygårdsgaten 112, 5008 Bergen, Norway
[2]Center for Alcohol & Drug Research, Stavanger University Hospital, Stavanger, Norway
Full list of author information is available at the end of the article

revealing that ED symptoms were associated with lower physical activity levels specifically among adolescents with higher BMI scores.

Introduction

Although eating disorders are rare in the general population, they are relatively more common among adolescent girls and young women compared with boys and young men [1, 2]. In a large, representative sample of US adolescents aged 13 to 18 years, the lifetime prevalence of anorexia nervosa (AN), bulimia nervosa (BN), and binge-eating disorders (BED) were estimated to be 0.3, 0.9 and 1.6%, respectively [3], with higher prevalence in girls compared with boys [3]. Hence, BED is the most common eating disorder, both in adolescence [3] and adulthood [4]. Importantly, there is a considerable heterogeneity in the symptom expression across different subtypes of eating disorders. Individuals with AN are underweight [5, 6]; individuals with BN have higher body mass index (BMI) than those without any eating disorder [6]; and over 65% of individuals with BED have a BMI > 30 [7].

The link between eating disturbances (ED) and physical activity is well documented (e.g. [8, 9]), and several studies have demonstrated associations between symptoms of eating disorders and excessive exercise (for a review, see [10]). Particularly, high levels of exercise are linked with both AN and BN [11]. One study found that excessive physical activity was highest among those with purging type AN [11], while another study reported the highest levels of compulsive exercise in AN restrictive type [12]. However, weight-related differences may have relevance for physical activity levels, as several studies have demonstrated negative associations between BMI and physical activity [13–15]. BED in females was in one study found to be associated with lower physical activity levels compared with counterparts without the disorder [16]. Another study found that high BMI individuals with BED had significantly lower physical activity levels compared with BMI-matched individuals without BED [17]. On the other hand, a recent study by Barber and colleagues [14] with overweight adults showed low levels of physical activity in this group, while BED symptoms were unrelated to physical activity amongst the overweight individuals. Thus, the literature is inconclusive to whether or not symptoms of eating disorders are independently related to physical activity levels when also weight/BMI is taken into account.

Most previous studies on associations between eating disorders and physical activity have been occupied with excessive or compulsive physical activity. Less attention has been given to how symptoms of eating disorders may also be linked with frequency of physical activity. Moreover, a large proportion of previous studies have used data from clinical samples, in which female patients are overrepresented, and in which eating disorders are often restricted to only include individuals suffering with AN/BN [10]. Only a minority of people who meet stringent diagnostic criteria for eating disorders are, however, seen in mental health care [2], and there is a need to supplement studies based on clinical population with data from more general populations. Although few in number, there are some studies that have explored associations between symptoms of ED and frequency of physical activity employing non-clinical, population-based samples of adolescents. Hay and colleagues [6] found no significant differences in amount of physical activity in adolescents with symptoms of eating disorders compared with the general adolescent population. An interesting, but small study from Gomes and colleagues [18] found that adolescents who exercised regularly showed fewer symptoms of eating disordered behaviors.

The existing scientific knowledge base is also rather scarce in regards to whether associations between symptoms of ED and physical activity differ across sexes, something that was investigated in the present study. Previous publications show that girls more frequently exhibit symptoms of eating disorders [3], and also display lower levels of overall physical activity than boys [19]. In addition, expression of eating disorders may vary across sexes [20, 21], to the extent that it has been suggested that eating disorders differ structurally among boys and girls [21–24]. All these findings highlight the possibility that symptoms of ED may be differentially associated with physical activity among respectively boys and girls.

In the present study, we investigated how symptoms of ED – using the five-item Eating Disturbance Scale (EDS-5) [25] – were associated with frequency of physical activity in a general adolescent population, and to what extent these associations varied across sexes. Importantly, we also analyzed the potential confounding effects from sociodemographic variables and BMI, as well as the potential moderating effects of BMI on the associations between symptoms of ED and physical activity. Based on the previous findings from Gomes and colleagues [18] we hypothesized that total symptoms of ED would be overall negatively associated with frequency of physical activity. However, we expected to find moderating effects from BMI on these associations, as BED has been linked with overweight and lower physical activity [17], while AN has been linked with underweight and excessive exercise [11, 12].

Method

Participants

This study used data from the youth@hordaland survey. This is a total population study aimed at all adolescents in the county of Hordaland born between 1993 and 1995. The aim of the youth@hordaland survey was to obtain information to improve children and adolescents' mental health care, as well as knowledge about life style, school function and family situation. The present study includes data collected in 2012 from the youth@hordaland survey. Ten thousand two hundred fifty-seven adolescents aged 16–18 years answered the questionnaire. As previous studies frequently apply 15 as a lower and 50 as the upper limit of BMI ranges [26], we excluded participants with outlier scores on BMI (< 15 or > 50, $N = 85$), and the final sample therefore comprised 10,172 individuals.

Materials

Eating disturbance (ED) symptoms

In the youth@hordaland survey, the Eating Disorders Scale (EDS-5) was used as a measure of symptoms of ED. The EDS-5 is based on self-report and consists of five questions considering eating, developed by Rosenvinge and colleagues [25]. Although the instrument has not been specifically validated in adolescents, it has shown adequate discriminative validity in detecting symptoms of eating disorders in students (mean age 25.6 years) [25]. Particularly, the EDS-5 score demonstrated high correlations with concern about weight (R = 0.89) and concern about shape (R = 0.85), and also adequate correlations with concern about eating (R = 0.70), dietary restraint (R = 0.61) and overeating/bulimia (R = 0.60) [25].

The EDS-5 items address discontent with own eating habits (item 1), comfort eating (item 2), feelings of guilt related to eating (item 3), strict dieting in order to gain control over eating (item 4), and thoughts of being too fat (item 5). The answers of each item were rated on a Likert scale from 0 ("not true"), 1 ("sometimes true") and 2 ("certainly true"). In order to calculate a total score, we reversed the first item of the EDS-5 questionnaire ("I am satisfied with my eating habits"), which was the only variable in which the response "not true" represented an indication of ED. Other items were indicative of a problem score when the response was "certainly true", for example "I have feelings of guilt related to eating." We then summed the items of each EDS-5 item into a continuous variable for total EDS-5 score, which indicated total levels of ED. The summed variable was used in our analyses as a continuous measure of ED ranging from 0 to 10 ($M = 2.23$, $SD = 0.23$).

The EDS-5 instrument has previously been shown to have a high sensitivity (.90) and specificity (.88) to the fourth edition of the Diagnostic and Statistical Manual for Mental Disorders (DSM-IV) criteria for eating disorders in the general young adult population, while internal reliability analyses showed a Cronbach's alpha of 0.83 [25].

We conducted a principal component analysis on the EDS-5 questionnaire in our sample. This analysis was conducted in order to indicate if symptoms of ED were best represented as a one-factor construct, as well as to evaluate the factor loading of each item. The results from this analysis informed the further operationalization of ED symptoms in this study. We found only one factor with an eigenvalue of 1 or higher, accounting for a total of 52% of the variance for girls and 46% of the variance for boys (Table 1). The factor loadings were overall strong for each of the five items (ranging from 0.60 to 0.84 for girls, and from 0.71 to 0.82 for boys). The only exception was item 1 (discontent with own eating habits) that had a considerably lower factor loading for boys (0.35), and below the threshold of .50 indicated by Hair et al. [27] of being acceptable. In our population, the EDS-5 demonstrated acceptable reliability for girls, measured by an overall Cronbach's Alpha of 0.76. For boys the reliability was somewhat lower for the five-item EDS-5 scale ($\alpha = 0.64$). Therefore, we also constructed a revised EDS total score for boys, which only EDS-items 2, 3, 4 and 5 (item 1 was omitted). This four-item scale performed acceptable for boys ($\alpha = 0.71$), and was used for boys in the secondary analyses.

Physical activity

The youth@hordaland survey included a question to investigate levels of physical activity. Specifically, the adolescents were asked to respond to how many of the past 7 days they engaged in physical activity for at least 60 min. The answers on this item ranged from 0 to 7. A continuous variable spanning from 0 to 7 was constructed ($M = 3.15$, $SD = 0.02$), and was used in all our analyses.

Body mass index (BMI)

Data on height in cm and weight in kg were collected by self-report, and body mass index (BMI) was calculated by dividing the adolescent's weight in kilograms by his/her height in meters squared. We also standardized BMI scores separately for each sex.

Table 1 Principal component analysis of the five items in the EDS-5 questionnaire

	Factor loadings on 1 component	
	Girls ($n = 5266$)	Boys ($n = 4611$)
EDS Item 1	0.68	0.35
EDS Item 2	0.60	0.71
EDS Item 3	0.84	0.82
EDS Item 4	0.67	0.71
EDS Item 5	0.79	0.71
Total variance accounted for by component	51.8	46.0

Eigenvalue for 1 factor: 2.59 for girls, 2.30 for boys

Sociodemographic variables

We collected information on sex and age of the participants from the National Population registry. Socioeconomic status (SES) was measured in the youth@hordaland survey by three separate variables: mother's education, father's education and perceived family financial circumstances. Responses on both the variables of mother's and father's education which were categorized as "primary school", "secondary school" and "college or university" Perceived family financial circumstances (i.e. how well off the adolescent perceived their family to be) were assessed by asking the adolescents about their family financial circumstances compared with most others. The response options were [1] "better financial circumstances", [2] "approximately like most others" and [3] "poorer financial circumstances". The three SES variables were included separately in the regression analyses.

Procedure

The youth@hordaland study is a cross-sectional population-based study carried out during early 2012, and data was collected from adolescents in upper secondary school. The adolescents received information per email and one school hour was used to complete the questionnaires at school. In addition, adolescents not going to school received the questionnaires by mail at their home address, and mental health services and other institutions were contacted to let adolescents from these settings participate. The questionnaires used in the youth@hordaland study were web-based, and electronic informed consent was obtained from all participants. The Regional Committee for Medical Research in Western Norway approved the study.

Design and analyses

First, we conducted descriptive analyses of the sample. We used t-tests for independent samples and Pearson chi-square tests to indicate sex differences in the participants' age, SES, BMI, weekly physical activity levels, and symptoms of ED. In addition, Cohens' d effect size of mean differences across sex were reported where applicable. Second, mean BMI levels were calculated for individuals with problem scores on each of the EDS-items, stratified by sex. Third, linear regression models were conducted for associations between continuous levels of symptoms of ED (i.e. EDS-5 total scores) and mean number of days with physical activity per week, stratified by sex. Specifically, we analyzed the associations between ED symptoms and physical activity in an unadjusted model, and after adjustment for sociodemographic variables and BMI. Finally, we analyzed interactions between ED symptoms and BMI scores for each sex in the linear prediction of physical activity. The results were visualized with margins plot of the predicted number of days with physical activity per week across increasing symptoms of ED stratified by high and low BMI scores. Specifically, symptoms of ED spanned from 0 to 10 on the EDS-5 scale. We used standardized BMI scores, in which low BMI scores were defined as two standard deviations below sex-specific mean and high BMI scores were defined as two standard deviations above the sex-specific mean. All data were analyzed using Stata version 14.

Results

As outlined in Table 2, the sample comprised significantly more girls (52.8%), and girls were slightly older compared with boys (17.45 versus 17.41 years, $d = 0.04$, $p < 0.05$). Girls reported somewhat lower levels of perceived family economic resources ($p < 0.001$) and had significantly lower mean BMI compared with boys (22.58 versus 21.96, $d = -0.17$, $p < 0.001$). Girls also reported lower mean number of days with physical activity per week (3.46 versus 2.88, $d = -0.28$, $p < 0.001$), and had considerably higher mean levels on symptoms of ED compared with boys (3.02 versus 1.32, $d = 0.80$, $p < 0.001$). Figure 1 outlines the distribution of positive scores on each individual EDS-5 item stratified by sex.

As highlighted in Table 3, individuals that reported symptoms of ED had higher mean levels of BMI compared with individuals with non-problem scores in the adolescent sample. This pattern was identified for each of the included EDS-5 items across sex.

Table 4 outlines results from linear regression analyses of associations between symptoms of ED and number of days with physical activity per week. Symptoms of ED were negatively associated with physical activity in unadjusted models for both girls (mean diff. = -0.04, $p < 0.001$) and boys (mean diff. = -0.09, $p < 0.001$), and in the adjusted model accounting for the potential confounding effects from age, SES and BMI, for both girls (adj. mean diff $= -0.03$, $p < 0.05$) and boys (adj. mean diff $= -0.08$, $p < 0.05$). Secondary analyses were conducted for boys with the ED scale that omitted item 1, and the results were very similar to the results using the full EDS-5 scale (not shown).

Moderation analyses showed that the interaction between total symptoms of ED and BMI was significant for both girls ($p < 0.01$) and boys ($p < 0.05$). Figures 2 and 3 illustrate that symptoms of ED were negatively associated with physical activity at the higher end of BMI scores. In addition, ED symptoms among girls in the lower end of BMI showed a tendency of a positive association with physical activity. In secondary analyses, we used the four-item ED symptoms scale for boys, and the interaction between symptoms of ED and physical activity remained significant ($p < 0.01$) (figure not shown).

Table 2 Descriptive characteristics of the sample ($N = 10,172$)

	Girls ($n = 5371$)	Boys ($n = 4801$)	Cohens d	p-value
Sociodemographic variables and BMI				
Sex, N (%)	5371 (52.8)	4801 (47.2)	–	<.001
Age, M (SD)	17.45 (0.85)	17.41 (0.84)	.04	.039
Perceived family economic resources, N (%)			–	<.011
- Poorer financial circumstances	413 (7.9)	289 (6.2)		
- Approximately like most others	3670 (70.1)	2968 (64.0)		
- Better financial circumstances	1150 (22.0)	1378 (29.7)		
Mother's education, N (%)[a]			–	.157
- Primary school	1664 (40.3)	1470 (42.4)		
- Secondary school	447 (10.8)	336 (9.7)		
- University / college	2021 (48.9)	1663 (47.9)		
Father's education, N (%)[b]			–	.272
- Primary school	1786 (45.8)	1670 (47.3)		
- Secondary school	425 (10.9)	367 (10.4)		
- University / college	1688 (43.3)	1496 (42.3)		
Body mass index, M (SD)	21.96 (3.58)	22.58 (3.56)	−.17	<.001
Physical activity				
Mean number of days per week, M (SD)	2.88 (0.03)	3.46 (0.03)	−.28	<.001
Eating disturbance				
EDS-5 total score, M (SD)	3.02 (2.49)	1.32 (1.64)	.80	<.001

[a]Includes only 7.601 individuals, due to $n = 2571$ having answered that they don't know
[b]Includes only 7.432 individuals, due to $n = 2740$ having answered that they don't know

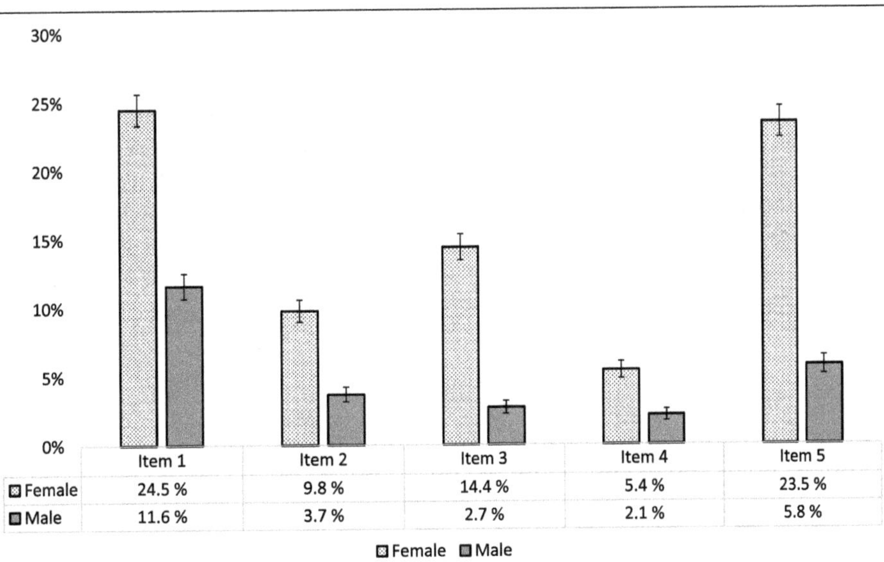

	Item 1	Item 2	Item 3	Item 4	Item 5
Female	24.5 %	9.8 %	14.4 %	5.4 %	23.5 %
Male	11.6 %	3.7 %	2.7 %	2.1 %	5.8 %

Fig. 1 Distribution of positive scores on single symptoms of eating disturbance stratified by sex ($N = 10,172$)[1]. [1] The error bars indicate the 95% confidence interval of each estimate. Includes items 1–5 on the EDS-5 questionaire

Table 3 Mean body mass index levels across problem scores on symptoms of eating disturbance in the sample ($N = 10{,}172$)

	Girls ($n = 5371$) M (SD)	Boys ($n = 4801$) M (SD)
Full sample	22.0 (0.05)	22.6 (0.05)
Item 1: Discontent with own eating habits[a]	22.7 (0.12)[b]	23.4 (0.20)[b]
Item 2: Comfort eating[a]	23.2 (0.20)[b]	24.1 (0.39)[b]
Item 3: Feelings of guilt related to eating[a]	23.1 (0.16)[b]	24.7 (0.48)[b]
Item 4: Strict dieting to gain control over eating[a]	23.1 (0.28)[b]	24.2 (0.53)[b]
Item 5: Thoughts of being too fat[a]	24.2 (0.13)[b]	27.2 (0.30)[b]

[a]Include individuals with problem scores on the indicated EDS-5 item
[b]Problem scores on each of the EDS-5 items were significantly associated ($p < 0.001$) with higher mean BMI compared with non-problem scores

Discussion

The present study demonstrates that despite considerable sex differences in levels of physical activity and symptoms of ED in a general sample of adolescents, associations between symptoms of ED and physical activity were overall similar for boys and girls. For both sexes, symptoms of ED were negatively associated with physical activity. However, these associations were significantly moderated by BMI. Specifically, for adolescents with higher BMI, symptoms of ED were negatively associated with physical activity, while this pattern was not observed for adolescents with lower BMI. On the contrary, symptoms of ED tended to be positively associated with physical activity for girls with lower BMI.

Eating disturbance and physical activity

The findings from the present study underscore the multifaceted relationship between disturbed eating symptoms and physical activity. We found an overall *negative* association between symptoms of ED and physical activity, corresponding with a similar study by Gomes and colleagues [18]. They reported lower levels of ED symptoms in adolescents that were regularly physical active compared with those with lower physical activity. On the other hand, our results provide less support to findings from Hay and colleagues [6] that reported no significant differences in amount of physical activity in adolescents with symptoms of eating disorders compared with the general adolescent population. As BED is the most prevalent eating disorder among adolescents [3], and is related to overweight as well as lower physical activity levels [17], it is possible that BED may account for this negative association entirely. However, our lack of data on specific eating disorders in the sample makes this assumption difficult to validate.

The present study demonstrates that associations between symptoms of ED and physical activity differ considerably across the weight-spectrum. The interaction analyses demonstrated that negative associations between symptoms of ED and physical activity were seen specifically among individuals with high BMI scores. These findings may be interpreted in the context of the large heterogeneity between different types of eating disorders, and their potentially differential associations with physical activity. Previous studies have demonstrated that dietary constraints are often observed in individuals with AN [28] and BN [29], and that higher levels of eating disorder symptoms [11], drive for thinness [30], and body dissatisfaction [30, 31] are other features among eating disordered individuals that are associated with excessive exercise. On the other hand, lower physical activity levels are previously demonstrated in relation to BED for females [16]. The present study adds to this knowledge base by demonstrating that ED was negatively associated with physical activity across sexes, and that BMI scores were an important moderator in the association between symptoms of ED and frequency of physical activity.

As expected from previous findings [3, 19], a range of sex differences were found in both the distribution of physical activity levels, symptoms of ED, and mean BMI scores. Boys had significantly higher frequency of physical activity compared with girls, lower mean symptoms of ED, and a somewhat higher mean BMI. Hence, the present study confirms the need to target girls selectively in interventions aiming at promoting physical activity in

Table 4 Associations between total symptoms of eating disturbance and levels of physical activity ($N = 10{,}172$)[a]

	Girls (n=5,371) Mean diff / adj. mean diff (95% CI)	p-value	Boys (n=4,801)[a] Mean diff / adj. mean diff (95% CI)	p-value
Unadjusted model				
- Symptoms of eating disturbance (ED)	-0.04 (-0.07, -0.02)	<.001	-0.09 (-0.13, -0.04)	<.001
Adjusted model				
- Symptoms of eating disturbance (ED)	-0.03 (-0.05, -0.01)	.049	-0.08 (-0.14, -0.02)	.013
- (+) adjusted for BMI[b]	-0.01 (-0.03, 0.01)	.168	-0.02 (-0.04, 0.01)	.197

[a] Excluding item 1 from total EDS-5 score due to low factor loading of item on eating disturbance concept
[b] The adjustment for BMI follows the additional adjustment for age and socioeconomic status (not shown)

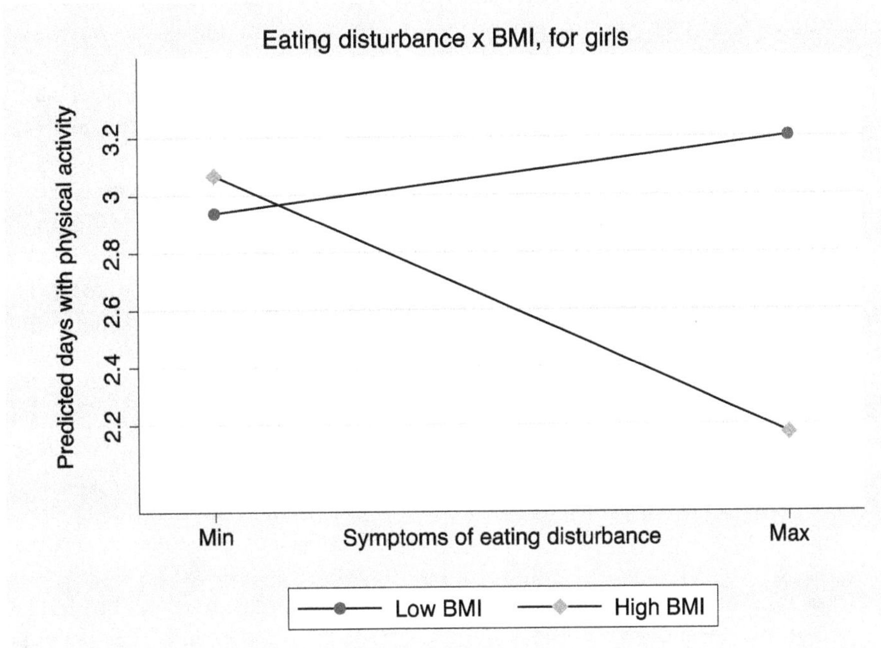

Fig. 2 Number of days with physical activity predicted from symptoms of eating disturbance across BMI scores, for girls ($n = 5371$)[1]. [1] Presents the predicted mean number of days with physical activity from symptoms of eating disturbance, stratified by high versus low BMI scores. Low BMI is defined here as two standard deviations below the sex-specific mean BMI, while high BMI is defined by two standard deviations above the mean BMI

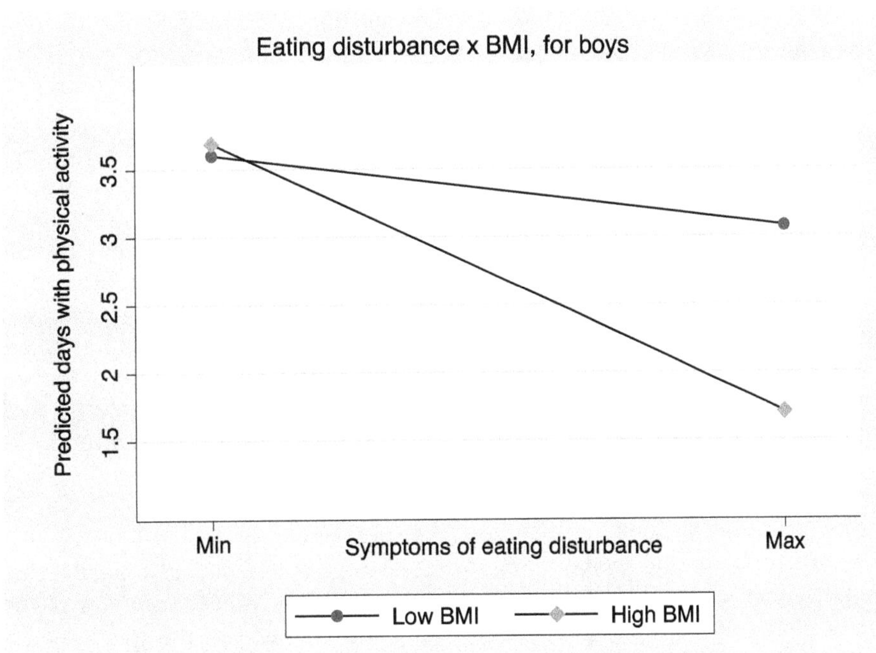

Fig. 3 Number of days with physical activity predicted from symptoms of eating disturbance (EDS-5, full scale) across BMI scores, for boys ($n = 4801$)[1]. [1] Presents the predicted mean number of days with physical activity from symptoms of eating disturbance, stratified by high versus low BMI scores. Low BMI is defined here as two standard deviations below the sex-specific mean BMI, while high BMI is defined by two standard deviations above the mean BMI

adolescents. On the other hand, both boys and girls with high BMI in combination with symptoms of ED had marked lower frequency of physical activity.

Our findings may suggest that symptoms of ED exacerbate sedentary lifestyle problem characterized by a general lack of physical activity among overweight individuals. These findings are aligned with previous studies that reported lower physical activity among individuals with BED [16, 17]. Individuals with BED typically exhibit excessive concerns with their body shape and lack of thinness and spend more time on dieting efforts than healthy controls [32]. Interestingly, all the distinct symptoms of ED included in the present study were associated with higher BMI. Future studies should therefore also investigate how features of eating disorders that correlate with lower BMI are associated with frequency of physical activity in non-clinical, population-based samples.

Strengths and limitations

A considerable strength of the present study is the application of a large, population-based sample. These data provided a promising approach to disentangle the multifaceted relationship between symptoms of eating disorders and physical activity in samples that is not biased by selection into mental health services [2]. Sex-specific analyses add as another strength of the study. We included frequency of physical activity as our outcome measure, something that seem important in light of previous literature that demonstrate significant links between symptoms of eating disorders and physical activity in both ends of the physical activity continuum. In addition, we adjusted our analyses for BMI, something that is useful in light of the likely correlation between BMI and physical activity levels [13–15]. Not least, BMI scores were also used in moderation analyses, highlighting the important role of weight characteristics in associations between symptoms of ED and frequency of physical activity.

The present study also has some limitations. First, the EDS-5 questionnaire applied in the present study is highly correlated with DSM-IV-defined eating disorders [25], but do not imply the presence of eating disorder diagnoses. Although the EDS-5 scale has been validated among young adults [25], there is still a need for studies that provide firm support of the suitability of the questionnaire in even younger adolescent populations. A principal component analysis of the five items in the EDS-5 in our sample supported a one-factor model of ED for both sexes, and the reliability of the five-factor scale were acceptable for girls, while the reliability was lower for boys. However, a four-item scale for symptoms of ED in boys (omitting item 1 from the EDS-5), provided an acceptable reliability, and supported the findings from analyses done with the full EDS-5 scale. Future studies should aim to replicate our findings using more rigorous measures of ED. Moreover, all the single symptoms of ED were associated with higher BMI and it is likely that they primarily represent non-restrictive patterns of eating disturbances. Thus, there is a need for future investigations into associations between specific symptoms of ED and physical activity that apply comprehensive measures of symptoms of ED including restrictive psychopathology. Second, the study has a cross-sectional design and we cannot conclude the directionality of the associations between symptoms of ED and physical activity. It is likely that physical activity levels as well as other lifestyle factors are reciprocally associated with symptoms of ED, and longitudinal studies on this subject are needed. Third, we only used one self-reported measure of weekly frequency of physical activity, in which the subjects reported days with physical activity "at least 60 minutes" per day. Some adolescents may exercise regularly but for shorter periods than an hour. In addition, girls may potentially be more reluctant to endorse that they were physically active over this cut-off compared with boys. Furthermore, we did not have any possibility to evaluate the quality of physical activity. More comprehensive physical activity instruments assessing both the frequency, duration and intensity of physical activity would have added strength to our findings. Associations between ED and the quality and character of exercise remain to be studied in large, population-based samples of adolescents.

Implications

The present study highlight the importance of being aware of reduced levels of physical activity among adolescents with symptoms of ED, specifically in the higher end of the weight-spectrum. The literature has previously highlighted that excessive physical activity is an important correlate of ED, as it can be viewed as a risk- and maintaining factor [31], as well as a symptom of some types of eating disorders [5]. The present study adds to this knowledge base, supporting previous findings that also pointed to low physical activity as a correlate of ED [16, 18].

Conclusions

The present study underscores the close relationship between symptoms of ED and low physical activity among adolescents, and that this was moderated by BMI.

Abbreviations

BMI: Body mass index; DSM-IV: Diagnostic and Statistical Manual of Mental Disorders, fourth edition; ED: Eating disturbance; EDS-5: Five-item Eating Disturbance Screening questionnaire; SES: Socioeconomic status

Acknowledgements
We thank Regional Centre for Child and Youth Mental Health and Child Welfare at NORCE Norwegian Research Centre for making the collection of data, and making the data available for this study.

Authors' contributions
OH analyzed and interpreted the data, and wrote the manuscript. EH, HK and BSø wrote an early version of the manuscript and were involved in the conduct of the statistical analyses. LS were involved in planning the study and in revising the manuscript. BSi was involved in statistical analyses and revising the manuscript. All authors read and approved the final manuscript.

Competing interests
The authors declare that they have no competing interests.

Author details
[1]Regional Centre for Child and Youth Mental Health and Child Welfare, Ove Heradstveit, NORCE Norwegian Research Centre, RKBU, Nygårdsgaten 112, 5008 Bergen, Norway. [2]Center for Alcohol & Drug Research, Stavanger University Hospital, Stavanger, Norway. [3]Faculty of Psychology, University of Bergen, Bergen, Norway. [4]Department of Health Promotion, Norwegian Institute of Public Health, Bergen, Norway. [5]Department of Research & Innovation, Helse Fonna HF, Haugesund, Norway. [6]Department of Mental Health, Norwegian University of Science and Technology, Trondheim, Norway.

References
1. Murnen SK, Smolak L. Gender and Eating Disorders. The Wiley Handbook of Eating Disorders. Chichester: Wiley; 2015. p. 352-366.
2. Hoek HW, Van Hoeken D. Review of the prevalence and incidence of eating disorders. Int J Eat Disord. 2003;34(4):383–96.
3. Swanson SA, Crow SJ, Le Grange D, Swendsen J, Merikangas KR. Prevalence and correlates of eating disorders in adolescents: results from the national comorbidity survey replication adolescent supplement. Arch Gen Psychiatry. 2011;68(7):714–23.
4. Hudson JI, Hiripi E, Pope HG Jr, Kessler RC. The prevalence and correlates of eating disorders in the National Comorbidity Survey Replication. Biol Psychiatry. 2007;61(3):348–58.
5. American Psychiatric Association. Feeding and eating disorders. Diagnostic and statistical manual of mental disorders. 5th ed. Washington, DC: American Psychiatric Publishing; 2013.
6. Hay P, Mitchison D, Collado AEL, González-Chica DA, Stocks N, Touyz S. Burden and health-related quality of life of eating disorders, including avoidant/restrictive food intake disorder (ARFID), in the Australian population. J Eat Disord. 2017;5(1):21.
7. Yager J. Binge eating disorder: the search for better treatments. Focus. 2009; 7(4):499–501.
8. Davis C, Katzman DK, Kirsh C. Compulsive physical activity in adolescents with anorexia nervosa: a psychobehavioral spiral of pathology. J Nerv Ment Dis. 1999;187(6):336–42.
9. Peñas-Lledó E, Vaz Leal FJ, Waller G. Excessive exercise in anorexia nervosa and bulimia nervosa: relation to eating characteristics and general psychopathology. Int J Eat Disord. 2002;31(4):370–5.
10. Meyer C, Taranis L, Goodwin H, Haycraft E. Compulsive exercise and eating disorders. Eur Eat Disord Rev. 2011;19(3):174–89.
11. Shroff H, Reba L, Thornton LM, Tozzi F, Klump KL, Berrettini WH, et al. Features associated with excessive exercise in women with eating disorders. Int J Eat Disord. 2006;39(6):454–61.
12. Dalle Grave R, Calugi S, Marchesini G. Compulsive exercise to control shape or weight in eating disorders: prevalence, associated features, and treatment outcome. Compr Psychiatry. 2008;49(4):346–52.
13. Sallis JF, Prochaska JJ, Taylor WC. A review of correlates of physical activity of children and adolescents. Med Sci Sports Exerc. 2000;32(5):963–75.
14. Barber J, Ivezaj V, Barnes R. Comparing physical activity in individuals with overweight/obesity with and without binge eating disorder. Obes Sci Pract. 2018;4(2):134 40.
15. Stovitz SD, Steffen LM, Boostrom A. Participation in physical activity among Normal-and overweight Hispanic and non-Hispanic White adolescents. J Sch Health. 2008;78(1):19–25.
16. Crandall KJ, Eisenman PA, Ransdell L, Reel J. Exploring binge eating and physical activity among community-dwelling women. Int J Psychol Behav Sci. 2011;1(1):1–8.
17. Vancampfort D, De Herdt A, Vanderlinden J, Lannoo M, Soundy A, Pieters G, et al. Health related quality of life, physical fitness and physical activity participation in treatment-seeking obese persons with and without binge eating disorder. Psychiatry Res. 2014;216(1):97–102.
18. Gomes R, Gonçalves S, Costa J. Exercise, eating disordered behaviors and psychological well-being: a study with Portuguese adolescents. Revista Latinoamericana de Psicología. 2015;47(1):66–74.
19. Vilhjalmsson R, Kristjansdottir G. Gender differences in physical activity in older children and adolescents: the central role of organized sport. Soc Sci Med. 2003;56(2):363–74.
20. McCreary DR, Sasse DK. An exploration of the drive for muscularity in adolescent boys and girls. J Am Coll Heal. 2000;48(6):297–304.
21. Anderson CB, Bulik CM. Gender differences in compensatory behaviors, weight and shape salience, and drive for thinness. Eat Behav. 2004;5(1):1–11.
22. Furnham A, Badmin N, Sneade I. Body image dissatisfaction: gender differences in eating attitudes, self-esteem, and reasons for exercise. J Psychol. 2002;136(6):581–96.
23. Strong SM, Williamson DA, Netemeyer RG, Geer JH. Eating disorder symptoms and concerns about body differ as a function of gender and sexual orientation. J Soc Clin Psychol. 2000;19(2):240–55.
24. Striegel-Moore RH, Rosselli F, Perrin N, DeBar L, Wilson GT, May A, et al. Gender difference in the prevalence of eating disorder symptoms. Int J Eat Disord. 2009;42(5):471–4.
25. Rosenvinge JH, Perry JA, Bjørgum L, Bergersen TD, Silvera DH, Holte A. A new instrument measuring disturbed eating patterns in community populations: development and initial validation of a five-item scale (EDS-5). Eur Eat Disord Rev. 2001;9(2):123–32.
26. Flegal KM, Kit BK, Graubard BI. Body mass index categories in observational studies of weight and risk of death. Am J Epidemiol. 2014;180(3):288–96.
27. Hair J, Black W, Babin B, Anderson R. Multivariate Data Analysis. 7th Edition ed. Essex: Pearson Education Limited; 2014.
28. Fairburn CG. Eating disorders. e LS; 2001.
29. Steiger H, Lehoux PM, Gauvin L. Impulsivity, dietary control and the urge to binge in bulimic syndromes. Int J Eat Disord. 1999;26(3):261–74.
30. Solenberger SE. Exercise and eating disorders: a 3-year inpatient hospital record analysis. Eat Behav. 2001;2(2):151–68.
31. Brewerton TD, Stellefson EJ, Hibbs N, Hodges EL, Cochrane CE. Comparison of eating disorder patients with and without compulsive exercising. Int J Eat Disord. 1995;17(4):413–6.
32. Grilo CM, White MA, Masheb RM. DSM-IV psychiatric disorder comorbidity and its correlates in binge eating disorder. Int J Eat Disord. 2009;42(3):228–34.

2

Canadian practice guidelines for the treatment of children and adolescents with eating disorders

Jennifer Couturier[1*], Leanna Isserlin[2], Mark Norris[2], Wendy Spettigue[2], Melissa Brouwers[2], Melissa Kimber[1], Gail McVey[3], Cheryl Webb[1], Sheri Findlay[1], Neera Bhatnagar[1], Natasha Snelgrove[1], Amanda Ritsma[1], Wendy Preskow[4], Catherine Miller[5], Jennifer Coelho[6], Ahmed Boachie[3], Cathleen Steinegger[3], Rachel Loewen[7], Techiya Loewen[8], Elizabeth Waite[8], Catherine Ford[9], Kerry Bourret[10], Joanne Gusella[11], Josie Geller[6], Adele LaFrance[12], Anick LeClerc[13], Jennifer Scarborough[5], Seena Grewal[3], Monique Jericho[14], Gina Dimitropoulos[14] and David Pilon[11]

Abstract

Objectives: Eating disorders are common and serious conditions affecting up to 4% of the population. The mortality rate is high. Despite the seriousness and prevalence of eating disorders in children and adolescents, no Canadian practice guidelines exist to facilitate treatment decisions. This leaves clinicians without any guidance as to which treatment they should use. Our objective was to produce such a guideline.

Methods: Using systematic review, the Grading of Recommendations Assessment, Development, and Evaluation (GRADE) system, and the assembly of a panel of diverse stakeholders from across the country, we developed high quality treatment guidelines that are focused on interventions for children and adolescents with eating disorders.

Results: Strong recommendations were supported specifically in favour of Family-Based Treatment, and more generally in terms of least intensive treatment environment. Weak recommendations in favour of Multi-Family Therapy, Cognitive Behavioural Therapy, Adolescent Focused Psychotherapy, adjunctive Yoga and atypical antipsychotics were confirmed.

Conclusions: Several gaps for future work were identified including enhanced research efforts on new primary and adjunctive treatments in order to address severe eating disorders and complex co-morbidities.

Keywords: Guidelines, Adolescent, Anorexia nervosa, Bulimia nervosa, Avoidant/restrictive food intake disorder

Plain English summary

The objective of this project was to develop Canadian Practice Guidelines for the treatment of children and adolescents with eating disorders. We reviewed the literature for relevant studies, rated the quality of the scientific information within these studies, and then reviewed this information with a panel of clinicians, researchers, parents and those with lived experience from across the country. The panel came up with a list of recommendations regarding specific treatments. These recommendations included strong recommendations for the provision of Family-Based Treatment, as well as care provided in a least intensive environment. Weak recommendations were determined for Multi-Family Therapy, Cognitive Behavioural Therapy, Adolescent Focused Psychotherapy, adjunctive Yoga, and atypical antipsychotics. The panel also identified several areas for future research including the development of new treatments for severe and complex eating disorders.

* Correspondence: coutur@mcmaster.ca
[1]McMaster University, Hamilton, Canada
Full list of author information is available at the end of the article

Introduction

Eating disorders are common and serious conditions affecting up to 4% of the population [1]. The mortality rate, particularly for Anorexia Nervosa (AN) is high [2, 3], and has been shown to increase by 5.6% for each decade that an individual remains ill [4, 5]. It is well-documented that interventions targeted at earlier stages of illness are critically important, given the evidence showing that earlier treatment leads to better outcomes [6, 7]. Despite the seriousness and prevalence of eating disorders in children and adolescents, no Canadian practice guidelines exist to facilitate treatment decisions. This leaves clinicians without any guidance as to which treatment they should use. We systematically reviewed and synthesized the knowledge available on treatments for children and adolescents with eating disorders to develop our guidelines.

Review of existing guidelines

In the United States, practice parameters have been published by the American Academy of Child and Adolescent Psychiatry for youth with eating disorders [8]. These parameters reflect good clinical practice rather than making statements as to the strength of the evidence to support the recommendations. Clinical practice guidelines have also been developed by the National Institute of Health and Care Excellence [9], however, grading of the evidence is also not presented in these guidelines. The Academy for Eating Disorders has also published guidelines on their website that focus on medical management, but do not focus on psychotherapeutic/psychopharmacological interventions, nor the strength of the evidence (http://aedweb.org/web/downloads/Guide-English.pdf). In summary, guidelines that are currently available tend to focus on medical stabilization, and neglect psychotherapeutic/psychopharmacological approaches to treating eating disorders. Furthermore, they do not rate the strength of evidence. No Canadian guidelines focused on eating disorders in the pediatric age group exist.

Objectives

Our aim was to synthesize the best available evidence on treatments for children and adolescents with eating disorders resulting in the production of a practice guideline. The research questions to drive this knowledge synthesis were discussed by our research team and guideline development panel, and are listed below.

Research questions

What are the best treatments available for children and adolescents diagnosed with eating disorders?

a) How effective is Family-Based Treatment for Anorexia Nervosa?
b) How effective is Family-Based Treatment for Bulimia Nervosa?
c) How effective is Cognitive Behavioural Therapy for Bulimia Nervosa?
d) How effective is Dialectical Behaviour Therapy for Bulimia Nervosa?
e) How effective are Atypical Antipsychotics for Anorexia Nervosa?
f) How effective are Selective Serotonin Reuptake Inhibitors for Bulimia Nervosa?
g) How effective is day treatment for any type of eating disorder?
h) How effective is inpatient treatment for any type of eating disorder?

Methods

Overview

We used systematic review of the literature to arrive at a knowledge synthesis of the best treatments for children and adolescents with eating disorders. This was followed by a grading of the evidence using the Grading of Recommendations Assessment, Development, and Evaluation (GRADE) system [10–12]. These evidence profiles were then presented to a panel of stakeholders from across Canada, followed by a voting system and arrival at consensus on the recommendations. The Appraisal of Guidelines, Research, and Evaluation (AGREE II) tool was used to inform guideline development and reporting [13].

Synthesis methods

Eligibility criteria

Following the principles outlined in the Cochrane Reviewer's Handbook [14] and the Users' Guides to Medical Literature [15], our inclusion criteria were:

A) Criteria pertaining to study validity: i) meta-analyses, randomized controlled trials, open trials, case series, and case reports,
B) Criteria pertaining to the subjects: i) involving children and adolescents (under age 18 years), ii) with eating disorders (Anorexia Nervosa, Bulimia Nervosa, Eating Disorder Not Otherwise Specified, Other Specified Feeding and Eating Disorder, Avoidant/Restrictive Food Intake Disorder, Binge Eating Disorder),
C) Criteria pertaining to the intervention: i) focusing on treatments including, but not limited to, Family-Based Treatment, Cognitive Behavioural Therapy, Dialectical Behavioural Therapy, Atypical Antipsychotics, Selective Serotonin Reuptake Inhibitors, Day Treatment, and Inpatient Treatment,
D) Criteria pertaining to the Outcome: i) weight (along with variants of weight such as BMI, treatment goal weight (TGW), etc.), ii) binge/purge frequency, iii) psychological symptoms such as drive for thinness, weight/shape preoccupation, and
E) Articles written in any language.

Exclusion criteria included: i) studies involving primarily adults (18 years or above), ii) studies focusing on medical management, iii) studies focusing on medical outcomes such as bone density, heart rate, iv) studies examining medical treatments such as hormone therapy, calcium, nutrition therapy, v) studies examining other medications. These exclusion criteria were developed for several reasons. We wanted to focus on treatments that were psychopharmacological and psychological in nature, along with outcomes that were central to the core features of eating disorders. We were trying to keep things as simple as possible when thinking of outcomes, especially with the goal of trying to combine studies in a narrative summary or even in a meta-analysis if possible. We focused on a couple of core outcomes with these goals in mind, so therefore excluded papers focusing on other physical outcomes (although these outcomes may indeed be related to weight status).

Identifying potentially eligible studies

Databases

A literature search was completed using the following databases: Medline, PsycINFO, EMBASE, Cochrane Database of Systematic Reviews, Cochrane Central Register of Controlled Trials (CENTRAL) and CINAHL. The references of relevant articles obtained were also reviewed. This was an iterative process, such that search terms were added based on developing ideas and articles obtained.

Literature search strategy

Initially, an environmental scan of existing guidelines for children and adolescents with eating disorders was completed by the core research team using search terms "guidelines" and "eating disorders" in children and adolescents. Our library scientist then designed and executed comprehensive searches in the databases listed above to obtain evidence to align with each of the guideline questions. The searches included a combination of appropriate keyword and subject heading for each concept. The sample search strategy included, but was not limited to, various combinations of the following terms as appropriate for the questions being addressed: Anorexia nervosa OR bulimia nervosa OR eating disorder not otherwise specified OR other specified feeding and eating disorder OR avoidant/restrictive food intake disorder; AND family-based treatment OR cognitive behavioural therapy OR dialectical behavioural therapy OR atypical antipsychotics OR selective serotonin reuptake inhibitors OR day treatment OR day hospital OR inpatient treatment. The search string was developed further and was modified for each database as appropriate. The search strategy was completed in August 2016. The screening and reviewing process then ensued. Some treatments emerged as important through our search strategy that were not initially identified by our research team and guideline panel as interventions to evaluate. We later included these treatments through panel discussions.

Forward citation chaining

In November 2018 we used a forward citation chaining process to search each included article to see if it had been cited by any additional articles since August 2016 up until November 2018. We then screened the newly found articles to decide whether to include them. The forward chaining process involved the use of Google Scholar to locate all articles citing our included articles from the primary search.

Other strategies

Grey literature was also reviewed, including conference proceedings from the International Conference on Eating Disorders dating back the last 10 years (2008–2018). Databases of ongoing research were searched including The Cochrane Central Register of Controlled Trials (CENTRAL). We also hand searched the International Journal of Eating Disorders from the last 10 years for relevant articles (2008–2018).

Applying eligibility criteria and extracting data

Two team members independently evaluated the results generated by our searches and came to consensus on which studies met eligibility criteria. We used the software Endnote and DistillerSR to organize our studies. DistillerSR was used for article screening and data extraction. Duplicate records identifying the same study were removed. Titles and abstracts were used to exclude obviously irrelevant reports by two reviewers. Potentially relevant articles were reviewed in full text by two reviewers who had to agree on inclusion, with a third resolving disputes. Authors of publications were contacted if any ambiguity existed about inclusion or exclusion. Data abstraction included the number of subjects, sex and/or gender of subjects, age range, type of treatment, type of control group if any, methodology (blinding, allocation concealment, intent-to-treat analysis), types of outcomes, and results. Sex was defined as biological sex, categorized into male or female. Gender was defined as the individual's self-identified gender role/identity, categorized as girl, boy, or transgendered.

Appraising studies

The Grading of Recommendations Assessment, Development, and Evaluation (GRADE) system explicitly describes how to rate the quality of each study, as well as how to synthesize the evidence and grade the strength of a recommendation [10–12]. Using this system, we developed an evidence profile of each included study that detailed all of the relevant data about the quality and strength of evidence for that particular study. Each evidence profile was created using GRADEpro software. We then used the GRADE system to synthesize and classify the overall quality of evidence for each intervention based on the quality of all of the studies using that intervention combined, taking into account risk of bias, inconsistency, indirectness, imprecision, publication bias, dose-response, and effect size. Although we looked at each outcome independently, when the rating of the evidence was the same, we collapsed the outcomes in the GRADEpro tables for the sake of efficiency.

Guideline-related frameworks

The Appraisal of Guidelines, Research, and Evaluation (AGREE II) tool is an international standard of practice guideline evaluation that was used to inform our guideline development and reporting, and was developed by a co-author (MB) [13]. The Guideline Implementability for Decision Excellence Model (GUIDE-M) is a recent model that identifies factors to create recommendations that are optimally implementable [16]. We used these models to guide our methodological processes in the development of our practice guideline.

The guideline team

The Guideline Team was comprised of a core research team and a larger guideline development panel (GDP). The core team presented the research questions to the GDP, reviewed evidence summaries, formulated practice recommendations, drafted the guideline, and limited biases that could impeach upon the guideline development process [17–19]. The chair of the GDP (MB) is an expert in guideline development having produced the AGREE framework [13]. She is a non-expert in the field of eating disorders, and as such, was an impartial chair. She led the consensus discussions of the GDP and she oversaw conflict-of-interest disclosures and management. A multidisciplinary GDP of 24 diverse stakeholders from across Canada was established including members from academic centres who are experts in the field of eating disorders, multi-disciplinary front-line clinicians/knowledge users from community settings, parent and patient representatives, hospital administrators, and policy-makers (all authors on this guideline).

Procedures

An initial teleconference was held on May 18, 2016 with the core research team and the GDP to confirm the research questions prior to starting the systematic reviews. The initial teleconference oriented GDP members to the guideline development process, the roles and responsibilities of the GDP, as well as reviewed all conflicts of interest. The research questions were refined, the clinical population and outcomes were discussed, and the target audience reviewed.

Once the reviews were completed and the evidence profiles were generated, an in-person meeting was held at a central location on December 20, 2018. The core research team presented their evidence profiles for discussion with the GDP. The in-person meeting focused on a facilitated discussion of the evidence profiles and draft recommendations generated by the core team. For each question, the panel reviewed the evidence, and discussed: i) whether the interpretation of the evidence put forward by the core team aligned with that of the GDP, ii) strengths and limitations of the evidence base, iii) considerations of the generalizability of the studies, precision of the estimates, and whether the evidence aligned with values and preferences of Canadian patients and clinicians. Alternative interpretations and suggestions for further research were discussed. Minority or dissenting opinions were noted. Issues regarding implementability of the recommendations were considered, and suggestions for dissemination of the guideline were elicited.

Following the in-person meeting, GDP members were provided with the draft guidelines for review and approval. Group consensus on recommendations and strength of recommendations was obtained using a modified Delphi method [20], with voting by all GDP members using an anonymous web-based survey platform, Lime Survey (www.limesurvey.com). For a recommendation to be approved, at least 70% of the GDP were required to identify their agreement with the recommendation [12]. Consensus was achieved in the first round of voting. The GDP agreed to review and update the guideline every 5 years.

External review

The purpose of the external review was to add validity to our guideline, but also initiate the dissemination process and elicit suggestions for dissemination and implementation. We invited review from four clinical and research experts in the area of pediatric eating disorders. Upon receiving external review, a summary of the review comments and suggestions was circulated to the GDP, along with a final version of the guideline for approval. The panel again discussed and voted on the changes suggested by the reviewers which included the addition of one further recommendation.

Results

Family therapy

Three thousand, five hundred and twenty-two abstracts were identified for review within the family therapy section of our guideline (see PRISMA flow diagram, Fig. 1). Nineteen additional abstracts were identified through citation chaining (up to November 23, 2018) and review of reference lists. Two additional papers were identified through external review. After duplicates were removed, abstracts screened, and full text articles reviewed, 74

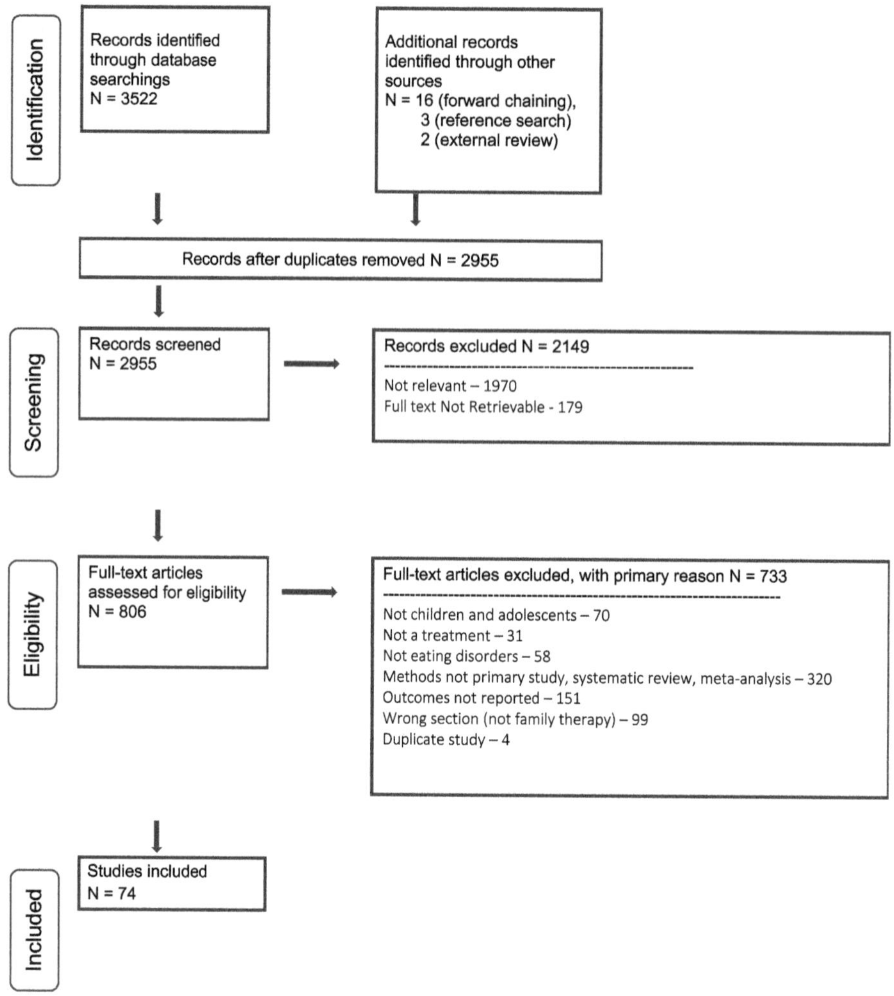

Fig. 1 PRISMA flow diagram for family therapy

studies were included within the family therapy section of our guideline.

Family-based treatment

Anorexia nervosa Of all treatments examined, Family-Based Treatment (FBT), in which parents are placed in charge of the refeeding process, had the most evidence to support its use in children and adolescents with Anorexia Nervosa (AN). One meta-analysis [21] and three high quality RCTs have demonstrated that greater weight gain and higher remission rates are achieved in FBT compared to individual treatment, especially when looking at 1 year follow up [6, 22, 23] (Table 1). One RCT compared a similar behavioural family systems therapy to Cognitive Behavioural Therapy (CBT) and found no significant differences [24], however the sample size was small (Table 1).

In terms of nonrandomized studies, a case-control study of 34 patients treated with FBT compared to 14 treated with "nonspecific therapy" indicated that those in FBT made greater gains in body weight and were less likely to be hospitalized [25]. Seven case series (223 patients) also showed improvement in weight following treatment with FBT [26–32]. Eleven additional case reports (number of total patients = 29) are described showing benefit of FBT in terms of weight gain [33, 35–38, 40–44]. Some of these focus on twins [35, 42, 44], comorbid conversion disorder [43], FBT in a group home setting [38], FBT started on a medical unit [39], and FBT combined with medication [42].

Parent-Focused Family Therapy; a type of FBT in which most of the session is spent with the parents alone, may be just as effective as traditional FBT where the family is seen together [45–47] (Table 2).

Bulimia nervosa Three high quality RCTs for Bulimia Nervosa (BN) have been completed and compared FBT

Table 1 Family-based treatment – anorexia nervosa

Certainty assessment							Impact	Certainty	Importance
№ of studies	Study design	Risk of bias	Inconsistency	Indirectness	Imprecision	Other considerations			
FBT vs supportive/dynamic individual– outcomes - Remission (assessed with: attaining target weight, good outcome category) Weight gain									
3	randomised trials	not serious	not serious	not serious	not serious	none	One meta-analysis indicated superiority of FBT at 6- and 12- month follow up. Three RCTs 43/90 (47.8%) with good outcome or in full remission with FBT, compared to 26/89 (29.2%) in Individual group. Total $n = 179$.	⊕⊕⊕⊕ HIGH	CRITICAL
		not serious	not serious	not serious	not serious	none	Weight gain greater in the FBT group compared to individual therapy group at end of treatment.	⊕⊕⊕⊕ HIGH	CRITICAL
RCT (FBT vs CBT) Remission/Good Outcome (assessed with: Morgan Russell Scale)									
1	randomised trials	not serious	not serious	not serious	not serious	none	7/13 (53.8%) had a good outcome in FBT group vs. 7/12 (58.3%) in the CBT group. No significant difference.	⊕⊕⊕⊕ HIGH	CRITICAL
Weight Gain (assessed with: kg and %IBW)									
1	Case control	serious [b]	not serious	not serious	not serious	none	One case control retrospective chart review. 32 treated with FBT model compared to 14 in nonspecific therapy. Those in FBT made greater gains in weight.	⊕◯◯◯ VERY LOW	CRITICAL
Weight (assessed with: kg)									
7	Case series	very serious [a,b]	not serious	not serious	not serious	none	7 large case series (total $n = 223$). Of these, 32 were children under age 13. Weight was significantly improved, pre to post.	⊕◯◯◯ VERY LOW	CRITICAL
Weight (assessed with: kg)									
11	Case reports	very serious [a,b]	not serious	not serious	not serious	none	11 case reports detailing 29 patients who restored weight with FBT. Some described twins, comorbid conversion disorder, FBT within a group home setting, or FBT starting on a medical unit or use of FBT combined with medication.	⊕◯◯◯ VERY LOW	CRITICAL

Bibliography:
RCTs - Russell 1987 [6], Lock 2010 [23], Robin 1999 [22] (compared to psychodynamic individual)
RCT – Ball 2004 [24] (compared to CBT)
Case Control -Gusella 2017 [25]
Case Series - Paulson-Karlsson 2009 [26], Lock 2006 [27], Le Grange 2005 [28], Loeb 2007 [29], Goldstein 2016 [30], Couturier 2010 [31], Herscovici 1996 [32]
Case Reports – Le Grange 1999 [33], Le Grange 2003 [34], Loeb 2009 [35], Sim 2004 [36], Krautter 2004 [37], Aspen 2014 [38], Matthews 2016 [39], Turkiewicz 2010 [40], O'Neil 2012 [41], Duvvuri 2012 [42], Goldstein 2013[43]

Table 2 Parent focused FBT compared to standard FBT for children and adolescents with anorexia nervosa

Certainty assessment							Impact	Certainty	Importance
№ of studies	Study design	Risk of bias	Inconsistency	Indirectness	Imprecision	Other considerations			
Remission (assessed with: Weight greater than 95% and EDE score within 1 SD), Weight (kg), Psychological symptoms (EDI score)									
3	Randomized Trials	not serious	not serious	not serious	not serious	none	one RCT ($n = 107$) adolescents aged 12–18. Remission higher in Separated FBT (43% vs. 22%) compared to Standard FBT at end of treatment.	⊕⊕⊕⊕ HIGH	CRITICAL
		not serious	not serious	not serious	not serious	none	one RCT ($n = 40$), found no differences in weight outcome at end of treatment, except when subgroups analyzed. Those with high expressed emotion did better in separated family therapy in terms of weight gain. One pilot RCT ($n = 18$) found no differences in weight outcome at the end of treatment; both groups improved.	⊕⊕⊕⊕ HIGH	CRITICAL
		not serious	not serious	not serious	not serious	none	Improvement in EDI score was greater in the standard FBT group compared to the separated group. One pilot RCT ($n = 18$) found both groups improved in EAT scores with no difference between groups.	⊕⊕⊕⊕ HIGH	CRITICAL

Bibliography:
RCTs - Eisler 2000 [45], Le Grange 1992 [47], Le Grange 2016 [46]

to varying groups [48–50]. When FBT was compared to CBT, remission rates were significantly higher in the FBT group (39% versus 20%) [50]. Remission rates were also significantly better in the FBT group compared to supportive psychotherapy (39% versus 18%)[48]. However, when family therapy (with some elements consistent with FBT) was compared to guided self-help CBT, there were no significant differences (10% versus 14%) [49]. The adolescents in this study were slightly older and had the option to involve a "close other" rather than a parent, which may have resulted in lower remission rates. A case series and case report also support the use of FBT for BN [34, 51] (Table 3).

Family-based treatment with other populations

Family-Based Treatment has been used for children and adolescents with atypical AN [52]. This case series of 42 adolescents who were not underweight but had lost a significant amount of weight, indicated that there were significant improvements in eating disorder and depressive symptoms, but no improvement in self-esteem (Table 4).

Two case reports describe the application of FBT for children with Avoidant/Restrictive Food Intake Disorder (ARFID) [53, 54]. These case reports ($n = 7$ cases total) indicate that weight improved in all cases (Table 4).

Family-Based Treatment and other family therapies for children and adolescents with eating disorders across the gender spectrum, including those who are gender variant or nonconforming requires more study. However, there is one case report describing the application of FBT with a transgendered youth, along with complexities that arose [55] (Table 4).

Adaptations to family-based treatment for anorexia nervosa

Adaptations to FBT, such as shorter or longer treatment [56], removal of the family meal [57], guided self-help [58], parent to parent consult [59], adaptive FBT involving extra sessions and another family meal [60], short term intensive formats [61, 62] and delivery of FBT by telehealth [63, 64], appear promising, but require more study (Table 5).

Adjuncts to family-based treatment for anorexia nervosa

Adjuncts to FBT, in which additional treatments have been added to FBT, such as cognitive remediation therapy versus art therapy [65], parental skills workshops [66] and Dialectical Behavioural Therapy (DBT) [67] for

Table 3 Family-based treatment for bulimia nervosa

Certainty assessment							Impact	Certainty	Importance
№ of studies	Study design	Risk of bias	Inconsistency	Indirectness	Imprecision	Other considerations			
Remission (assessed with: Abstinence from binge or purge behaviour for 4 weeks) Psychological Symptoms (assessed with: EDE), Depression (assessed with: BDI),									
3	randomised trials	not serious	serious [a,b,c]	not serious	not serious	none	one RCT ($n = 130$) compared FBT to CBT for adolescents with BN. FBT group achieved significantly higher remission rates (39% vs. 20%) at end of study. One RCT (n-85) compared FBT to CBT guided self care and found no difference in BP remission (although Binge alone was decreased in the CBT group). One RCT randomized 80 patients to FBT or supportive psychotherapy. 39% in FBT vs. 18% in supportive therapy were in remission at end of treatment; a significant difference.	⊕⊕⊕◯ MODERATE	CRITICAL
		not serious	serious [a,b,c]	not serious	not serious	none	one RCT ($n = 130$) did not find any differences in EDE score at end of treatment for FBT vs. CBT for adolescents with BN. The other RCT ($n = 80$) also showed all EDE scores were more improved in the FBT group compared to supportive group.	⊕⊕⊕◯ MODERATE	CRITICAL
		not serious	serious [a,b,c]	not serious	not serious	none	One RCT ($n = 130$) showed a decrease in depression scores that was greater in the FBT group compared to the CBT group at the end of the study. Another RCT ($n = 80$) did not show any differences in depression scores between FBT and supportive group.	⊕⊕⊕◯ MODERATE	CRITICAL
Binge Purge Frequency (assessed with: Frequency Scores)									
2	Case Reports	very serious [d,e]	not serious	not serious	not serious	none	Two case reports of 9 patients in total describe decreases in binge and purge behaviours with FBT pre compared to post.	⊕⊕⊕◯ VERY LOW	CRITICAL

[a]one of three RCTs did not find a difference at end of treatment
[b]one RCT found a difference in psychological symptoms and the other did not
[c]one RCT showed a difference in depression scores and the other did not
[d]no randomization
[e] no control condition
Bibliography:
RCTs – Le Grange 2015 [50], Le Grange 2007 [48], Schmidt 2007 [49]
Case Reports - Dodge 1995 [51], LeGrange 2003 [34]

children and adolescents with AN show promise, but require further study (Table 6).

Two case reports describe the application of adjunctive emotion coaching and attachment based strategies to FBT for one male and one female patient with AN [68, 69] (Table 6).

Cognitive Behavioural Therapy has also been added as an adjunct to FBT for young patients with AN or BN. For AN, three case series [70–72] and two case reports [73, 74] indicate improved weight and psychological symptoms with added modules on perfectionism or exposure (Table 7). For BN, one case control study exists that compared one patient treated with FBT plus CBT to another patient treated with FBT alone, finding that both patients improved in terms of binge/purge symptoms and Eating Disorder Examination (EDE) scores [75] (Table 8).

Multi-family therapy

One large high quality RCT ($n = 169$) found that Multi-Family Therapy (MFT) conferred additional benefits compared to single family therapy (FT) in terms of remission rates for adolescents with AN (75% in MFT versus 60% in FT), although no differences were found on the EDE [76]. There is one case control study examining MFT versus

Table 4 Family-based treatment for other populations

Certainty assessment							Impact	Certainty	Importance
№ of studies	Study design	Risk of bias	Inconsistency	Indirectness	Imprecision	Other considerations			
Atypical AN - Depressive symptoms - Hughes 2017 (atypical AN) [52]									
1	Case series	very serious [a,b]	not serious	not serious	not serious	none	Case series of 42 adolescents (age 12 to 18 years) with Atypical AN, that is adolescents who had lost a significant amount of weight, but were not currently underweight. There were significant decreases in eating disorder and depressive symptoms during FBT but no improvement in self esteem.	⊕◯◯◯ VERY LOW	CRITICAL
Case Reports - Spettigue 2018 [53], Murray 2012 [54] (ARFID)									
ARFID - Food Variety (assessed with: clinical impression), Weight									
2	Case Reports	very serious [a,b]	not serious	not serious	not serious	none	Two case reports describe 7 cases in total (2 male, 5 female) in which ARFID was treated using a combination of FBT techniques, as well as some behavioural rewards and cognitive strategies. Food variety improved by clinical impression.	⊕◯◯◯ VERY LOW	CRITICAL
		very serious [a,b]	not serious	not serious	not serious	none	Weight improved in all cases.	⊕◯◯◯ VERY LOW	CRITICAL
Case Report - Strandjord 2015 (transgendered youth) [55]									
Transgendered Youth -BMI									
1	Case Report	very serious [a,b]	not serious	not serious	not serious	none	16 yo female sex assigned at birth treated with FBT to weight restoration then disclosed gender dysphoria with a desire to transition to male gender. BMI 14.9 before treatment, and 19 with treatment.	⊕◯◯◯ VERY LOW	CRITICAL

[a]no control condition
[b]no randomization

treatment as usual (TAU) in 50 female adolescents with AN [77]. Those in the MFT group had a higher percent body weight (99.6%) versus the TAU group (95.4%) at the end of the study. Two case series have also demonstrated a benefit of MFT for adolescents with AN [78, 79], and one case series with a mixed sample of adolescents with AN or BN showed benefit in psychological symptoms [80]. There is also one small case series examining MFT for adolescents with BN that found improvements in eating disorder symptoms [81] (Table 9).

Other forms of family therapy

Systemic Family therapy has been used in one RCT [82] and three case reports [83–85] for AN. The high quality RCT compared Systemic Family Therapy to FBT and found no significant differences in terms of remission rates, however, rate of weight gain was greater in the FBT group and the use of hospitalization was also significantly lower in the FBT group (Table 10). Structural Family Therapy has been studied within two case series [86, 87] and two case reports [88, 89]. Remission rates in the case series were 75% (38/51) by clinical impression (Table 11). Both of these types of family therapy (Systemic and Structural) might be helpful for children and adolescents with AN, but the evidence generally does not indicate superiority to FBT, especially when costs are taken into consideration.

When looking at other nonspecific, family therapies in which family dynamics were examined, there is one high quality RCT which compared family therapy plus TAU to TAU alone [90] and three case reports [91–93] indicating a benefit of family therapy (Table 12). Family therapy has also been compared to family group psychoeducation with no significant differences in

Table 5 FBT adaptations for children and adolescents with anorexia nervosa

Certainty assessment							Impact	Certainty	Importance
№ of studies	Study design	Risk of bias	Inconsistency	Indirectness	Imprecision	Other considerations			
Weight and Psychological Symptoms									
1	randomised trials 10 vs 20 sessions	not serious	not serious	not serious	not serious	none	RCT comparing 10 sessions of FBT to 20 sessions of FBT ($n = 86$). No differences in weight seen at 1 year. Those with nonintact families and severe eating related obsessive-compulsive features fair better in FBT.	⊕⊕⊕⊕ HIGH	IMPORTANT
		not serious	not serious	not serious	not serious	none	No differences in psychological symptoms (EDE) seen at 1 year. Those with nonintact families and severe eating related obsessive-compulsive features fair better in FBT.	⊕⊕⊕⊕ HIGH	IMPORTANT
1	randomised trials Adaptive vs. Standard FBT	not serious	not serious	not serious	not serious	none	45 adolescents in RCT comparing Adaptive FBT (3 extra sessions) to Standard FBT. No differences in outcomes in terms of weight.	⊕⊕⊕⊕ HIGH	CRITICAL
1	Randomized trial FBT +/− family meal	not serious	not serious	not serious	not serious	none	One RCT examined FBT with and without the family meal intervention ($n = 23$). No differences were found in weight at the end of the study.	⊕⊕⊕⊕ HIGH	CRITICAL
1	randomised trials FBT alone vs. FBT plus parent consultation	not serious	not serious	not serious	not serious	none	RCT of 20 adolescents aged 12–16 all female. 10 received FBT plus parent to parent consultation and 10 received FBT alone. Small increase in rate of weight restoration was seen in FBT plus consultation group.	⊕⊕⊕⊕ HIGH	CRITICAL
Weight									
4	Case Series guided self help, short term intensive, telemedicine	very serious [a,b]	not serious	not serious	not serious	none	Uncontrolled feasibility study looked at Parental guided self help FBT for AN ($n = 19$). Improvement in weight was seen at the end of the study. Uncontrolled Short-Term Intensive Family Based Treatment for AN ($n = 19$). 18/19 patients gained and maintained weight. 30 month outcome of 74 patients treated with this Short Term Intensive Modal indicated 61% remained in full remission. One case series ($n = 10$) showing benefit of FBT delivery via telemedicine.	⊕◯◯◯ VERY LOW	CRITICAL
Weight									
1	Case Report telemedicine	very serious [a,b]	not serious	not serious	not serious	none	One case report of FBT delivered by telehealth. Weight improved pre to post treatment.	⊕◯◯◯ VERY LOW	CRITICAL

Explanations
[a] **no control condition**
[b] **no randomization**
Bibliography:
RCT - Lock 2005 [56], Lock 2015 [60] Herscovici 2017 [57] Rhodes 2008 [59]
Case Series - Lock 2017 [58], Anderson 2017 [64], Marzola 2015 [62], Rockwell 2011 [61]
Case Report - Goldfield 2003 [63]

Table 6 FBT adjuncts for children and adolescents with anorexia nervosa

Certainty assessment							Impact	Certainty	Importance
№ of studies	Study design	Risk of bias	Inconsistency	Indirectness	Imprecision	Other considerations			
Psychological symptoms (EDE)									
1	randomised trials Art therapy vs. CRT	not serious	not serious	not serious	not serious	none	RCT examining FBT plus either Art Therapy or Cognitive Remediation Therapy. Global EDE score was slightly more improved in the Art Therapy Group ($p < 0.03$, $n = 30$).	⊕⊕⊕⊕ HIGH	CRITICAL
Weight Restoration (assessed with: Median BMI)									
1	Case control FBT +/−skills workshop	serious [a]	not serious	not serious	not serious	none	One case control study described 45 families who had FBT with 45 families who had FBT plus a parent education and skills workshop. Week 4 weight gain was higher in those with the workshop, but there were no significant differences at the end of the study.	⊕◯◯◯ VERY LOW	CRITICAL
Weight (assessed with: pounds and %expected body weight)									
1	Case series DBT added	very serious [a,b]	not serious	not serious	not serious	none	One case series ($n = 11$) of DBT added to FBT in a community-based clinic. 2/11 achieved full weight restoration at end of treatment	⊕◯◯◯ VERY LOW	CRITICAL
		very serious [a,b]	not serious	not serious	not serious	none	6/11 had normal EDE scores at the end of the study.	⊕◯◯◯ VERY LOW	CRITICAL
Weight									
2	Case reports Emotion coaching	very serious [a,b]	not serious	not serious	not serious	none	Two case reports of two patients with AN (one male) treated with adjunctive emotion coaching and the other with Attachment Based Family Therapy during a course of FBT. Both improved in weight to be fully weight restored.	⊕◯◯◯ VERY LOW	CRITICAL

[a]no randomization
[b]no control condition
Bibliography:
RCT – Lock 2018 [65]
Case Control – Ganci 2018 [66]
Case Series - Accurso 2018 [67]
Case Reports - Peterson 2016 [68], Wagner 2016 [69]

Table 7 FBT plus CBT for children and adolescents with anorexia nervosa

Certainty assessment							Impact	Certainty	Importance
№ of studies	Study design	Risk of bias	Inconsistency	Indirectness	Imprecision	Other considerations			
Weight (assessed with: percent ideal body weight) Psychological Symptoms of ED (assessed with: EDE and EDI)									
3	Case series adding CBT to FBT	very serious [a,b]	not serious	not serious	not serious	none	Total $n = 78$. Three case series looked at a perfectionism module added to FBT, or an exposure component to FBT. Weight increased significantly. One case series looked at Acceptance-Based Separated Family Treatment ($n = 47$), and also noted weight improved to ideal weight in about 50% of cases from pre to post treatment (20 sessions over 24 weeks).	⊕○○○ VERY LOW	CRITICAL
		very serious [a,b]	not serious	not serious	not serious	none	In one study 2/3 in full remission, 1/3 in partial remission.	⊕○○○ VERY LOW	CRITICAL
		very serious [a,b]	not serious	not serious	not serious	none	Decreases in EDE scores and EDI scores reported.	⊕○○○ VERY LOW	CRITICAL
Perfectionism (assessed with: Child and Adolescent Perfectionism Scale)									
2	Case reports	very serious [a,b]	not serious	not serious	not serious	none	Two case reports ($n = 9$ total) report on decreased perfectionism scores with the addition of a CBT perfectionism module or the addition of acceptance-based strategies	⊕○○○ VERY LOW	IMPORTANT

Explanations
[a]no randomization
[b]no control condition
Bibliography:
Case Series - Hurst 2019 [72], Hildebrandt 2014 [70], Timko 2015 [71]
Case Reports - Hurst 2015 [74], Merwin 2013 [73]

Table 8 FBT plus CBT for children and adolescents with Bulimia Nervosa

Certainty assessment							Impact	Certainty	Importance
№ of studies	Study design	Risk of bias	Inconsistency	Indirectness	Imprecision	Other considerations			
Binge Purge Frequency (assessed with: frequency diary), Psychological symptoms (EDE)									
1	Case control	serious [a]	not serious	not serious	not serious	none	One 15 yo female treated with FBT alone, compared to one 15 yo female treated with FBT and CBT (1 h sessions were split into 30 min of FBT and 30 min of CBT). Both improved significantly - BP episodes decreased from 10 to 12 episodes per week to 0.	⊕○○○ VERY LOW	IMPORTANT
		serious [a]	not serious	not serious	not serious	none	EDE scores were collected at end of this CBT plus FBT compared to FBT alone study ($n = 2$). EDE scores were similar in these two patients and demonstrated normal scores (in remission).	⊕○○○ VERY LOW	IMPORTANT

Explanations
[a]no randomization
Bibliography:
Case Control - Hurst 2017 [75]

Table 9 Multi family therapy for eating disorders

Certainty assessment							Impact	Certainty	Importance
DE	Study design	Risk of bias	Inconsistency	Indirectness	Imprecision	Other considerations			
Good Outcome at End of Treatment (assessed with: Morgan Russell Scale), Psychological Symptoms (EDE)									
1	randomised trials	not serious	not serious	not serious	not serious	none	RCT ($n = 169$) of adolescents with AN aged 11–18 comparing MFT to FBT (91% female). 65/86 (75.6%) good outcome at end of treatment in MFT versus 48/83 (57.8%) in the FBT group - significant difference. No differences between groups seen on the EDE. Both groups improved over time on the EDE.	⊕⊕⊕⊕ HIGH	CRITICAL
		not serious	not serious	not serious	not serious	none	No differences between groups seen on the EDE. Both groups improved over time on the EDE.	⊕⊕⊕⊕ HIGH	CRITICAL
Weight (assessed with: Percent ideal body weight)									
1	Case control	serious [a]	not serious	not serious	not serious	none	Retrospective case control study looking at MFT versus TAU for AN. 50 female adolescents aged 11–18 were included (25 in MFT group and 25 in TAU group). Those in MFT restored weight to a higher percentage (99.6% vs. 95.4%).	⊕○○○ VERY LOW	CRITICAL
Weight (assessed with: kg and BMI) Psychological Symptoms (assessed with: EDE, EDI)									
4	Case Series	very serious [a,b]	not serious	not serious	not serious	none	Four studies without a control condition. Total $n = 142$ adolescents (5 males, 137 females), Diagnoses were mixed including AN, EDNOS and BN. Significant improvements in weight were reported.	⊕○○○ VERY LOW	CRITICAL
		very serious [a,b]	not serious	not serious	not serious	none	Improvements in psychological symptoms were seen pre to post MFT. In a case series of 10 adolescents aged 13 to 18 years, EDE scores decreased from 4.31 to 3.41 (cohen's d 0.82).	⊕○○○ VERY LOW	CRITICAL

[a]no randomization
[b]no control condition
Bibliography:
RCT – Eisler 2016 [76]
Case control - Gabel 2014 [77]
Case Series - Gelin 2015 [80], Hollesen 2013 [78], Salaminiou 2017 [79], Stewart 2015 [81]

Table 10 Systemic family therapy for anorexia nervosa

Certainty assessment							Impact	Certainty	Importance
№ of studies	Study design	Risk of bias	Inconsistency	Indirectness	Imprecision	Other considerations			
Systemic Family Therapy vs. FBT- Remission (assessed with: greater than 95% IBW)									
1	randomised trials	not serious	not serious	not serious	not serious	none	One RCT $n = 164$ (82 in each group, 141 were female). Remission rates were 27/82 in the FBT group and 21/82 in the Systemic Group - not significantly different.	⊕⊕⊕⊕ HIGH	CRITICAL
		not serious	not serious	not serious	not serious	none	Rate of weight gain were significantly faster in the FBT group compared to the Systemic Group.	⊕⊕⊕⊕ HIGH	CRITICAL
		not serious	not serious	not serious	not serious	none	No differences were seen in EDE score at end of treatment between FBT and Systemic Therapy	⊕⊕⊕⊕ HIGH	CRITICAL
Weight (assessed with: kg)									
3	Case Reports	very serious [a,b]	not serious	not serious	not serious	none	Three case reports describe the use of systemic family therapy to good effect in terms of weight restoration. One case was a 14 yo male in which only the parents came to some of the sessions, another was a 15 yo female with comorbid osteosarcoma, and another is a 15 yo male.	⊕○○○ VERY LOW	IMPORTANT

Explanations
[a]no control condition
[b]no randomization
Bibliography:
RCT - Agras 2014 [82]
Case Reports - Carr 1989 [83], De Benedetta 2011 [85], Merl 1989 [84]

outcomes [94]. Both groups were recruited through an inpatient program. Both groups gained weight and were receiving other forms of treatment including medical monitoring and nutritional advice, in addition to the interventions of interest (Table 13).

Emotion focused family therapy (EFFT) was compared in a randomized trial to CBT for 13 adolescents with BN [95] (Table 14). No differences were found in terms of binge/purge symptoms or psychological symptoms at the end of the study, however, the study was likely underpowered to detect differences.

Individual and group outpatient psychotherapies

Twelve thousand and eleven abstracts were identified in our database searches for the individual and group psychotherapy section of our guideline (see PRISMA flow diagram, Fig. 2). Twenty-five were added with forward chaining up to November 21, 2018, and 15 more through reference list review. Nine thousand, two hundred and eight abstracts were excluded during the abstract screening phase, and a further 1457 were excluded based on full article review, leaving a total of 48 articles included.

Cognitive Behavioural therapy

Anorexia nervosa A small RCT ($n = 22$) did not show any difference between CBT and Behavioural Family Therapy (similar to FBT) in terms of weight, or psychological symptoms on the EDE for children and adolescents with AN, however, both groups improved [24] (Table 15). One large case series [96] indicated that CBT resulted in weight gain and improvement in eating disorder psychological symptoms for children and adolescent with AN

Table 11 Structural family therapy for children and adolescents with Anorexia Nervosa

Certainty assessment							Impact	Certainty	Importance
№ of studies	Study design	Risk of bias	Inconsistency	Indirectness	Imprecision	Other considerations			
Recovery (assessed with: clinical impression), Weight Gain									
2	Case series	very serious [a,b]	not serious	not serious	not serious	none	Two large case series of 51 female adolescents total used structural family therapy. 38/51 (75%) were deemed recovered by clinical impression.	⊕○○○ VERY LOW	CRITICAL
		very serious [a,b]	not serious	not serious	not serious	none	One of these case series reported between 5 and 31 kg of weight gain with the treatment ($n = 25$).	⊕○○○ VERY LOW	CRITICAL
Weight Gain (assessed with: kg)									
2	Case reports	very serious [a,b]	not serious	not serious	not serious	none	Two case reports ($n = 2$ both female) report weight restoration - one of these cases had co-morbid asthma.	⊕○○○ VERY LOW	CRITICAL

Explanations
[a]no randomization
[b]no control condition
Bibliography:
Case Series - Minuchin 1975 [86], Wallin 2002 [87]
Case Reports - Combrinck-Graham 1974 [88], Liebman 1974 [89]

($n = 49$). Eight additional case reports [97–104] support these results as well. Improvements have also been shown when CBT is delivered in a group setting for AN in a case control design involving 22 patients [105], and in a case series of 29 adolescents [106] (Table 16).

Bulimia nervosa For BN, three high quality RCTs were found examining CBT (Table 17). One RCT compared CBT to psychodynamic therapy in primarily adolescents, but also some young adults. This trial did not find any difference in terms of remission from BN. There were

Table 12 Family therapy (dynamic) for children and adolescents with Anorexia Nervosa

Certainty assessment							Impact	Certainty	Importance
№ of studies	Study design	Risk of bias	Inconsistency	Indirectness	Imprecision	Other considerations			
RCT - Good Outcome (assessed with: Morgan Russell)									
1	randomised trials	not serious	not serious	not serious	not serious	none	one RCT involving 60 adolescents randomized to TAU or TAU plus Family Therapy looking at family dynamics. 12/30 had a good outcome in the FT group compared to 5/30 in the TAU group ($p < 0.05$).	⊕⊕⊕⊕ HIGH	CRITICAL
Weight (assessed with: kg)									
3	Case Reports	very serious [a,b]	not serious	not serious	not serious	none	three case reports looking at 4 female patients (one set of twins) treated with family therapy (one solution focused). Weight improved in all cases.	⊕○○○ VERY LOW	IMPORTANT

Explanations
[a]no randomization
[b]no control group
Bibliography:
RCT - Godart 2012 [90]
Case Reports - Debow 1975 [91], Lane 1987 [92], O'Halloran 1999 [93]

Table 13 Family therapy compared to family group psychoeducation for adolescents with Anorexia Nervosa

Certainty assessment							Impact	Certainty	Importance
№ of studies	Study design	Risk of bias	Inconsistency	Indirectness	Imprecision	Other considerations			
Weight Restoration (assessed with: kg)									
1	randomised trials	not serious	not serious	not serious	not serious	none	No differences in weight restoration were seen at the end of the study between treatments. Both groups gained weight. ($n = 25$).	⊕⊕⊕⊕ HIGH	IMPORTANT

Bibliography:
Geist 2000 [94]

small differences in terms of a greater reduction in binge-purge frequency in the CBT group [107]. There were also two high quality RCTs identified comparing CBT to family-based approaches for BN [49, 50]. There are conflicting results between these two studies, with the study by Le Grange and colleagues [50] indicating significantly greater remission rates in the FBT group compared to the CBT group, whereas the study by Schmidt and colleagues [49] showed no significant difference between the groups with only a small proportion remitted in each group. Two large case series indicate significant decreases in binge-purge frequency pre to post treatment [108, 109]. Several case reports indicating improvement in binge-purge symptoms exist [110–114].

Avoidant/restrictive food intake disorder There were 13 case reports identified in which CBT was used to treat ARFID [115–127]. One of these described the delivery of CBT by telemedicine [127]. One case described the combined treatment of CBT with fluoxetine for a significant choking phobia [120]. Although these reports are preliminary, improvements in food avoidance were noted in all cases (Table 18).

Adolescent focused psychotherapy

Anorexia nervosa Adolescent Focused Psychotherapy (AFP: based on psychodynamic principles) [22, 23, 128] and other psychodynamic treatments [129] have some evidence to support their use (Table 19). Remission rates were not significantly different between AFP and FBT in two RCTs involving a total sample of 158 adolescents with AN [22, 23]. Rates of 20% (12/60) remitted in AFP compared to 34% (21/60) in FBT were found in a study by Lock and colleagues [23], whereas 41% in the AFP group met the weight goal of the 50th percentile in a study by Robin and colleagues [22] compared to 53% in the FBT group. Differences between AFP and FBT became more apparent at 1 year follow-up with FBT demonstrating an advantage [23]. Group analytic psychotherapy also has some evidence to support its use for AN [130] (Table 20).

Table 14 Emotion focused family therapy compared to cognitive behavioural therapy for children and adolescents with Bulimia Nervosa

Certainty assessment							Impact	Certainty	Importance
№ of studies	Study design	Risk of bias	Inconsistency	Indirectness	Imprecision	Other considerations			
Binge Purge Frequency (assessed with: frequency), Psychological Symptoms (assessed with: EDI)									
1	randomised trials	not serious	not serious	not serious	serious[a]	none	$n = 13$ adolescents with BN randomly assigned to EFFT or CBT. No differences in terms of binge purge frequency at end of study.	⊕⊕⊕◯ MODERATE	CRITICAL
		not serious	not serious	not serious	serious[a]	none	No differences in terms of psychological symptoms at end of study. Very small sample size.	⊕⊕⊕◯ MODERATE	CRITICAL

Explanations
[a]very small sample size
Bibliography:
RCT - Johnson 1998 [95]

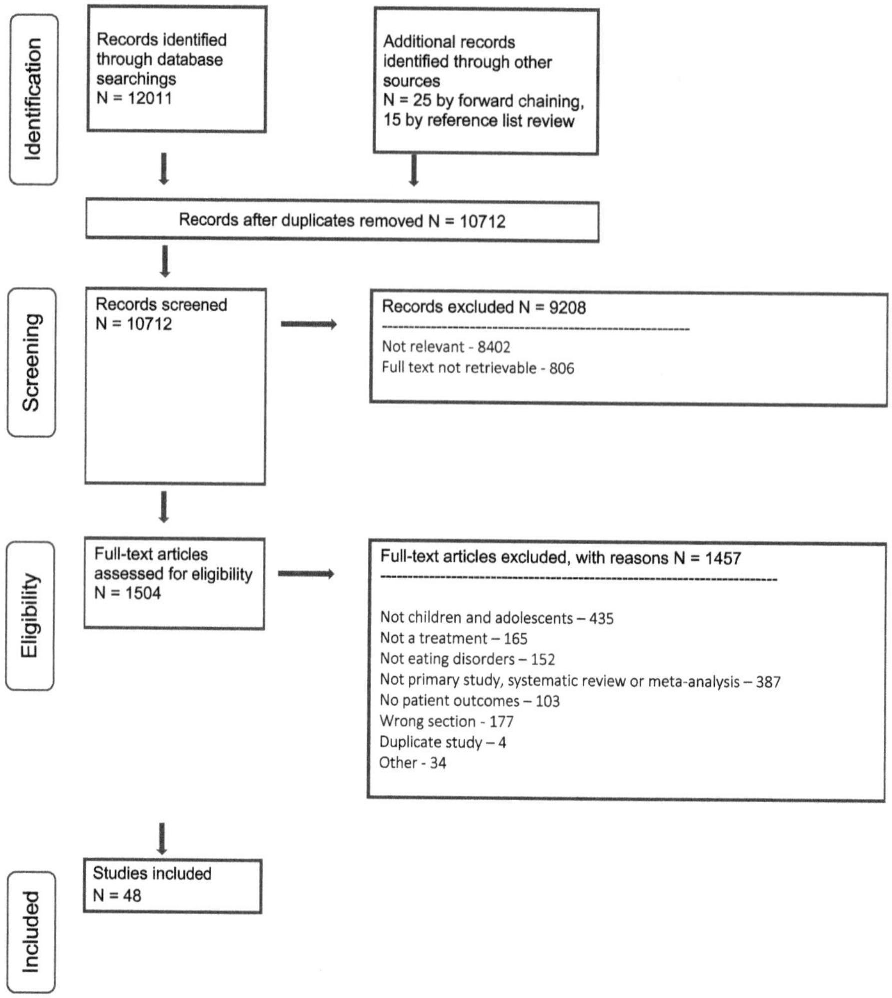

Fig. 2 PRISMA flow diagram for individual and group psychotherapy

Psychodynamic Therapy (group or individual) for AN may be beneficial, however other treatments have some advantages over psychodynamic therapy in terms of cost and more rapid improvement in symptoms.

Dialectical Behavioural therapy

Dialectical Behavioural Therapy (DBT) for eating disorders has been applied for youth with AN, BN, Eating Disorder Not Otherwise Specified (EDNOS) and Binge Eating Disorder (BED) with promising results [131–133]. Two case series report decreases in binge-purge symptoms, and improvements in psychological eating disorder symptoms [131, 133], along with reductions in frequency of self-harm in multi-diagnostic youth [131] (Table 21).

Adjunctive treatments

Cognitive Remediation Therapy (CRT) has been mentioned in the family therapy section of this guideline as an adjunct to FBT [65], however, it has also been studied as an adjunct to other therapies in a case series [134] and a case report [135] for AN (Table 22). It has been used in multiple settings and will be touched upon again within the level of care section of this guideline.

One high quality study suggests some benefits of adjunctive yoga in terms of psychological symptoms of eating disorders, as well as depression and anxiety [136]. In this study, 50 girls and 4 boys were randomly assigned to an 8-week trial of yoga plus standard care versus standard care alone. The majority of the participants had AN (29/54), and others were diagnosed with BN (9/54) and EDNOS (15/54). Eating disorder symptoms measured by the EDE decreased more significantly in the yoga group. Both groups demonstrated maintenance of body mass index (BMI), along with decreases in anxiety and depression scores (Table 23).

Table 15 Cognitive behavioural therapy for Anorexia Nervosa

Certainty assessment							Impact	Certainty	Importance
№ of studies	Study design	Risk of bias	Inconsistency	Indirectness	Imprecision	Other considerations			
Weight (assessed with: BMI), Psychological symptoms (EDE)									
1	randomised trials	not serious	not serious	not serious	not serious	none	RCT with 11 adolescents and young adults in CBT group compared to 11 in the Behavioural Family Therapy group (age range 13–23). There were no significant differences in terms of weight.	⊕⊕⊕⊕ HIGH	CRITICAL
		not serious	not serious	not serious	not serious	none	No differences seen in the eating psychopathology on the EDE between treatment groups.	⊕⊕⊕⊕ HIGH	CRITICAL
Weight (assessed with: kg), psychological symptoms with EDE									
1	Case Series	very serious [a,b]	not serious	not serious	not serious	strong association	This was a large case series of 49 adolescents age 13 to 17 years, all female. 40 sessions weekly for 45 min. Weight was significantly increased by an average of 8.6 kg comparing pre to post weight.	⊕◯◯◯ VERY LOW	CRITICAL
		very serious [a,b]	not serious	not serious	not serious	strong association	EDE scores were substantially decreased by a score of 2.03 (range 0–6) indicating psychological symptoms were much improved from pre to post treatment.	⊕◯◯◯ VERY LOW	CRITICAL
Weight (assessed with: kg), psychological symptoms									
8	Case Reports	very serious [a,b]	not serious	not serious	not serious	none	8 case reports describing 8 adolescents (7 females, 1 male) with AN treated with CBT. One case had comorbid OCD. Weight improved with treatment. Age range 11.5 to 17 years.	⊕◯◯◯ VERY LOW	CRITICAL
		very serious [a,b]	not serious	not serious	not serious	none	Improved EDE scores and EDI scores as well as improved eating behaviours in terms of a reduction in restricted eating.	⊕◯◯◯ VERY LOW	CRITICAL

Explanations

[a]no randomization

[b]no control condition

Bibliography:

RCT - Ball 2004 [24]

Case Series - Dalle Grave 2013 [96]

Case Reports - Cowdrey 2016 [97], Cooper 1984 [98], Martin-Murcia 2011 [99], Heffner 2002 [100], Scrignar 1971 [101], Fundudis 1986 [102], Ollendick 1979 [103], Wildes 2011 [104]

Table 16 Group cognitive behavioural therapy for children and adolescents with Anorexia Nervosa

Certainty assessment							Impact	Certainty	Importance
№ of studies	Study design	Risk of bias	Inconsistency	Indirectness	Imprecision	Other considerations			
Weight (assessed with: kg) Psychological Symptoms of ED (assessed with: EDE)									
1	Case Control	serious [a]	not serious	not serious	not serious	none	This controlled study involved 11 adolescents in the CBT group condition compared to 11 adolescents in the treatment as usual condition. CBT group involved 24 sessions (90 min each) over a six-month period. There were no significant differences in terms of weight at the end of treatment.	⊕○○○ VERY LOW	CRITICAL
		serious [a]	not serious	not serious	not serious	none	Significant difference on the EDE subscale of Restraint (0.56 vs. 0.70 - clinical significance questionable).	⊕○○○ VERY LOW	CRITICAL
Weight (assessed with: BMI) Psychological Symptoms of ED (assessed with: EDE)									
1	Case Series	very serious [a,b]	not serious	not serious	not serious	none	Case series of 29 adolescent females (22 AN-R, 7 AN-BP). No control group. 40 sessions of group CBT over 40 weeks. Weight (BMI) improved pre to post treatment. EDE restraint and EDE weight concern improved Pre to Post treatment.	⊕○○○ VERY LOW	CRITICAL

Explanations
[a]no randomization
[b]no control condition
Bibliography:
Case Control – Pegado 2018 [105]
Case Series - Ohmann 2013 [106]

Medications

Atypical antipsychotics

Two hundred and thirty-six abstracts were identified through database searching for the atypical anti-psychotic section of our guideline (see PRISMA flow diagram Fig. 3). Seven additional articles were found through citation chaining and reference list review. After excluding 97 abstracts and then excluding 73 full text articles we arrived at 32 included studies for the atypical antipsychotic section. We then divided up the antipsychotics into their respective categories – Olanzapine, Risperidone, Quetiapine, and Aripiprazole.

Olanzapine

Anorexia nervosa Olanzapine has been the most commonly studied psychotropic medication for children and adolescents with AN (Table 24). At present, only one double blind placebo-controlled trial in this population has been published. Kafantaris and colleagues [137] examined olanzapine in 20 underweight adolescents being treated in inpatient ($n = 9$), day treatment ($n = 6$) and outpatient ($n = 5$) settings (age range 12.3 to 21.8 years). In a 10-week pilot study, they found no differences in beneficial effect between the olanzapine and placebo groups in the 15 subjects who completed the trial; however, the treated group showed a trend towards increasing fasting glucose and insulin levels by the end of the study. The mean dose of olanzapine was 8.5 mg daily. Of note, only 21% of eligible patients were recruited into the study and there was a high attrition rate. Although other research teams have also attempted RCTs using olanzapine in this population, trials have been hampered by a myriad of confounding and recruitment issues [155].

Three case control studies have examined the use of olanzapine in children and adolescents with AN [138–140]. The most recent of these studies enrolled 38 patients with AN; 22 of whom took olanzapine and 10 who declined medication and were retained as a comparison group [138]. The mean dose of medication was 5.28 mg daily over a 12-week trial period. Those in the medication group demonstrated a significantly higher rate of weight gain in the first 4 weeks, although approximately one third of participants discontinued olanzapine early due to side effects [138]. Norris and colleagues [139] completed a retrospective chart

Table 17 Cognitive behavioural therapy for Bulimia Nervosa

Certainty assessment							Impact	Certainty	Importance
№ of studies	Study design	Risk of bias	Inconsistency	Indirectness	Imprecision	Other considerations			
CBT vs FBT - Remission (assessed with: abstinence from BP for 4 weeks)									
2	randomised trials	not serious	not serious	not serious	not serious	none	RCT $n = 130$ aged 12–18 years. 18 sessions over 6 months. 20% remitted in CBT group versus 39% remitted in FBT group ($p <$ 0.04, NNT = 5). RCT $n = 85$ (guided self care CBT) remitted 6/44 in CBT group versus 4/41 in family group. no significant difference.	⊕⊕⊕⊕ HIGH	CRITICAL
CBT vs. Psychodynamic - Remission Rates (assessed with: Diagnostic Criteria)									
1	randomised trials	not serious	not serious	not serious	not serious	none	one RCT 81 females mean age 18.7 years (range 14–20). 33.3% remitted in the CBT group and 31.0% in the psychodynamic group. No significant differences. Mean of 37 sessions. Both groups improved, there were small between groups effect sizes for binge eating (d = 0.23) and purging (d = 0.26) in favour of CBT and for eating concern (d = 0.35) in favour of PDT.	⊕⊕⊕⊕ HIGH	CRITICAL
Binge Purge Behaviour (assessed with: EDE)									
2	Case Series	very serious [a,b]	not serious	not serious	not serious	none	Two large case series ($n = 68$ including 2 males, 66 females, and $n = 34$ all female). Total age range 12–19. Number of sessions 16–20. Frequency of binge and purge episodes decreased significantly pre to post treatment.	⊕◯◯◯ VERY LOW	CRITICAL
		very serious [a,b]	not serious	not serious	not serious	none	Case series of 68 adolescents - EDE significantly improved global EDE score from 3.6 to 1.8 from pre to post treatment.	⊕◯◯◯ VERY LOW	CRITICAL
Binge Purge Frequency (assessed with: Frequency), Psychological Symptoms (EDE or EAT)									
5	Case Reports	very serious [a,b]	not serious	not serious	not serious	none	Case reports involving 9 patients in total. Frequency of binge and purge behaviours described as decreased.	⊕◯◯◯ VERY LOW	CRITICAL
		very serious [a,b]	not serious	not serious	not serious	none	7 cases -EDE or EAT significantly improved.	⊕◯◯◯ VERY LOW	CRITICAL

Explanations
[a]no randomization
[b]no control condition
Bibliography:
RCT – Le Grange 2015 [50], Schmidt 2007 [49] (CBT vs. FBT) Stefini 2017 [107] (CBT vs. psychodynamic)
Case Series - Dalle Grave 2015 [108], Lock 2005 [109]
Case Reports – Schapman-Williams 2006 [110], Cooper 2007 [111], Anbar 2005 [112], Schapman-Williams 2007 [113], Sysko 2011 [114]

Table 18 Cognitive behavioural therapy for ARFID

Certainty assessment							Impact	Certainty	Importance
№ of studies	Study design	Risk of bias	Inconsistency	Indirectness	Imprecision	Other considerations			
Avoidance of Food (assessed with: clinical impression)									
12	Case Reports	very serious [a,b]	not serious	not serious	not serious	none	28 cases are described in which various cognitive behavioural strategies including systematic desensitization (17), hypnosis (6) and EMDR (4) were used. Patients were aged 3 to 16 years (12 male, 16 female). Improvement in food avoidance behaviour was reported in all cases.	⊕◯◯◯ VERY LOW	IMPORTANT
Telemedicine - Increased food variety (assessed with: bites of nonpreferred food)									
1	Case Report	very serious [a,b]	not serious	not serious	not serious	none	Case report with CBT delivered by teleconsultation to parents of 8 year old boy with ARFID. Increased frequency of bites of nonpreferred food was noted.	⊕◯◯◯ VERY LOW	IMPORTANT

Explanations
[a]no randomization
[b]no control condition
Bibliography:
Case Reports - Murphy 2016 [125], Fischer 2015 [124], Nock 2002 [119], Okada 2007 [122], Ciyiltepe 2006 [121], de Roos 2008 [123], Culbert 1996 [117], Siegel 1982 [115], Reid 2016 [126], Chatoor 1988 [116], Chorpita 1997 [118], Bloomfield 2018 [127], Bailly 2003 [120]

Table 19 Adolescent focused psychotherapy/psychodynamic for Anorexia Nervosa

Certainty assessment							Impact	Certainty	Importance
№ of studies	Study design	Risk of bias	Inconsistency	Indirectness	Imprecision	Other considerations			
Remission (assessed with: normal weight and EDE score)									
2	randomised trials	not serious	not serious	not serious	not serious	none	RCT of Adolescent Focused Psychotherapy versus FBT ($n = 121$, 11male, 110 female, age 12–18). 12/60 (20%) remitted at end of treatment in AFT group versus 21/61 (34.4%) in FBT group. No significant differences in terms of remission. No differences in remission in another RCT ($n = 37$). 52.6% in FBT reached 50th percentile weight vs. 41.2 in individual ($p < 0.05$).	⊕⊕⊕⊕ HIGH	CRITICAL
		not serious	not serious	not serious	not serious	none	Those in FBT had greater change on EDE scores at end of treatment.	⊕⊕⊕⊕ HIGH	CRITICAL
Weight									
2	Case Reports	very serious [a,b]	not serious	not serious	not serious	none	Two case reports describing three cases total (age 12–16 years, all female) in which psychodynamic therapy over 1–2 years of therapy resulted in weight restoration.	⊕◯◯◯ VERY LOW	CRITICAL

Explanations
[a]no control condition
[b]no randomization
Bibliography:
RCT - Lock 2010 [23], Robin 1999 [22]
Case Reports - Fitzpatrick 2010 [128], Pharis 1984 [129]

Table 20 Group analytic therapy for children and adolescents with AN and BN

Certainty assessment							Impact	Certainty	Importance
№ of studies	Study design	Risk of bias	Inconsistency	Indirectness	Imprecision	Other considerations			
Psychological Symptoms (assessed with: EDI, SEED-short evaluation eating disorders)									
1	Case Reports	very serious [a]	not serious	not serious	not serious	none	8 female adolescents aged 15–17 (3 with AN, 5 with BN). SEED AN and EDI maturity fears significantly decreased from pre to post. Setting was outpatient - 2 years 1.5 h per week	⊕○○○ VERY LOW	IMPORTANT

Explanations
[a]no control condition
Bibliography:
Case Report - Prestano 2008 [130]

review of 22 inpatients treated with olanzapine compared to an untreated age-matched group. The rate of weight gain was not significantly different, however, the treated group had more psychiatric co-morbidities than those not taking olanzapine and experienced side effects of sedation and dyslipidemia [139]. Hillebrand and colleagues [140] also reported on olanzapine use in seven patients (mean age 16.0 years) with AN. Most were taking 5 mg of olanzapine, with one patient receiving 15 mg once daily. The authors found reductions in activity levels in the adolescents taking olanzapine in comparison to 11 adolescents not treated with olanzapine. All patients were receiving either inpatient or day hospital care and there were no significant differences in weight [140].

In terms of case series, Leggero and colleagues [142] reported on 13 young patients (age 9.6 to 16.3 years) treated with a mean dose of 4.13 mg daily of olanzapine. Significant improvements were seen in weight, functioning, eating disorder symptoms and hyperactivity. Similarly, Swenne and Rosling [141] reported on 47 adolescents with AN treated with a mean dose of 5.1 mg daily. A mean weight gain of 9 kg was noted. The patients were treated for a mean of 228 days with olanzapine and were followed for three months following medication discontinuation. Biochemical side effects were closely monitored and were felt to be more related to refeeding processes than to medication [141].

Table 21 Dialectical behavioural therapy for eating disorders

Certainty assessment							Impact	Certainty	Importance
№ of studies	Study design	Risk of bias	Inconsistency	Indirectness	Imprecision	Other considerations			
Binge Frequency (assessed with: number per month) Purge Frequency									
2	Case Series	very serious [a]	not serious	not serious	not serious	none	Two case series and one case report for a total of 22 patients (10 EDNOS, 6 AN, 6 BN) reported a significant decrease in binge frequency. Reduction in vomiting pre and post treatment.	⊕○○○ VERY LOW	IMPORTANT
		very serious [a]	not serious	not serious	not serious	none	There were decreases in psychological symptoms.	⊕○○○ VERY LOW	IMPORTANT
		very serious [a]	not serious	not serious	not serious	none	A decrease in self harm also noted.	⊕○○○ VERY LOW	IMPORTANT
Binge Frequency, EDE scores									
1	Case Report	very serious [a]	not serious	not serious	not serious	none	*N* = 1 female with BED – decreased frequency of binge episodes	⊕○○○ VERY LOW	IMPORTANT
		very serious [a]	not serious	not serious	not serious	none	improvement in EDE scores.	⊕○○○ VERY LOW	IMPORTANT

Explanations
[a]no control group
Bibliography:
Case Series – Salbach-Andrae 2008 [133], Fischer 2015 [131]
Case Report - Safer 2007 [132]

Table 22 Cognitive remediation therapy for children and adolescents with Anorexia Nervosa

Certainty assessment							Impact	Certainty	Importance
№ of studies	Study design	Risk of bias	Inconsistency	Indirectness	Imprecision	Other considerations			
ART vs. CRT - Weight (assessed with: BMI), ED symptoms, depression, anxiety									
1	randomised trials	not serious	not serious	not serious	not serious	none	RCT comparing Art Therapy and CRT (both receiving FBT) $n = 30$ (3 male, 27 female). BMI not significantly different.	⊕⊕⊕⊕ HIGH	CRITICAL
		not serious	not serious	not serious	not serious	none	Art Therapy significantly better than CRT in terms of global EDE score at the end of 15 sessions.	⊕⊕⊕⊕ HIGH	CRITICAL
		not serious	not serious	not serious	not serious	none	No difference between CRT and Art Therapy with respect to depression scores.	⊕⊕⊕⊕ HIGH	CRITICAL
		not serious	not serious	not serious	not serious	none	No difference between CRT and Art Therapy with respect to Anxiety scores	⊕⊕⊕⊕ HIGH	CRITICAL
Weight (assessed with: BMI), Depression (BDI), Anxiety (STAI)									
1	Case Series	very serious [a,b]	not serious	not serious	not serious	none	One open trial of 20 patients (10 inpatients, 10 outpatients) describes weight improvement with 10 sessions of CRT. Open trial was pre post CRT.	⊕◯◯◯ VERY LOW	CRITICAL
		very serious [a,b]	not serious	not serious	not serious	none	Depression scores decreased significantly following CRT (pre compared to post)	⊕◯◯◯ VERY LOW	CRITICAL
		very serious [a,b]	not serious	not serious	not serious	none	No differences pre and post were seen in terms of Anxiety.	⊕◯◯◯ VERY LOW	CRITICAL
Weight									
1	Case Report	very serious [a,b]	not serious	not serious	not serious	none	Case report – 12 year old female with AN - pre post and 7 month follow up after 10 sessions CRT. Weight improved at the follow up assessment to a healthy weight range.	⊕◯◯◯ VERY LOW	IMPORTANT

Explanations
[a]no control group
[b]no randomization
Bibliography:
RCT - Lock 2018 [65]
Case Series -Dahlgren 2013 [134]
Case Report - van Noort 2015 [135]

Thirteen case reports (Table 24) have also been published [42, 143–154]. Pisano and colleagues [143] reported on five cases of adolescents with AN treated with 2.5 to 7.5 mg of olanzapine. At 6 month follow-up these patients demonstrated increased oral intake and improved BMI. Dennis, Le Grange, and Bremer [144] used olanzapine at a dose of 5 mg daily in five adolescent females with AN and found an increase in BMI, reduction of body concerns, and improvements in sleep and anxiety surrounding food and weight. Another case series involving four young patients aged 10 to 12 years reported on the use of olanzapine at a dose of 2.5 mg daily to treat AN [145]. These authors reported improvements in compliance and weight gain, as well as decreases in agitation. Mehler et al. [146] reported on five female patients aged 12 to 17 years on a dose range of 5 mg to 12.5 mg daily of olanzapine. They found improvements in body image distortion and rigidity. La Via, Gray, and Kaye [147] described two females with AN who experienced reduction of inner tension and "paranoid ideas" with use of 10 mg daily of olanzapine. Finally, there is a case report using olanzapine 5 mg daily to treat a 17 year old girl with AN and co-morbid pervasive developmental disorder not otherwise specified [150]. These authors reported weight restoration and improvements in eating behavior within 5 months of initiating treatment.

Table 23 Yoga for eating disorders

Certainty assessment							Impact	Certainty	Importance
№ of studies	Study design	Risk of bias	Inconsistency	Indirectness	Imprecision	Other considerations			
Psychological Symptoms (assessed with: EDE), weight, anxiety, depression									
1	randomised trials	not serious	not serious	not serious	not serious	none	In this RCT 50 girls and 4 boys were randomized to yoga plus standard treatment, or standard treatment alone.. There were no differences in weight between the yoga group and the no yoga group at the end of the study.	⊕⊕⊕⊕ HIGH	CRITICAL
		not serious	not serious	not serious	not serious	none	The yoga group demonstrated greater decreases in EDE score at 12 weeks.	⊕⊕⊕⊕ HIGH	CRITICAL
		not serious	not serious	not serious	not serious	none	Anxiety scores improved over time in the yoga group and were significantly improved compared to the no yoga group.	⊕⊕⊕⊕ HIGH	CRITICAL
		not serious	not serious	not serious	not serious	none	Depression scores were significantly improved in the yoga group compared to the control group.	⊕⊕⊕⊕ HIGH	CRITICAL

Bibliography:
RCT - Carei 2010 [136]

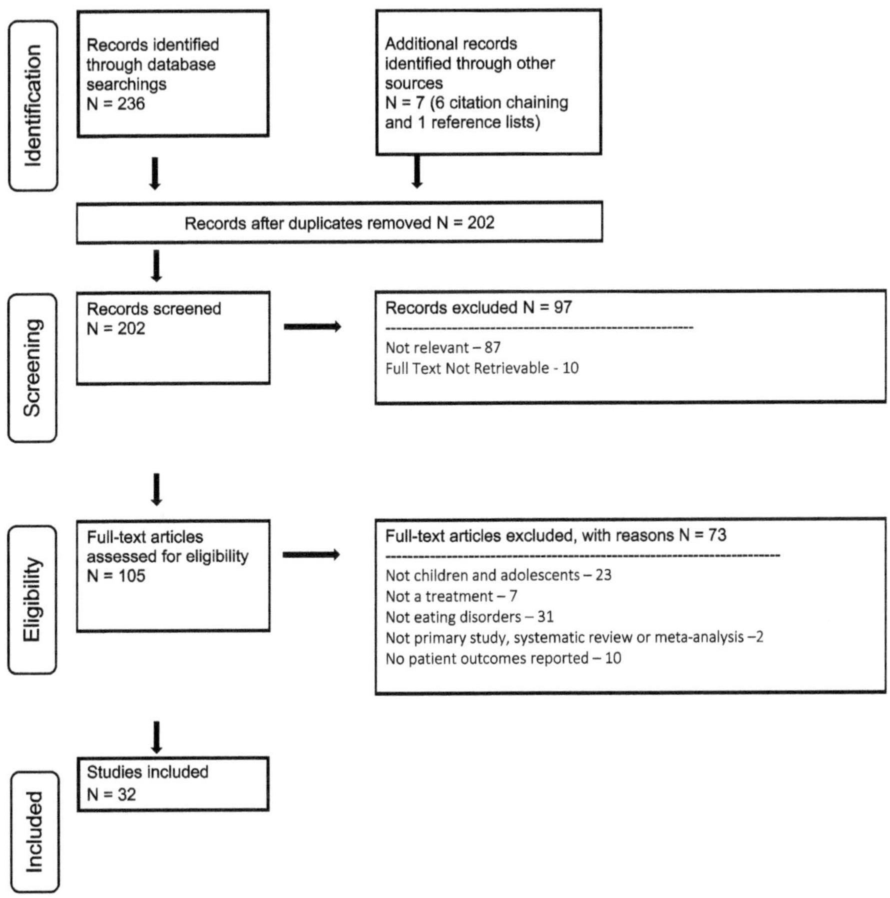

Fig. 3 PRISMA flow diagram for antipsychotics

Table 24 Olanzapine for children and adolescents with Anorexia Nervosa

Certainty assessment							Impact	Certainty	Importance
№ of studies	Study design	Risk of bias	Inconsistency	Indirectness	Imprecision	Other considerations			
Weight (assessed with: BMI), Psychological Symptoms, Side Effects									
1	randomised trials	not serious	not serious	not serious	not serious	none	RCT with 10 subjects in olanzapine group and 10 in placebo group. No differences were found between groups in rate of weight restoration or final weight. Difference in BMI was 0.4 kg/m2 and was not significant. Mean dose was 8.5 mg/day.	⊕⊕⊕⊕ HIGH	CRITICAL
		not serious	not serious	not serious	not serious	none	No differences in eating disorder symptoms or psychological functioning.	⊕⊕⊕⊕ HIGH	CRITICAL
		not serious	not serious	not serious	not serious	none	A trend of increasing fasting glucose and insulin levels were found in the olanzapine group.	⊕⊕⊕⊕ HIGH	CRITICAL
Weight gain, activity levels, side effects									
3	Case Control	serious [a]	not serious	not serious [a]	not serious	none	There are three non randomized case control studies. One of the studies found the rate of weight gain was greater in the olanzapine group, while another study found no differences between cases and controls in terms of weight gain.	⊕◯◯◯ VERY LOW	CRITICAL
		serious [a]	not serious	not serious [a]	not serious	none	Reduced activity levels were observed in one study.	⊕◯◯◯ VERY LOW	CRITICAL
		serious [a]	not serious	not serious [a]	not serious	none	Sedation and dyslipidemia was found in 56% of patients in one study. One study found that 32% of patients discontinued the treatment due to a side effect.	⊕◯◯◯ VERY LOW	CRITICAL
Weight, hyperactivity, side effects									
2	Case Series	very serious [a]	not serious	not serious	not serious	none	60 patients total involved in these two case series. Improvements in weight noted.	⊕◯◯◯ VERY LOW	CRITICAL
		very serious [a]	not serious	not serious	not serious	none	Improvements in hyperactivity are noted.	⊕◯◯◯ VERY LOW	CRITICAL
		very serious [a]	not serious	not serious	not serious	none	No long term adverse effects were seen 3 months after discontinuing medication.	⊕◯◯◯ VERY LOW	CRITICAL
Weight, side effects									
13	Case Reports	very serious [a]	not serious	not serious	not serious	none	Thirteen studies report on 30 cases. All studies report improvement in weight.	⊕◯◯◯ VERY LOW	CRITICAL
		very serious [a]	not serious	not serious	not serious	none	One case study reports on QTc prolongation (a problem on the ECG), another reports a case with neuroleptic malignant syndrome.	⊕◯◯◯ VERY LOW	CRITICAL

Explanations
[a]observational study, non randomized
Bibliography:
RCT - Kafantaris 2011 [137]
Case Control - Spettigue 2018 [138], Norris 2011 [139], Hillebrand 2005 [140]
Case Series -Swenne 2011 [141], Leggero 2010 [142]
Case Reports - Pisano 2014 [143], Duvvuri 2012 [42], Dennis 2006 [144], Boachie 2003 [145], Mehler 2001 [146], La Via 2000 [147], Dadic-Hero 2009 [148], Hein 2010 [149], Tateno 2008 [150], Ercan 2003 [151], Dodig-Curkovic 2010 [152], Ayyildiz 2016 [153], Ritchie 2009 [154]

Table 25 Olanzapine for children and adolescents with OSFED/EDNOS

Certainty assessment							Impact	Certainty	Importance
№ of studies	Study design	Risk of bias	Inconsistency	Indirectness	Imprecision	Other considerations			
Global improvement (assessed with: Clinical Global Impressions Scale)									
1	Case Report	very serious [a]	not serious	serious [b]	not serious	none	Single case report of 12 year old female with EDNOS. CGI improved with olanzapine 10 mg daily.	⊕◯◯◯ VERY LOW	IMPORTANT

Explanations
[a]single case report, no control
[b]outcome measured does not really answer our clinical question
Bibliography:
Case Report - Bozabali 2002 [156]

Eating disorder not otherwise specified Olanzapine was used in a case report of a 12 year old female with EDNOS with improvements on the clinical global impressions scale at a dose of 10 mg daily [156] (Table 25).

Avoidant/restrictive food intake disorder In a recent case series, Spettigue and colleagues [53] described six patients with ARFID and co-morbid anxiety (median age 12.9 years) who were treated with a combination of family therapy plus pharmacotherapy (Table 26). All patients were treated with olanzapine in combination with other medications, making interpretation of the results difficult: three cases were treated with a combination of olanzapine and fluoxetine, one case was treated with olanzapine followed by fluvoxamine, and two cases were treated with a combination of olanzapine, cyproheptadine and fluoxetine. All six cases reached their treatment goal weights.

Another recent case series reported beneficial effects from olanzapine in the treatment of patients with ARFID [157]. These authors completed a retrospective chart review and described a significant increase in weight, as well as improvements in anxiety and depressive symptoms in nine patients with ARFID treated with olanzapine. The mean final dose of olanzapine was 2.8 mg daily. All nine patients had comorbid mental health diagnoses including separation

Table 26 Olanzapine for children and adolescents with avoidant/restrictive food intake disorder

Certainty assessment							Impact	Certainty	Importance
№ of studies	Study design	Risk of bias	Inconsistency	Indirectness	Imprecision	Other considerations			
Weight (assessed with: lbs), Anxious/Depressive Symptoms									
2	Case Reports	very serious [a]	not serious	not serious	not serious	none	*N* = 15 total in two studies. Nine patients aged 9–19 years in this pre-post- study. Rate of weight gain increased significantly with olanzapine treatment from 3.3lbs to 13.1 lbs. All patients were in a residential treatment facility. Another case series of 6 patients indicated all patients gained to their target weight with olanzapine (2.5 to 7.5 mg daily) in combination with SSRIs and family therapy.	⊕◯◯◯ VERY LOW	IMPORTANT
		very serious [a]	not serious	not serious	not serious	none	The Clinical global impressions scale was used to rate anxious/depressive symptoms for 9 patients pre and post. The rating changed from markedly ill to mildly ill. All patients were in a residential treatment facility.	⊕◯◯◯ VERY LOW	IMPORTANT

Explanations
[a]small sample size, no control group
Bibliography:
Case Reports - Brewerton 2017 [157], Spettigue 2018 [53]

Table 27 Risperidone for children and adolescents with anorexia nervosa

Certainty assessment							Impact	Certainty	Importance
№ of studies	Study design	Risk of bias	Inconsistency	Indirectness	Imprecision	Other considerations			
Weight (assessed with: kg), Psychological Symtpoms, Side Effects									
1	randomised trials	not serious	not serious	not serious	not serious	none	There were no significant differences in weight at end of study (risperidone $n = 18$, placebo $n = 22$). Even when just data from those under age 18 (placebo 18, risperidone 12) were analyzed separately, there were no differences. Mean dose 2.5 mg over 9 weeks.	⊕⊕⊕⊕ HIGH	CRITICAL
		not serious	not serious	not serious	not serious	none	There were no significant differences at end of study on any subscale of the EDI (Eating Disorders Inventory).	⊕⊕⊕⊕ HIGH	CRITICAL
		not serious	not serious	not serious	not serious	none	ECG, bloodwork (prolactin, lipids, liver enzymes, glucose) no differences. Patient in the treated group reported fatigue and dizziness.	⊕⊕⊕⊕ HIGH	CRITICAL
Weight (assessed with: kg), Psychological Symptoms									
4	Case Reports	very serious [a]	not serious	not serious	serious [a]	none	Weight generally increased pre to post study period by several kg in 4 cases.	⊕○○○ VERY LOW	CRITICAL
		very serious [a]	not serious	not serious	serious [a]	none	Psychological symptoms including willingness to eat improved over the study period. Rigidity decreased. ($n = 4$)	⊕○○○ VERY LOW	CRITICAL

Explanations
[a]These are four case reports with no comparison condition
Bibliography:
RCT - Hagman 2011 [158]
Case Reports - Fisman 1996 [159], Kracke 2014 [160], Umehara 2014 [161], Newman-Toker 2000 [162]

anxiety, obsessive-compulsive disorder, posttraumatic stress disorder, generalized anxiety disorder, and social anxiety disorder. Six of the nine also had significant major depressive symptoms.

Risperidone

Anorexia nervosa The use of risperidone for AN has been studied in one high quality RCT and four case reports (Table 27). Hagman and colleagues [158] conducted a double-blind placebo-controlled trial of risperidone in adolescents and young adults with AN (age range 12 to 21 years). These authors randomized 40 patients to risperidone or placebo. The mean dose of risperidone was 2.5 mg daily over a mean duration of 9 weeks. There were no differences found between the groups at the end of the study [158]. Personal communication with the primary author indicates that even when the subgroup of patients under age 18 years was examined, no differences were found. These authors concluded that their results do not support the use of risperidone in the weight restoration phase of treatment for young patients with AN [158].

Four case reports were found on the use of risperidone in the treatment of AN [159–162]. Weight generally increased in all four cases described, and willingness to eat increased. Of these was a case report of a 12 year old girl with autism and AN who is described as benefitting from treatment with risperidone at a dose of 0.5 mg twice daily [159]. One of these cases describes the use of risperidone long-acting injection [161].

Avoidant/restrictive food intake disorder Pennell and colleagues [163] described two cases of ARFID where significant weight loss occurred with stimulant treatment for Attention Deficit Hyperactivity Disorder (ADHD), resulting in the need for hospitalization. These cases were managed by temporarily stopping the stimulant and adding risperidone to help with appetite and behaviour (Table 28).

Table 28 Risperidone for children and adolescents with avoidant/restrictive food intake disorder

Certainty assessment							Impact	Certainty	Importance
№ of studies	Study design	Risk of bias	Inconsistency	Indirectness	Imprecision	Other considerations			
Weight, psychological symptoms									
1	Case Report	very serious [a]	not serious	not serious	not serious	none	In two cases of ARFID on dose of 1 mg daily of risperidone. Weight gain was observed to target weight over several weeks.	⊕◯◯◯ VERY LOW	IMPORTANT
		very serious [a]	not serious	not serious	not serious	none	Oppositional behaviour and rigidity around eating improved.	⊕◯◯◯ VERY LOW	IMPORTANT

Explanations
[a]two case reports with no control group
Bibliography:
Case Report - Pennell 2016 [163]

Quetiapine

Anorexia nervosa Very few studies could be found on the treatment of AN with quetiapine (Table 29). One case series described quetiapine use in three subjects, aged 11 to 15 years with severe AN (lengthy hospitalization, use of nasogastric tubes, and BMI 12.3 to 13.9) [164]. Two of these patients were treated with quetiapine 100 mg twice daily, and one patient was treated with 250 mg twice daily. Authors reported improvements in body image disturbance, weight phobia, and "paranoid ideas". Sedation and constipation were noted as side effects.

Aripiprazole

Anorexia nervosa One case control study and two case reports were found on the use of aripiprazole in AN (Table 30). Frank and colleagues completed a retrospective case control study [165] and a case report [166] on the use of aripiprazole in adolescents with AN. The chart review described 22 adolescents with AN taking aripiprazole at a mean dose of 3.59 mg daily compared to an untreated comparison group of 84 adolescents with AN. These authors found a greater increase in BMI in the treated group [165]. The case report described four adolescents who benefitted in terms of weight and improved eating disorder cognitions [166]. One other case report was found on the use of aripiprazole [167]. The adolescent received a dose of 5 mg daily. The authors report an improvement in anxiety and rigidity around eating with aripiprazole.

Avoidant/restrictive food intake disorder One case report described the beneficial use of fluoxetine (20 mg daily) in combination with aripiprazole (2.5 mg daily) for a 15 year old girl with severe choking phobia [168] (Table 31).

Antidepressants

Nine hundred and ninety-six abstracts were identified through our database searches along with six additional articles through citation chaining and reference list searching for the antidepressant section of our guideline (see PRISMA flow diagram Fig. 4). Six hundred and fifty-seven citations were excluded on screening. On full text review, 197 articles were excluded, leaving 19 papers for data extraction.

Table 29 Quetiapine for children and adolescents with Anorexia Nervosa

Certainty assessment							Impact	Certainty	Importance
№ of studies	Study design	Risk of bias	Inconsistency	Indirectness	Imprecision	Other considerations			
Weight, fear of weight gain, side effects									
1	Case Report	very serious [a]	not serious	not serious	not serious	none	Three cases described in which weight increased.	⊕◯◯◯ VERY LOW	CRITICAL
		very serious [a]	not serious	not serious	not serious	none	Fear of weight gain improved.	⊕◯◯◯ VERY LOW	CRITICAL
		very serious [a]	not serious	not serious	not serious	none	Side effects - Initial Fatigue, constipation.	⊕◯◯◯ VERY LOW	CRITICAL

Explanations
[a]this a series of three cases with no control group
Bibliography:
Case Report - Mehler-Wex 2008 [164]

Table 30 Aripiprazole for children and adolescents with Anorexia Nervosa

Certainty assessment							Impact	Certainty	Importance
№ of studies	Study design	Risk of bias	Inconsistency	Indirectness	Imprecision	Other considerations			
Weight									
1	Case Control	serious [a]	not serious	not serious	not serious	none	Retrospective case-control study with 22 subjects treated with aripiprazole, 84 no treatment. BMI was slightly different between groups 18.8 vs. 17.9 $p < 0.35$.	⊕◯◯◯ VERY LOW	CRITICAL
Weight									
2	Case Reports	very serious [a,b]	not serious	not serious	not serious	none	5 cases report a benefit in terms of weight gain	⊕◯◯◯ VERY LOW	CRITICAL

Explanations
[a]the study was not randomized
[b]there are five cases reported on in total with no comparison group
Bibliography:
Case Control - Frank 2017 [165]
Case Reports - Frank 2016 [166], Trunko 2011 [167]

Selective serotonin reuptake inhibitors

Anorexia nervosa In terms of Selective Serotonin Reuptake Inhibitors (SSRIs) for AN, one case control study and five case reports were found (Table 32). One retrospective study compared 19 adolescent patients with AN taking SSRIs to 13 patients with AN not treated with SSRIs [169]. These authors found no differences between groups in terms of BMI, eating disorder psychopathology, or depressive and obsessive-compulsive symptoms after evaluating patients on admission, discharge and one-year follow-up. The SSRIs involved in this study included fluoxetine ($n = 7$, mean dose 35 mg daily), fluvoxamine ($n = 8$, mean dose 120 mg daily), and sertraline ($n = 4$, mean dose 100 mg daily).

Five adolescent case reports have been published on the use of SSRIs in AN. One of these focused on the use of sertraline in an adolescent with AN and symptoms of purging [170], another on the use of fluoxetine in an adolescent with AN and depressive features [171], and another on the use of fluoxetine for comorbid obsessive compulsive disorder [172]. All of these cases described a benefit in terms of anxiety, mood and weight restoration. Two additional case reports examined SSRIs in combination with antipsychotics [151, 162]. Newman-Toker [162] described two cases of adolescents with AN in which risperidone (1.5 mg daily) was added to antidepressant treatment, with improvements in anxiety and weight gain. Similarly, Ercan and colleagues [151] described a case of a 15 year old female with severe AN treated with olanzapine, fluoxetine, alprazolam, and thioridazine, demonstrating that polypharmacy is sometimes needed for severe symptoms of AN including agitation and fear of weight gain. These authors also reported that once stabilized in terms of agitation, a maintenance dose of 10 mg of olanzapine daily resulted in an

Table 31 Aripiprazole for children and adolescents with avoidant/restrictive food intake disorder

Certainty assessment							Impact	Certainty	Importance
№ of studies	Study design	Risk of bias	Inconsistency	Indirectness	Imprecision	Other considerations			
Weight (assessed with: kg), psychological Symptoms									
1	Case Report	very serious [a]	not serious	not serious	not serious	none	Only one case report. Patient gained 10 kg. Also on fluoxetine.	⊕◯◯◯ VERY LOW	IMPORTANT
		very serious [a]	not serious	not serious	not serious	none	Psychological symptoms including anxiety and rigidity improved.	⊕◯◯◯ VERY LOW	IMPORTANT

Explanations
[a]one case report, no comparison
Bibliography:
Case Report - Sivri 2018 [168]

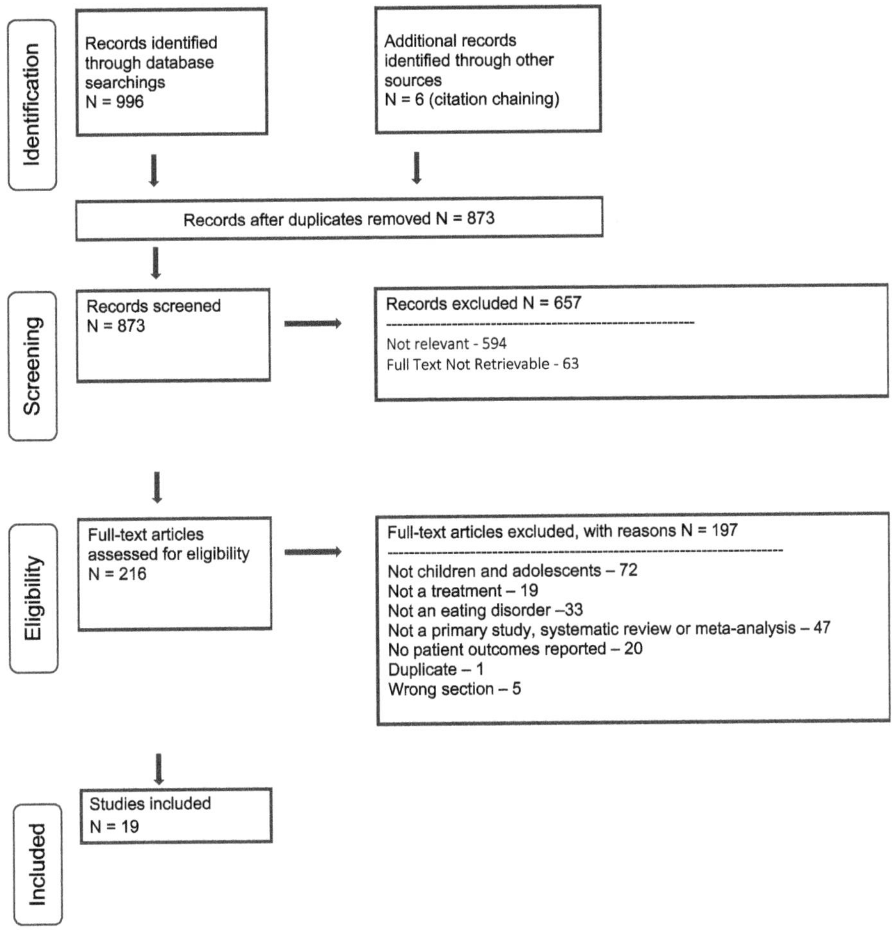

Fig. 4 PRISMA flow diagram for antidepressants

increase in BMI, along with a reduction of obsessive-compulsive symptoms, exercising, and eating disorder cognitions [151].

Bulimia nervosa Selective serotonin reuptake inhibitors have been studied in children and youth with BN, although the evidence is scant (Table 33). One open trial of fluoxetine in ten adolescents aged 12 to 18 years [173] reported on 8 weeks of a titrating dose of fluoxetine (maximum 60 mg daily) along with supportive psychotherapy. Frequencies of binge episodes decreased significantly from a mean of 4.1 to zero episodes per week, and weekly purges decreased from 6.4 to 0.4 episodes per week [173]. Seventy percent of patients were rated as improved or much improved on the clinical global impressions-improvement scale. No significant side effects were noted. Whether patients maintained these benefits over the long term is unknown.

One case report describes the use of valproate 200 mg twice daily following onset of mania felt to be related to the use of fluoxetine in an adolescent female with BN. In this report mood stabilized and binge eating and purging symptoms resolved once the fluoxetine had been stopped and valproate was initiated [174].

Other specified feeding and eating disorders Our review identified one case report of a patient with Other Specified Feeding and Eating Disorder (OSFED), atypical AN, whose depressive symptoms were treated with escitalopram with improvement noted [175]. She had lost almost 40 kg over a period of 4 months, but remained within a normal weight range (Table 34). Body image concerns remained.

Avoidant/restrictive food intake disorder In terms of the 'post-traumatic' subtype of ARFID where there has been a choking event followed by refusal to eat and drink, the SSRIs have been described in case reports as being helpful (Table 35). Several SSRIs have been mentioned in case reports including; escitalopram [177] and fluoxetine [120, 178]. Of note, Celik and colleagues reported a case of two 2-year old twins who were treated with fluoxetine 5 mg daily for a severe posttraumatic food avoidance, with good effect [178]. Similarly, a case

Table 32 SSRIs for children and adolescents with Anorexia Nervosa

Certainty assessment							Impact	Certainty	Importance
№ of studies	Study design	Risk of bias	Inconsistency	Indirectness	Imprecision	Other considerations			
Weight (assessed with: BMI), Core Eating disorder Symptoms (assessed with: ANIS), Depression (assessed with: DIJK)									
1	Case Control	serious [a]	not serious	not serious	not serious	none	Retrospective chart review - 19 patients on SSRIs (7 fluoxetine 20-60 mg, 8 fluvoxamine 100-150 mg, 4 sertraline 50-150 mg) compared to 13 on no medication. No differences in BMI.	⊕○○○ VERY LOW	CRITICAL
		serious [a]	not serious	not serious	not serious	none	No differences in core ED pathology.	⊕○○○ VERY LOW	CRITICAL
		serious [a]	not serious	not serious	not serious	none	No difference in depression scores between treated and untreated groups.	⊕○○○ VERY LOW	CRITICAL
		serious [a]	not serious	not serious	not serious	none	No difference in obsessive compulsive symptoms between treated and untreated groups.	⊕○○○ VERY LOW	CRITICAL
Weight (assessed with: kg)									
5	Case Reports	very serious [a,b]	not serious	not serious	not serious	none	Five case reports (3 fluoxetine 20 mg, 2 sertraline 75-100 mg) are described in which patients had a good response to various SSRIs and gained weight.	⊕○○○ VERY LOW	CRITICAL

Explanations
[a]Non randomized study
[b]No control condition
Bibliography:
Case Control - Holtkamp 2005 [169]
Case Report - Frank 2001 [170], Newman Toker 2000 [162], Lyles 1990 [171], Ercan 2003 [151], Gee 1999 [172]

Table 33 SSRIs for children and adolescents with Bulimia Nervosa

Certainty assessment							Impact	Certainty	Importance
№ of studies	Study design	Risk of bias	Inconsistency	Indirectness	Imprecision	Other considerations			
Binge Frequency (assessed with: average weekly binges), purge frequency, psychological symptoms, depression (BDI)									
1	Case Series	very serious [a]	not serious	not serious	not serious	none	Ten subjects all female, no control group. 8 week study of fluoxetine 60 mg/day. Binge frequency decreased from 4.1 to 3.8 ($p < 0.01$). Purge frequency decreased from 6.4 to 5.2 ($p < 0.005$).	⊕○○○ VERY LOW	CRITICAL
		very serious [a]	not serious	not serious	not serious	none	EDI Bulimia Subscale decreased significantly from 10.6 to 4.2 ($P < 0.01$).	⊕○○○ VERY LOW	CRITICAL
		very serious [a]	not serious	not serious	not serious	none	BDI scores were not significantly different pre and post.	⊕○○○ VERY LOW	CRITICAL
Adverse Effect - Mania									
1	Case Report	very serious [a,b]	not serious	not serious	not serious	none	Case described of teen with BN treated with fluoxetine 20 mg who developed mania - fluoxetine stopped and valproate started.	⊕○○○ VERY LOW	CRITICAL

Explanations
[a]no control group
Bibliography:
Case Series - Kotler 2003 [173]
Case report - Tor 2008 [174]

Table 34 SSRIs for children and adolescents with OSFED/EDNOS

Certainty assessment							Impact	Certainty	Importance
№ of studies	Study design	Risk of bias	Inconsistency	Indirectness	Imprecision	Other considerations			
Depressive symptoms (assessed with: clinical impression)									
1	Case Report	very serious [a]	not serious	not serious	not serious	none	Single case report of adolescent female, initially overweight with depressive symptoms. Treated with escitalopram 10 mg and depressive symptoms improved.	⊕○○○ VERY LOW	IMPORTANT

Explanations
[a]no control group, single case report
Bibliography:
Case Report - Wolter 2009 [175]

series of three children with "severe choking phobias" were successfully treated with low-dose SSRIs (sertraline and paroxetine) [176]. Spettigue and colleagues [53] also described the treatment of six children with ARFID treated with combinations of SSRIs and antipsychotics (described above in more detail in the olanzapine section).

Other antidepressants - mirtazapine

Anorexia nervosa To date, one case control study as well as two case reports involving the use of mirtazapine in AN have been published (Table 36). Hrdlicka and colleagues [179] examined nine adolescent patients with AN who had been treated with mirtazapine for anxiety or depression compared to nine female controls with AN. The two groups were matched in terms of age and BMI. The mean dose of mirtazapine was 21.7 mg daily. There were no significant differences in terms of weight or BMI at the end of this study [179].

In terms of the case reports, the first case report described a 16 year old female hospitalized for AN and depression treated with mirtazapine [180]. These authors found positive results in terms of weight restoration and mood improvement, and suggested further study of the medication was needed. More recently, Naguy and Al-Mutairi [181] described the case of a 16 year old boy hospitalized for severe AN who responded well to mirtazapine 30 mg/day in terms of weight restoration.

Avoidant/restrictive food intake disorder For ARFID, mirtazapine has also been used to good effect, although the evidence is limited to one case series and one case report (Table 37). The case series described 14 cases with the rate of weight gain reported pre and post initiation of mirtazapine (average dose 25.5 mg daily) [182]. Rate of weight gain was significantly greater after the initiation of the medication. An additional case report described the treatment of a 10 year old girl with ARFID and Obsessive-Compulsive Disorder (OCD). Anxiety and eating improved with 15 mg daily [183].

Lack of evidence No studies could be found on the use of Selective Norepinephrine Reuptake Inhibitors (SNRIs)

Table 35 SSRIs for children and adolescents with avoidant/restrictive food intake disorder

Certainty assessment							Impact	Certainty	Importance
№ of studies	Study design	Risk of bias	Inconsistency	Indirectness	Imprecision	Other considerations			
Anxiety (assessed with: clinical impression)									
5	Case Reports	very serious [a]	not serious	not serious	not serious	none	13 patients (3 male, 10 female) treated with various SSRIs including fluoxetine (8), paroxetine (2), fluvoxamine (1), sertraline (1), escitalopram (1). All cases experienced an improvement in anxiety and improved eating.	⊕○○○ VERY LOW	CRITICAL

Explanations
[a]no control group
Bibliography:
Case Reports - Banerjee 2005 [176], Hosoglu 2018 [177], Spettigue 2018 [53], Celik 2007 [178], Bailly 2003 [120]

Table 36 Mirtazapine for children and adolescents with Anorexia Nervosa

Certainty assessment							Impact	Certainty	Importance
№ of studies	Study design	Risk of bias	Inconsistency	Indirectness	Imprecision	Other considerations			
Weight (assessed with: kg)									
1	Case Control	serious [a]	not serious	not serious	not serious	none	9 females with AN treated with mirtazapine (mean dose 21.7 mg/day) matched with 9 controls. No significant differences in weight or BMI at the end of 4 weeks of treatment.	⊕○○○ VERY LOW	CRITICAL
Weight (assessed with: kg) Depression (assessed with: clinical impression)									
2	Case Reports	very serious [a,b]	not serious	not serious	not serious	none	Two case reports (one male, one female) with AN and depression. Both improved in weight.	⊕○○○ VERY LOW	CRITICAL
		very serious [a,b]	not serious	not serious	not serious	none	One of these case reports mentioned remission of depression in the context of AN with treatment with mirtazapine (30 mg).	⊕○○○ VERY LOW	CRITICAL

Explanations
[a]subjects were not randomized
[b]no control condition
Bibliography:
Case Control - Hrdlicka 2008 [179]
Case Report - Jaafar 2007 [180], Naguy 2018 [181]

for this population. The same was true for Mood Stabilizers.

Level of care

The database search initially provided 7136 citations, as reported in the PRISMA flow diagram (Fig. 5). An additional 49 citations were added through review of references, and forward citation chaining. After removing the duplicates, 6426 records remained, of which 5881 were eliminated on screening given that they did not meet the inclusion criteria. Of the 545 full text articles assessed for eligibility, 440 full text articles were excluded because they were longitudinal follow-up studies, primarily adult studies, review or secondary analysis papers, book chapters or guidelines, did not provide sufficient description of the treatment provided, did not focus on inpatient treatment or otherwise did not meet the inclusion criteria. Ultimately, 105 studies were selected for inclusion in the level of care section of this guideline – 70 within the inpatient subsection, 29 within the day hospital subsection, and six within the residential subsection.

Table 37 Mirtazapine for children and adolescents with avoidant/restrictive food intake disorder

Certainty assessment							Impact	Certainty	Importance
№ of studies	Study design	Risk of bias	Inconsistency	Indirectness	Imprecision	Other considerations			
Mealtime Anxiety (assessed with: clinical impression)									
1	Case Series	very serious [a]	not serious	not serious	not serious	none	Retrospective chart review of 14 cases pre and post documentation of rate of weight gain pre and post mirtazapine. Rate of gain significantly greater after mirtazapine (mean dose 25.5 mg).	⊕○○○ VERY LOW	CRITICAL
Anxiety									
1	Case Report	very serious [a]	not serious	not serious	not serious	none	Single case report of 10 yo girl with ARFID and OCD treated with 15 mg/day of mirtazapine. Anxiety improved and she began to eat solid food within 1–2 weeks.	⊕○○○ VERY LOW	CRITICAL

Explanations
[a]no control condition
Bibliography:
Case series – Gray 2018 [182]
Case Report - Tanidir 2015 [183]

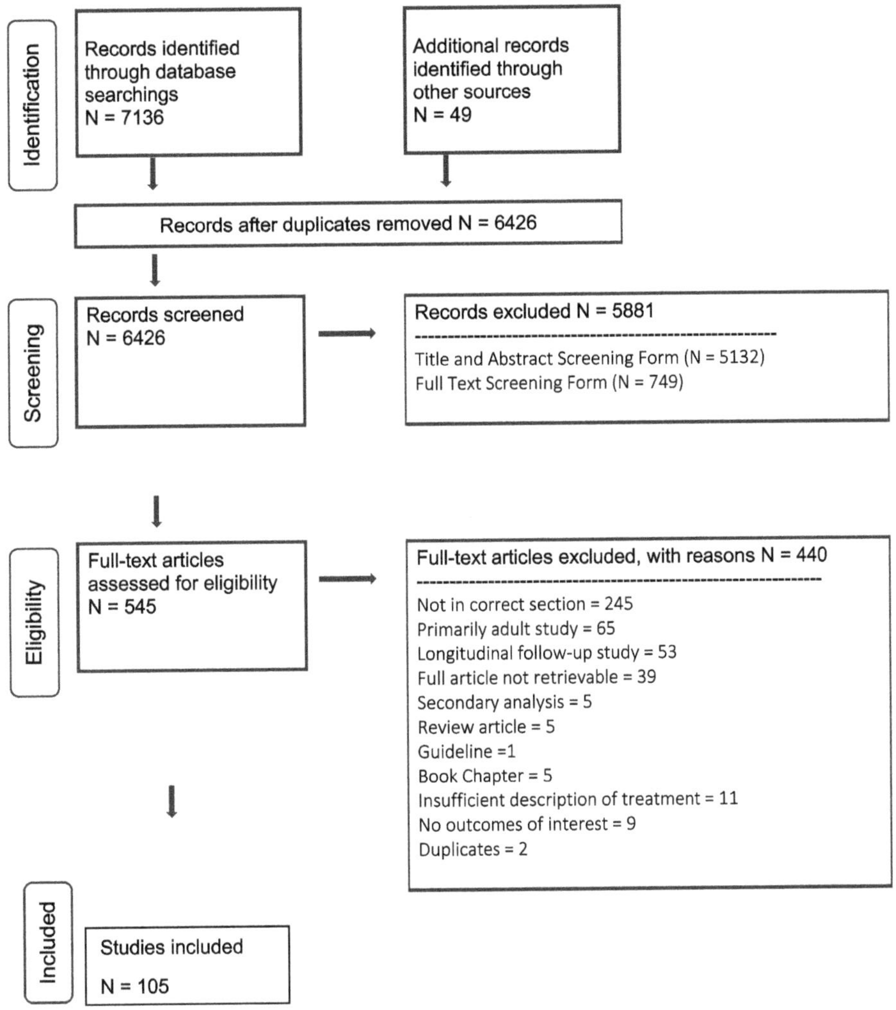

Fig. 5 PRISMA flow diagram for inpatient, day hospital and residential treatment

Inpatient

Multimodal treatment

Anorexia nervosa Twenty-one observational studies, none of which included control or comparison groups, have been published for a combined total of 1347 patients (Table 38) [184–191, 193–196, 198, 199, 201–207]. Various measures of change in weight were used across these studies including BMI, absolute weight in kg, percent Treatment Goal Weight (%TGW), weight gain per week and percent of patients attaining a predetermined discharge weight prior to discharge. Mean change in weight was positive in all studies. Mean length of stay ranged from 20.10 to 328.5 days.

While all of the observational studies of multimodal inpatient treatment reported on change in weight, fewer reported on change in eating disorder symptoms. Three studies (total $n = 88$) reported on Eating Disorders Examination-Questionnaire (EDE-Q) and one of the three studies reported significant change ($n = 44$, $p < 0.05$) [187, 201, 207]. This pre-post difference was attributed predominantly to the restraint and eating concerns subscales. Mean length of stay for these studies was between 203 and 115 days. Three studies (total $n = 126$) reported improvements in Eating Attitudes Test (EAT) scores at admission and discharge [186, 198, 203]. Length of stay varied between these three studies (29.8 days, 91 days and not reported). One study (total $n = 44$), with a mean LOS of 115 days reported on Eating Disorder Inventory (EDI) scores at admission and discharge [187]. This study found no significant change in total or subscales of the EDI. One study reported on frequency of binge, laxative and exercise symptoms, however the total number of patients reporting these symptoms at admission was small (i.e. laxatives 0, bingeing 3, exercise 5) [188]. Overall the study population was small (total $n = 11$ at admission and 7 at discharge). No statistical change was noted in any of these outcomes.

Table 38 Multimodal inpatient treatment for anorexia nervosa and/or low weight eating disorders

Certainty assessment							Impact	Certainty	Importance
№ of studies	Study design	Risk of bias	Inconsistency	Indirectness	Imprecision	Other considerations			
Weight (assessed with: Change in Weight Measures from Admission to Discharge), ED Symptoms (EDE-Q, EDI, EAT), motivational stage of change, laxative use, binge eating									
20	Case Series	very serious [a]	serious [b]	not serious	serious [c]	none	Twenty studies examined change in weight during inpatient treatment for total 1346 patients. Various measures of change in weight used across studies including BMI, absolute weight in KG, %TGW, weight gain per week and % of patients attaining predetermined D/C weight prior to d/c. Seventeen ($N = 1319$) used BMI as measure of weight. Mean BMI at admission varied from 13.2 to 16.3 between studies. Mean BMI at d/c varied from 16.3 to 19.49. Change in BMI from admission to d/c varied from 1.4 to 4.1. One study ($n = 40$) reported on mean BMI% change which rose from BMI 8.98 (+/−2.07) to 21.25 (+/− 3.13). Six studies ($n = 134$) reported mean absolute weight gain during admission which varied from 5.4 to 10.1 kg. Three studies ($N = 151$) reported mean %TGW change admission to discharge of 10.3 and 10.5%. One study ($n = 40$) only reported weight outcomes as rate of weight gain per week which was 1.86 kg/wk. with a mean LOS of 20.63 days (SD 13.03). Finally 2 studies reported on the % of patients attaining a pre-determined adequate weight as inpatients with 1 study reporting 76.1% ($n = 196$) reaching a mean BMI of > 17.63 and 1 study reporting 79.6% ($n = 108$) attaining > 90% TGW at time of d/c. LOS varied considerably which is likely related to difference in weight change as an inpatient. Mean LOS ranged from 20.10 to 328.5 days between studies. One study noted that longer LOS, lower age at admission and no previous inpatient treatment was associated with greater improvement in BMI.	⊕◯◯◯ VERY LOW	CRITICAL
		very serious [d]	serious [e]	not serious	serious [c]	all plausible residual confounding would reduce the demonstrated effect	Three studies - Two self-report measures of symptoms were used (EDI-3 and EDE-Q), change reported from admission to discharge. Treatment provided was multimodal. Three studies (total $n = 88$) reported on EDE-Q. Change in EDE-Q was found to be significant in one of these studies ($n = 44$, $p < 0.05$) - this difference was attributed to the restraint and eating concerns subscales. In the other 2 studies there was no difference in EDE scores from admission to discharge. LOS for	⊕◯◯◯ VERY LOW	CRITICAL

Table 38 Multimodal inpatient treatment for anorexia nervosa and/or low weight eating disorders *(Continued)*

Certainty assessment							Impact	Certainty	Importance
№ of studies	Study design	Risk of bias	Inconsistency	Indirectness	Imprecision	Other considerations			
							these studies was a mean of 203 and 115 days. BMI at discharge was higher in the study which found significant change in EDE-Q (ie BMI 19.49 vs 18.5 and BMI% 21.25 at discharge).		
		very serious [d]	serious [e]	not serious	serious [c]	all plausible residual confounding would reduce the demonstrated effect	All three studies (total $n = 126$) reported EAT scores at admission and discharge. Two studies used the EAT-26 and 1 study used the EAT-40. Treatment was multimodal and varied between studies. The difference in EAT score was noted to be statistically different in 2 studies ($p < 0.001$) and the third study reported a difference of 19 on the EAT-26 pre-post. LOS varied between studies (29.8 days, 91 days and not reported). Mean BMIs at discharge in these 3 studies were 19.2. 18.4 and 16.3.	⊕◯◯◯ VERY LOW	CRITICAL
		very serious [f]	serious [e]	not serious	serious [g]	all plausible residual confounding would reduce the demonstrated effect	One study - Number of patients reporting laxative use, binge/purge, exercise symptoms, even at admission were exceedingly small (ie laxatives 0, bingeing 3, exercise 5). Overall study small (total n = 11 at admission and 7 at discharge). No statistical change noted in any of these outcomes.	⊕◯◯◯ VERY LOW	IMPORTANT
		very serious [d]	not serious	not serious	serious [c]	all plausible residual confounding would reduce the demonstrated effect	One study with $n = 49$ patients and mean LOS 30 days. Change in mean ANSOCQ was statistically significant, however both admission and d/c scores fall into "preparation" phase of motivation and confidence intervals wide (ie admit score 53.6, SD 19.7 and d/c score 62.9, SD 24.5). During the course of the study BMI rose from 15.5 to 18.4.	⊕◯◯◯ VERY LOW	IMPORTANT
		very serious [d]	serious [e]	not serious	serious [c]	strong association all plausible residual confounding would reduce the demonstrated effect	Three studies ($n = 353$), mean LOS 115 days, 33.61 and 81.9 days respectively, reported on EDI-2 outcomes. One study (LOS 115 days) found no significant change in total or subscales of EDI-2 from admission to discharge. One study ($n = 71$ and LOS 33.61 days) found statistically significant improvement on Drive for Thinness (13.19 +/− 6.86 at admission and 11.23 +/− 6.52 at discharge, $p < 0.05$) and Bulimia (1.50 +/− 2.15 at admission and 0.66 +/− 1.08 at discharge, $p < 0.05$), but no change in Body Dissatisfaction. The final study ($n = 238$) found statistically significant improvements in global (ES 0.8) and all subscales of the EDI-2. The largest effect size was found for Drive for Thinness (ES = 1.1) and the lowest for	⊕◯◯◯ VERY LOW	CRITICAL

Table 38 Multimodal inpatient treatment for anorexia nervosa and/or low weight eating disorders *(Continued)*

Certainty assessment							Impact	Certainty	Importance
№ of studies	Study design	Risk of bias	Inconsistency	Indirectness	Imprecision	Other considerations			
							"Maturity Fears" (ES = 0.3).		
Weight									
1	Case Study	very serious [d]	serious [e]	not serious	serious [c]	strong association all plausible residual confounding would reduce the demonstrated effect	One case report describing a 17.1 kg wt gain	⊕○○○ VERY LOW	CRITICAL

Explanations
[a]Observational studies with no comparison group
[b]Multimodal treatment not well described/defined
[c]Confidence interval wide and cross over threshold for change
[d]Self-report measures and no control/comparison group
[e]Differing inclusion/exclusion criteria and treatments provided
[f]Unclear how these symptoms were measured and study took place over two sites which may have resulted in variation
[g]Number of patients in study small and numbers reporting these particular symptoms even smaller
Case Series – Anis 2016 [184], Ayton 2009 [185], Castro-Fornieles 2007 [186], Fennig 2017 [187], Goddard 2013 [188], Heinberg 2003 [189], Kalisvaart 2007 [190], Leon 1985 [191], Lievers 2009 [192], Mekori 2017 [193], Morris 2015 [194], Nova 2007 [195], Roux 2016 [196], Schlegl 2016 [197], Shugar 1995 [198], Tasaka 2017 [199], Treat 2008 [200], Vall 2017 [201], Bourion-Bedes 2013 [202], Rothschild-Yakar 2013 [203]
Case Reports – Toms 1972 [204]

Although not a focus of our guideline, one study measured motivation for change using the Anorexia Nervosa Stage of Change Questionnaire (ANSOCQ) at admission and then again at discharge [186]. The study included 49 patients whose mean length of stay was 30 days. Change in mean ANSOCQ score was noted to be statistically significant, however both admission and discharge scores fell into the "preparation" phase of motivation and the confidence intervals were wide.

Mixed diagnoses Two studies of multimodal inpatient treatment were found which reported on weight gain during inpatient treatment for patients with mixed eating disorder diagnoses (Table 39). One study differentiated between patients with AN restricting type versus those with AN binge-purge type or BN [203], and the other differentiated between those with AN restricting type or AN binge-purge type versus those with BN or Eating Disorder Not Otherwise Specified binge-purge type (EDNOS-B/P) [193]. Multimodal treatment was provided in both studies but varied between studies. Total number of patients studied was 150 across the two studies. In both cases there was a significantly greater increase in BMI for the group containing AN restricting type patients (total $n = 94$). In both cases this group started with a much lower BMI. Length of stay in these studies was approximately 6–7 months.

One of these studies compared symptom change using the EAT at admission to discharge in the group of patients with AN restricting type ($n = 33$) versus AN binge-purge type or BN ($n = 29$) [203]. Overall there was a statistically significant improvement in EAT scores over the course of the admission. There was no significant difference in change on EAT by diagnosis.

Avoidant/restrictive food intake disorder Four articles were found which reported on the inpatient treatment of a total of thirteen children treated using either a family-based or cognitive behaviour therapy approach [53, 208–210] (Table 40). Length of stay for these studies varied from 16 days to 60 days. In two of these studies weight gain was reported as an outcome and all patients gained weight [53, 208]. One of these studies reported on caloric intake in kcal/day which rose for all three patients [208]. The third study reported on two cases of females ages 17 and 13 years who were "severely underweight" due to the onset of vomiting and food refusal [209]. After admission, nasojejunum (NJ) tubes were placed to initiate refeeding when oral feeding was not tolerated. The authors reported that the use of an individualized behaviour plan for each patient providing reinforcements for eating was the critical factor which helped these patients to tolerate oral intake without vomiting and allowed for the removal of the NJ tubes.

Family-based inpatient care

Anorexia nervosa There were three studies found examining inpatient treatment utilizing a family-based

Table 39 Multimodal inpatient treatment for children and adolescents with eating disorders

Certainty assessment							Impact	Certainty	Importance
№ of studies	Study design	Risk of bias	Inconsistency	Indirectness	Imprecision	Other considerations			
Change in Weight (assessed with: Change in BMI from Admit to D/C)									
2	Case Series	very serious [a]	serious [b]	not serious	not serious	none	One study differentiated between patients with AN-R vs those with AN-B/P or BN and the other differentiated between those with AN-R or AN-B/P and those with BN or EDNOS-B/P. Multimodal treatment was provided in both studies, but varied between studies. Total n = 150 across the two studies. In both studies there was a significantly greater increase in BMI for the group containing AN-R patients (total n = 94). In both studies this group started with a much lower BMI (ie 14.94 and 15.78) and d/c BMI was 19.24 and 19.79. In the group containing only BN and EDNOS-B/P (n = 27) there was no change in BMI during admission. LOS in these studies was 6.25 +/− 2.28 months and 6.8 +/− 3 months.	⊕◯◯◯ VERY LOW	CRITICAL
		very serious [a,c]	not serious	not serious	serious [d]	all plausible residual confounding would reduce the demonstrated effect	Study compared EAT-26 at admission to discharge in group of patients with AN-R (n = 33) vs AN-B/P or BN (n = 29). Overall there was a statistically significant improvement in EAT-26 over the course of the admission (p < 0.001). In AN-R groups EAT-26 score decreased from 41.8 (SD 18.56) to 32.17 (SD 22.2) and in AN-B/P or BN group EAT-26 score decreased from 46.67 (SD 15) to 28.83 (SD 14.74). There was no significant difference in change on EAT-26 by diagnosis. LOS was 6.25 +/− 2.28 months.	⊕◯◯◯ VERY LOW	IMPORTANT

Explanations
[a]Observational Study with no control/comparison
[b]Differing inclusion/exclusion criteria and treatments provided
[c]Self-report scale
[d]Wide confidence intervals which cross over threshold of change
Bibliography:
Case Series - Rothschild-Yakar 2013 [203], Mekori 2017 [193]

approach, one of which included 37 patients [211], and the other two studies which included one patient each (i.e. case reports) [39, 63] (Table 41). Length of stay in hospital was a mean of 20.6 weeks (SD = 13.6, range 3–58) in the first study [211] and 10 days in one case report [39] and unclear in the second case report [63]. Mean weight gain was reported as 7.5 kg in the case series [211], a change in BMI from 16.32 to 17.5 in one case report [39], and a change in BMI of 15.4 to 19.5 in the other case report [63]. In the case report by Goldfield and Boachie [63], the family received eight sessions of family-based informed therapy via telepsychiatry as one parent and siblings were not local.

CBT-based inpatient care

Anorexia nervosa Three studies reported on inpatient treatment utilizing a CBT framework [197, 212, 213] (Table 42). These studies included two case series without a control group [197, 213] and one case study [212], for a total of 296 patients. Mean length of stay in these studies varied from 6 days to 90 days. In all studies patients gained weight in hospital.

One of these studies also reported on symptom change and included 238 patients [197]. Global EDI score and all subscales showed significant improvements. Forty-five percent showed "clinically significant" changes in EDI

Table 40 Inpatient Treatment for ARFID

Certainty assessment							Impact	Certainty	Importance
№ of studies	Study design	Risk of bias	Inconsistency	Indirectness	Imprecision	Other considerations			
Weight Change (assessed with: Pre-post weight in KG), caloric intake, ability to tolerate oral intake									
4	Case Reports	very serious [a,b]	not serious	not serious	not serious	none	Two articles reporting on case studies of 3 boys with ARFID ages 6–8 yrs. treated in an inpatient CBT-based treatment program and 2 studies reporting on a total of 5 children ages 9–13 yrs. treated in a family-based inpatient setting. LOS varied from 16 days to 112 days. All patients gained weight. For studies reporting on absolute weight gain the cases gained 2.7 kg in 60 days, 1.2 kg in 16 days and 0.3 kg in 19 days). At discharge these patients were at 97, 104 and 96%TGW. For the study reporting on change in %TGW, patients weight improved from 83 to 100%TGW (in 38 d), 75.8 to 100%TGW (in 2 months) and 72 to 88%TGW (in 2 months) and 69 to 86.8%TGW (LOS unclear).	⊕◯◯◯ VERY LOW	CRITICAL
		very serious [a]	not serious	not serious	not serious	none	One study reporting on 3 case studies on boys with ARFID ages 6–8 years treated in an inpatient CBT-based program. LOS varied from 16 to 60 days. Caloric intake in kcal/day rose for all 3 patients (from 1557 to 2208, 740 to 1300, and 1200 to 1500).	⊕◯◯◯ VERY LOW	CRITICAL
		very serious [b]	not serious	not serious	serious [c]	none	One study reporting on 2 cases of females ages 17 and 13 yrs. and one study describing two 9 yo girls. In the adolescent case reports both patients were severely underweight and due to the onset of vomiting and food refusal after admission NJ tubes were placed. Authors report that the use of an individualized behaviour plan for each patient providing reinforcements for eating was the critical factor in helping patients to tolerate oral intake without vomiting. The case reports involving the 9 yo girls, in both cases the patients were exclusively NGT fed due to a refusal of all oral nutrition, but with the addition of family therapy and mobilization from hospital the patients were able to resume eating orally.	⊕◯◯◯ VERY LOW	IMPORTANT

Explanations

[a]Observational study, no comparison/control

[b]Case studies only, likely biased reporting on patients with successful outcomes

[c]Results descriptive only, no quantitative outcomes re frequency of amount of food tolerated

Bibliography:

Case Reports - Pitt 2018 [209], Singer 1992 [208], Spettigue 2018 [53], Rhodes 2009 [210]

Table 41 Family-based inpatient treatment for children and adolescents with anorexia nervosa

Certainty assessment							Impact	Certainty	Importance
№ of studies	Study design	Risk of bias	Inconsistency	Indirectness	Imprecision	Other considerations			
Change in weight (assessed with: Absolute weight gain during admission in kg)									
1	Case Series	very serious[a]	not serious	not serious	not serious	none	One case series including 37 patients. LOS in hospital was a mean of 20.6 weeks (SD = 13.6, range 3–58) in this study. Weight gain was reported as 7.5 kg (SD 4.4, range – 1.1 to 14.8 kg)	⊕○○○ VERY LOW	CRITICAL
Weight									
2	Case Reports	very serious [a]	not serious	not serious	not serious	none	Two case reports – LOS in hospital was 10 days in one case report and unclear in the second case report. A change in BMI from 16.32 to 17.5 (ie 82%TGW to 85.8%TGW) in one case report, and a change in BMI of 15.4 to 19.5 in the second case report. In the second case report the family received 8 sessions of family-based informed therapy via telepsychiatry as one parent and siblings were not local.	⊕○○○ VERY LOW	CRITICAL

Explanations
[a]Observational study with no comparison or control
Bibliography:
Case Series - Halvorsen 2018 [211]
Case Reports - Goldfield 2003 [63], Matthews 2016 [39]

Global Scores, 23.6% showed "reliable" changes, 28% of patients remained "unchanged" and 3.7% "deteriorated".

Behaviour therapy based inpatient care

Anorexia nervosa Fifteen studies reported on inpatient treatment utilizing a behaviour therapy approach (4 case series and 11 case reports) [214–228] (Table 43). These studies included a total of 219 patients. Length of stay in these studies ranged from 13 days to 6.25 weeks [215, 217, 218]. In all studies patients gained weight.

Two of the case reports described change in intake as measured by kcal/day from admission to discharge. Only one of these studies reported the length of stay, which was 39 days. Calorie intake increased from 1600 kcal/d at admission to 3900 kcal/d at discharge in this study [214]. The other study did not report the length of stay, but stated that intake increased from 850 kcal/d at admission to 1700 kcal/d at discharge [221].

Several studies reported on symptom change during admission to hospital. One case report described a decrease in purging after meals from 48% of meals/week to 0% of meals per week, although the length of stay for this patient was not noted [221]. Two studies reported on EAT scores over the course of inpatient treatment. One was a case report describing that EAT scores remained high for the first 7 weeks of treatment and then dropped (from total score of 60 to 10) over the last 3 weeks of a 10-week admission [225]. The other study measured EAT scores in 24 patients at admission and discharge (mean length of stay 11 weeks) and reported a change from total mean EAT of 37.1 at admission to 12.7 at discharge ($p = 0.0001$) [224].

Bulimia nervosa Only one case series of 24 patients was found that examined inpatient treatment specifically for BN, and the treatment provided was based on behaviour therapy [229] (Table 44). The only eating disorder related outcome that was reported was weight. The mean LOS was 9.9 wks. (+/– 3.5 wks.). Weight decreased slightly over admission from a mean BMI of 20.6 to 20.5.

Psychodynamic based inpatient care

Anorexia nervosa Only two reports of a total of six patients being treated as inpatients using a psychodynamic based approach were found [230, 231] (Table 45). The length of stay for these patients varied between 1.5 months and 5 months. Patients were reported to have gained between 1.3 kg/month to 6 kg/month while admitted.

Admission to pediatric unit

Mixed diagnoses Four studies including a total of 200 patients, examined the effect of admission to a pediatric unit in terms of weight change in hospital [232–235] (Table 46). These studies did not include comparator groups and included patients with AN, BN and EDNOS. Mean length of stay varied between studies from 31 days to 85 days. In all studies weight improved.

Table 42 CBT-based inpatient treatment for children and adolescents with anorexia nervosa

Certainty assessment							Impact	Certainty	Importance
№ of studies	Study design	Risk of bias	Inconsistency	Indirectness	Imprecision	Other considerations			
Weight Change (assessed with: Pre-post weight measures), EDI-2 Scores pre and post									
2	Case Series	very serious [a]	not serious	not serious	serious [b]	none	Two studies - Total 295 patients. In all studies patients gained weight in hospital. Weight change reported differently across studies. One study reported BMI pre/post with BMI increasing from 14.83 (+/− 1.22) at admission to 17.34 (+/− 1.37) at discharge signifying an ES of 2.1. One study reported change in BMI % which rose from mean of 1.46 (+/− 2.41) at admission to 9.44 (+/− 6.68) at discharge.	⊕◯◯◯ VERY LOW	CRITICAL
		very serious [a]	not serious	not serious	serious [b]	all plausible residual confounding would reduce the demonstrated effect	One study which included 238 patients, mean LOS 81.9 (+/− 31.9) days. Global score and all subscales of the EDI-2 showed significant improvements. The ES of the Global score was 0.8. For subscales the highest ES was found for Drive for Thinness with an ES of 1.1, and the lowest ES was for Maturity Fears with an ES of 0.3. Forty-five % showed "clinically significant" changes in EDI-2 Global Scores, 23.6% showed "reliable" changes, 28% of patients remained unchanged and 3.7% deteriorated.	⊕◯◯◯ VERY LOW	IMPORTANT
Weight									
1	Case Report	very serious [a]	not serious	not serious	serious [b]	none	In the case study weight increased 1.1 kg in 6 days.	⊕◯◯◯ VERY LOW	CRITICAL

Explanations
[a]Observational study, no comparison/control
[b]Confidence intervals wide in some studies and overlapping with any true effect
Bibliography:
Case Series - Salbach-Andrae 2009 [213], Schlegl 2016 [197]
Case Report - Paul 2013 [212]

Inpatient adjunctive treatments

Adjunctive multi-family/parent group therapy

Mixed diagnoses One study with total 112 patients with various eating disorder diagnoses reported on symptom change as measured by the EDI during admission to a multimodal inpatient eating disorders unit in two groups of patients; those who received adjunctive multi-family group therapy (MFT, $n = 62$) and those who received adjunctive multi-parent group therapy (MPT, $n = 50$) [236] (Table 47). Both MPT and MFT interventions "promoted an autonomy-supportive parental attitude and the adolescents' autonomy and self-determination." Parents were encouraged to "create the conditions supporting their daughters' autonomy in establishing healthy eating at home to indirectly increase their daughters' motivation". Affected children were only included in the MFT group. Group format was one introductory 3-h session followed by five 2-h sessions every 2 weeks. Measures were taken pre/post of the intervention. Patients were not randomized, but rather were allocated to MFT versus MPT depending on the time of admission. Results reported a main effect of time on drive for thinness ($p < 0.001$) and body dissatisfaction ($p < 0.001$) as measured by EDI. Both scales improved independent of type of intervention. A separate case series of 32 inpatient adolescents (29 with AN, 3 with BN) described improvements in EDI score pre-post delivery of Family-Oriented Group Therapy [237].

Meal support

Mixed diagnoses Three studies were found that examined the effect of meal support/supervision as part of inpatient treatment for groups of patients with mixed eating disorders diagnoses [238–240] (Table 48). There were no significant differences between cohorts who

Table 43 Behaviour therapy based inpatient treatment for children and adolescents with anorexia nervosa

Certainty assessment							Impact	Certainty	Importance
№ of studies	Study design	Risk of bias	Inconsistency	Indirectness	Imprecision	Other considerations			
Change in Weight (assessed with: Pre-post measures of weight), Change in EAT scores, EDI Scores									
4	Case Series	very serious [a]	not serious	not serious	serious [b]	none	Four Case series utilizing a behaviour therapy approach. Total 198 patients. Various approaches to reporting change in weight. One study reported absolute weight change of 1.89 kg (+/− 1.41) over a mean of 23 days in hospital; one study reported a rise from a mean of 65.9%TGW to 87.4%TGW over 11 weeks. One study reported that patients admitted at > 75%TGW all reached 100%of their TGW by discharge, 91% of those admitted at < 75%TGW not requiring NGT feeds reached their TGW by discharge and only 62% of patients admitted at < 75%TGW and requiring NGT feeds reached 100% of their TGW at discharge. This study also noted that those admitted at > 75%TGW had a mean LOS of 20.8 d, those < 75%TGW at admission had a mean LOS of 18.4d and those < 75%TGW and NGT fed had a mean LOS of 32.7d. The final case series reported weight gain under 2 types of behaviour contracts, varying only with regards to the expected rate of weight gain (ie 0.36 kg/q4d vs 0.55 kg/q4d). Those treated under the contract requiring greater weight restoration gained weight at a faster rate (0.09 kg/d, range 0.04–0.4 kg/d vs 0.17 kg/d, range 0.01–0.64 kg/d), thereby attaining a greater weight gain overall during admission (LOS 28 days). Most case series reported weight gain observed while patients were adhering to a behaviour contract. LOS in these studies ranged from 13 days to 6.25 weeks. In all cases patients gained weight (ranging from 0.17 to 0.63 kg/day.	⊕○○○ VERY LOW	CRITICAL
		very serious [a]	not serious	not serious	serious [c]	all plausible residual confounding would reduce the demonstrated effect	One study measured EAT scores in 24 patients at admission and discharge (mean LOS 11 weeks) and reported a change from total mean EAT of 37.1 at admission to 12.7 at discharge ($p = 0.0001$).	⊕○○○ VERY LOW	IMPORTANT
		very serious [a]	not serious	not serious	serious [c]	all plausible residual confounding would reduce the demonstrated effect	One study of 24 patients, mean LOS 11 weeks. Reported a change in EDI score "Drive for Thinness" score of 8.0 at admission to 1.9 at discharge ($p = 0.02$). Other subscales and total EDI score not reported.	⊕○○○ VERY LOW	IMPORTANT

Table 43 Behaviour therapy based inpatient treatment for children and adolescents with anorexia nervosa *(Continued)*

Certainty assessment							Impact	Certainty	Importance
№ of studies	Study design	Risk of bias	Inconsistency	Indirectness	Imprecision	Other considerations			
Change in Weight, Change in EAT score, change in intake, change in rate of purging									
11	Case reports	very serious [a]	not serious	not serious	serious [b]	none	Case reports all described patients gaining weight in hospital ranging from 0.45 kg/wk. to 4.0 kg/wk. Two case reports did not note the LOS andstated that the patients gained 10 kg total and change in BMI from 13.5 to 16.5 during their admissions.	⊕○○○ VERY LOW	CRITICAL
		very serious [a]	not serious	not serious	serious [c]	all plausible residual confounding would reduce the demonstrated effect	One case report describing that EAT scores remained high for the first 7 weeks of treatment and weight restoration (4.5 kg over first 7 weeks) and then dropped (from total score of 60 to 10) over the last 3 weeks of 10 week admission.	⊕○○○ VERY LOW	IMPORTANT
		very serious [a]	not serious	not serious	not serious	strong association	Two case reports describing change in intake measured by kcal/day from admission to discharge. Only one study reported LOS of 39 days. Kcal/day increased from 1600 kcal/d at admission to 3900 kcal/d at discharge in this study. The other study did not report on LOS, but stated that intake increased from 850 kcal/d at admission to 1700 kcal/d at discharge.	⊕○○○ VERY LOW	CRITICAL
		very serious [a]	not serious	not serious	not serious	none	1 case report describing a decrease in purging after meals from 48% of meals/week to 0% of meals per week. LOS not noted.	⊕○○○ VERY LOW	IMPORTANT

Explanations
[a]Observational studies with no comparison group or control
[b]Wide confidence intervals in some studies, overlapping with any true effect
[c]Confidence intervals not noted
Bibliography:
Case series - Collins 1983 [222], Solanto 1994 [227], Steinhausen 1985 [224], Nygaard 1990 [226]
Case reports - Alessi 1989 [225], Blanchet-Collet 2016 [228], Blinder 1970 [215], Boey 1985 [223], Cinciripini 1983 [221], Clark 1981 [220], Garfinkel 1973 [216], Halmi 1975 [217], Leitenberg 1968 [214], Pertschuk 1978 [218], Poole 1978 [219]

Table 44 Behaviour therapy based inpatient treatment for children and adolescents with bulimia nervosa

Certainty assessment							Impact	Certainty	Importance
№ of studies	Study design	Risk of bias	Inconsistency	Indirectness	Imprecision	Other considerations			
Change in weight (assessed with: Pre/post BMI)									
1	Case Series	very serious [a]	not serious	not serious	not serious	none	One case series, including 24 patients. Mean LOS was 9.9 wks (+/−3.5 wks). Weight decreased slightly over admission from mean BMI of 20.6 +/− 4.3 to 20.5 +/− 2.7.	⊕○○○ VERY LOW	IMPORTANT

Explanations
[a]Observational study with no comparison/control
Bibliography:
Case Series - Wockel 2009 [229]

Table 45 Psychodynamic based inpatient treatment for children and adolescents with anorexia nervosa

Certainty assessment							Impact	Certainty	Importance
№ of studies	Study design	Risk of bias	Inconsistency	Indirectness	Imprecision	Other considerations			
Change in weight (assessed with: Pre/post measures of weight)									
2	Case Reports	very serious [a]	serious [b]	not serious	not serious	none	Two reports of 6 patients total. LOS varied between 1.5 months and 5 months. Patients were reported to have gained between 1.3 kg/month to 6 kg/month while admitted.	⊕◯◯◯ VERY LOW	CRITICAL

Explanations
[a]Case reports only, no comparison/control
[b]Large variation in results, likely due to individual factors of patients described in studies
Bibliography:
Case Reports - Kronenberg 1994 [231], Groen 1966 [230]

received meal support and those who did not on the rate of weight gain per day or week, although there was a trend towards greater weight gain in the group who received meal support. One of these studies reported on the difference in the rate of nasogastric tube (NGT) feeds in the cohort of patients treated on inpatient unit before the institution of consistent meal support versus after [238]. Eight of 12 patients not receiving meal support (66.7%) and 1 of 9 (11.1%) of those receiving meal support required NGT feeds as part of inpatient admission, which was a statistically significant difference.

Selective versus non-selective menus

Anorexia nervosa One study was found which included 22 patients with AN who received non-selective menus compared to 18 patients who received selective menus as part of their multimodal inpatient treatment [241] (Table 49). Length of stay varied between groups (although non-significantly) with patients on non-select menus remaining in hospital a mean of 60.3 (+/− 22.8) days vs 74.2 (+/− 28.7) days in the selective menus group. The non-selective menu group gained a significantly greater amount of weight. No significant differences were found on the EDE.

Table 46 Inpatient admission on pediatric unit for children and adolescents with eating disorders

Certainty assessment							Impact	Certainty	Importance
№ of studies	Study design	Risk of bias	Inconsistency	Indirectness	Imprecision	Other considerations			
Weight Change (assessed with: Pre-post weight measures)									
3	Case Series	very serious [a]	not serious	not serious	not serious	none	Three case series including a total of 195 patients. Mean LOS varied between studies from 31 days to 85 days. Two studies reported change in weight using %TGW. In both studies weight rose during admission from mean %TGW of 68% (+/− 5.5) to 99% (+/− 7.7); mean %TGW 75.8% (+/− 2.3) to 85.4% (+/− 1.7) and 73.7% (+/− 2.5) to 86.4% (+/− 3.0 kg) (note: results reported in two groups in second study based on whether the patients were followed after discharge).. The final study including 102 children aged 8–12 yrs. with diagnoses of restrictive ED (93.1%) or bulimia (7.1%). At admission the mean weight was 32.3 kg (SD 7.7) and at discharge mean weight was 35.4 kg (SD 8.9).	⊕◯◯◯ VERY LOW	CRITICAL
Weight Change (assessed with: Pre-post weight measures)									
1	Case Report	very serious [a]	not serious	not serious	not serious	none	In one case report ($n = 6$) study change in weight was reported in kg and rose a mean of 8.8 kg from admission to discharge ($n = 5$)	⊕◯◯◯ VERY LOW	CRITICAL

Explanations
[a]Observational study with no comparison/control
Bibliography:
Case Series - Lock 2003 [234], Jenkins 1987 [233], Meilleur 2012 [235]
Case Report - Maxmen 1974 [232]

Table 47 Multi-family therapy during inpatient treatment versus multi-parent therapy during inpatient treatment for children and adolescents with eating disorders

Certainty assessment							Impact	Certainty	Importance
№ of studies	Study design	Risk of bias	Inconsistency	Indirectness	Imprecision	Other considerations			
Change in eating disorder symptomatology (assessed with: Pre/post EDI-2)									
1	Case Control	serious [a]	not serious	not serious	not serious	none	One study with total 112 patients (MFT = 62 and MPT = 50). Intervention took place during inpatient multimodal treatment. Both MPT and MFT interventions "promoted an autonomy-supportive parental attitude and the adolescents' autonomy and self-determination." Parents were encouraged to "create the conditions supporting their daughters' auton omy in establishing healthy eating at home to indirectly increase their daughters' motivation". Group format was one introductory 3-h session followed by five 2-h sessions every 2 weeks. Measures were taken pre/post the intervention. Patients were not randomized, but rather allocation to MFT vs MPT depended on time of admission. Results reported a main effect of time for drive for thinness ($p < 0.001$) and body dissatisfaction ($p < 0.001$) as measured by EDI-2. Both scales improved independent of type of intervention.	⊕◯◯◯ VERY LOW	IMPORTANT
Change in EDI score									
1	Case series	very serious [a]	not serious	not serious	not serious	none	One case series describing the addition of Family-Oriented Group Therapy to an inpatient sample of 32 adolescent patients (29 with AN, 3 with BN). Improvements in EDI scores were noted.	⊕◯◯◯ VERY LOW	IMPORTANT

Explanations
[a]Due to design, no blinding possible
Bibliography:
Case Control - Depestele 2017 [236]
Case Series – Salbach 2006 [237]

Bright light therapy

Anorexia nervosa and major depressive disorder One study of patients with AN and depressive symptoms admitted to a CBT-based inpatient program and treated adjunctively with Bright Light Therapy was found [242] (Table 50). In this study patients were randomized to receive either daily 30 min Bright Light Therapy (BLT) + inpatient treatment ($n = 12$) for 6 weeks or inpatient treatment only for 6 weeks ($n = 12$). Patients in both groups had a significant change in their BMI during the 6-week study, however change from baseline was statistically significant by week 3 ($p = 0.038$) in BLT group versus by week 6 ($p = 0.048$) in the comparison group.

Cognitive remediation therapy

Anorexia nervosa Four studies reported on the addition of Cognitive Remediation Therapy (CRT) to multimodal inpatient treatment [243–246] (Table 51). One study described change in weight between patients who received 10 sessions of CRT over 10 weeks versus those who received TAU in a quasi-experimental design ($n = 24$ in each group) [244]. Both groups gained weight at a similar rate. The other studies reported on patients (total 79 patients) who received either 4 or 10 sessions of CRT provided as once weekly sessions. In all three studies patients gained weight. Given the design of these last three studies it was not possible to determine whether CRT had an impact on weight above and beyond what would have been expected by inpatient treatment alone.

Several studies of CRT added to inpatient treatment for AN reported on symptom change. One study included a description of two patients who received 10 sessions of CRT over 10 weeks in addition to multimodal inpatient treatment [243]. Scores on EAT decreased for one patient (30 to 16) and increased in the other patient (35 to 36). One study, including 125 hospitalized patients [246], received either group ($n = 55$) or individual ($n = 70$) CRT. Only those patients receiving individual

Table 48 Meal support during inpatient treatment versus no meal support be used in the treatment of children and adolescents with eating disorders

Certainty assessment							Impact	Certainty	Importance
№ of studies	Study design	Risk of bias	Inconsistency	Indirectness	Imprecision	Other considerations			
Rate of Weight Gain (assessed with: Measures of Weight Gain in Kg/Day), Need for NGT Feeds (assessed with: # of Patients Receiving NGT Feeds)									
3	Case Control	serious [a]	serious [b]	not serious	serious [c]	all plausible residual confounding would reduce the demonstrated effect	Three studies examined the effect of meal support/ supervision as part of inpatient treatment for a total number of patients receiving meal support of 88 patients. There were no significant differences between cohorts who received meal support and those who did not on the rate of weight gain per day or week,although there was a trend towards greater weight gain /day or week in the group who received meal support. Weight gain varied from 0.09 kg/day to 0.35 kg/day across studies.	⊕◯◯◯ VERY LOW	CRITICAL
		serious [d]	not serious	not serious	not serious	strong association all plausible residual confounding would reduce the demonstrated effect	One study of these studies reported on difference in the rate of NGT feeds in cohort of patients treated on inpatient unit before the institution of consistent meal support vs after. 8/12 patients not receiving meal support (ie 66.7%) and 1/9 (11.1%) of those receiving meal support required NGT feeds as part of inpatient admission.	⊕⊕⊕◯ MODERATE	IMPORTANT

Explanations
[a]Differences in LOS and age between those receiving meal support and those not receiving meal support may have affected outcomes
[b]Wide variation in # of meals/day supervised between various studies
[c]Wide confidence intervals in some studies/groups
[d]Criteria for initiating NGT feeds somewhat vague (ie "consistent failure" to meet expected weight gain and/or acute refusal of food
Bibliography:
Case Control - Kells 2013 [239], Kells 2017 [240], Couturier 2009 [238]

CRT completed the EDE-Q pre-post. Patients receiving individual CRT did not experience a change in their EDE-Q global score over the course of the 10 weeks they received CRT. One additional case report describes 10 sessions of CRT delivered to an inpatient with AN. Improvements on the EAT were observed [247].

One study, comprising 70 hospitalized patients who received multimodal inpatient treatment along with 10 individual sessions of CRT over 10 weeks reported on change in motivation as measured by the Motivational Stages of Change for Adolescents Recovering from an Eating Disorder (MSCARED) [246]. Patients completed the MSCARED before and after the course of CRT. There was a statistically significant improvement in motivation noted. Due to the design of this study it was not possible to differentiate the effect of inpatient treatment alone from inpatient treatment plus CRT.

Inpatient and day treatment combined

Anorexia nervosa Five reports on 265 patients with AN treated as inpatients followed immediately by day treatment were found [200, 248–251] (Table 52). In all five studies, patients were treated as inpatients and then transferred to day treatment once medically stable. Details regarding the number of hours/days spent in day treatment were not thoroughly reported, although mean length of stay varied from 7.9 weeks to 3.9 months. Weight change was reported in various ways, however, all studies indicated improvement in weight.

Symptom change was reported using various scales in these studies. One study included 35 patients with a mean length of stay of 15.1 weeks [251]. Change in EDI total, drive for thinness and body dissatisfaction were not significantly different between admission

Table 49 Non-selective menus during inpatient treatment versus selective menus for children and adolescents with anorexia nervosa

Certainty assessment							Impact	Certainty	Importance
№ of studies	Study design	Risk of bias	Inconsistency	Indirectness	Imprecision	Other considerations			
Rate of Weight Gain (assessed with: Weekly weight gain in kg/week), EDE Scores									
1	Case Control	serious [a,b]	not serious	not serious	serious [c]	all plausible residual confounding would reduce the demonstrated effect	One study including 22 patients who received non-selective menus compared to 18 patients who re ceived selective menus. LOS varied between groups (although non-significant) with non-select patients remaining in hospital a mean of 60.3 (+/− 22.8) days vs 74.2 (+/−28.7) days in selective menus group. Non-selective menu group gained a mean of 0.95 kg/wk (+/−0.35) and those in selective menu group gained a mean of 0.72 kg/wk (+/− 0.24) (p = 0.02).	⊕◯◯◯ VERY LOW	CRITICAL
		serious [a,b]	not serious	not serious	serious [c]	all plausible residual confounding would reduce the demonstrated effect	No significant differences were found on any of the EDE items related to eating concern. Overall change in EDE eating concern scores were low ranging from −0.6 to 1.1.	⊕◯◯◯ VERY LOW	IMPORTANT

Explanations
[a]Unclear whether groups differed at baseline as these details were not reported
[b]Cohort study design (pre/post introduction of non-selective menus), unclear if other aspects of care may have also varied between groups
[c]Confidence intervals relatively wide and overlap with actual difference in effect
Bibliography:
Case Control - Leacy 2012 [241]

Table 50 Bright light therapy during CBT-based inpatient treatment versus CBT-based inpatient treatment alone for children and adolescents with anorexia nervosa and major depressive disorder

Certainty assessment							Impact	Certainty	Importance
№ of studies	Study design	Risk of bias	Inconsistency	Indirectness	Imprecision	Other considerations			
RCT - Change in Weight (assessed with: Change in BMI per week)									
1	randomised trials	serious [a]	not serious	not serious	serious [b]	none	One study randomized patients with AN-R and depressive symptoms (> 17 on HDRS) admitted to CBT-based inpatient treatment to receive either daily 30 min BLT + inpatient treatment ($n = 12$) × 6 weeks or inpatient treatment only × 6 weeks ($n = 12$). Patients in both groups had a significant change in their BMI during 6 week study, however change from baseline was statistically significant by week 3 ($p = 0.038$) in BLT group vs only significant change from baseline at week 6 ($p = 0.048$) in TAU group.	⊕⊕◯◯ LOW	CRITICAL

Explanations
[a]No blinding of subjects to treatment group
[b]Confidence intervals overlapping with actual size of treatment effect
Bibliography
RCT - Janas-Kozik 2011 [242]

Table 51 Cognitive remediation therapy during inpatient treatment be used for the treatment of children and adolescents with anorexia nervosa

Certainty assessment							Impact	Certainty	Importance
№ of studies	Study design	Risk of bias	Inconsistency	Indirectness	Imprecision	Other considerations			
Change in Weight (assessed with: Pre/Post CRT Measures of Weight), change in EBRS, change in EDE-Q									
3	Case/control Case Series	very serious [a]	not serious	not serious	not serious	all plausible residual confounding would reduce the demonstrated effect	Three studies reported on addition of CRT to multimodal inpatient treatment. One study described change in weight between patients who received 10 sessions of CRT over 10 weeks vs those who received TAU in a quasi-experimental design ($n = 24$ in each group). Both groups gained weight at a similar rate (change from mean BMI% of 2.2 to 5.7 over 10 weeks in CRT group vs mean BMI% 5.5 to 7.6 over 10 weeks in TAU group). The other studies reported on patients (total 79 patients) who received either 4 or 10 sessions of CRT provided as once weekly sessions. In all 3 studies patients gained weight. Given the design of these studies it is not possible to deter mine whether CRT had an impact on weight above and beyond what would have been expected by in patient treatment alone.	⊕○○○ VERY LOW	CRITICAL
		very serious [b]	not serious	not serious	not serious	all plausible residual confounding would reduce the demonstrated effect	One study included description of 2 patients who received 10 sessions of CRT over 10 weeks in addition to multimodal inpatient treatment. EBRS scores decreased slight for both patients from 26 to 22 and 29 to 26 at end of 10 weeks.	⊕○○○ VERY LOW	IMPORTANT
		very serious [a]	not serious	not serious	serious [d]	all plausible residual confounding would reduce the demonstrated effect	One study, including 125 hospitalized patients. Received either group ($n = 55$) or individual ($n = 70$) CRT. Only those patients receiving individual CRT completed the EDE-Q. pre-post. Patients receiving individual CRT did not experience a change in their EDE-Q global score over the course of the 10 weeks where they received CRT.	⊕○○○ VERY LOW	IMPORTANT
		very serious [a]	not serious	not serious	not serious	all plausible residual confounding would reduce the demonstrated effect	One study, comprising 70 hospitalized patients who received multimodal inpatient treatment along with 10 individual sessions of CRT over 10 weeks. Patients completed the MSCARED before and after the course of CRT. There was a statistically significant shift in motivation noted ($p < 0.001$), where at initiation of CRT % of patients in each stages of change category were as follows: pre-contemplation 18.6%, contemplation 38.6%, prepar ation 28.6%, action 11.4%, mainten ance 2.9%. At the end of CRT % of patients in each stage of change were: pre-contemplation 0%, con templation 4.3%, preparation 31.4%, action 42.9%, maintenance 21.4%,	⊕○○○ VERY LOW	IMPORTANT

Table 51 Cognitive remediation therapy during inpatient treatment be used for the treatment of children and adolescents with anorexia nervosa *(Continued)*

Certainty assessment							Impact	Certainty	Importance
№ of studies	Study design	Risk of bias	Inconsistency	Indirectness	Imprecision	Other considerations			
							Due to the design of this study it is not possible to differentiate the effect of inpatient treatment alone from inpatient treatment + CRT.		
		very serious [b]	serious [c]	not serious	not serious	all plausible residual confounding would reduce the demonstrated effect	One study included description of 2 patients who received 10 sessions of CRT over 10 weeks in addition to multimodal inpatient treatment. Scores on EAT decreased for one patient (30 to 16) and increased in the other patient (35 to 36).	⊕○○○ VERY LOW	IMPORTANT
Weight, EAT-26									
2	Case reports	very serious [b]	serious [c]	not serious	not serious	all plausible residual confounding would reduce the demonstrated effect	One study involved 7 adolescents inpatients with AN using group CRT. Weight improved as did motivation.	⊕○○○ VERY LOW	IMPORTANT
		very serious [b]	serious [c]	not serious	not serious	all plausible residual confounding would reduce the demonstrated effect	Another study is a single case report describing improvement on the EAT-26 after 10 sessions of CRT with an inpatient with AN.	⊕○○○ VERY LOW	IMPORTANT

Explanations
[a]Not all studies had comparison group and were receiving inpatient treatment which could account for some of the differences observed/reported
[b]Case report design, no comparison/control
[c]Differing results between the 2 reports likely secondary to individual differences
[d]Wide confidence intervals, overlapping with with the size of the effect noted
Bibliography:
Case control - Herbrich 2017 [244], Harrison 2018 [246]
Case series – Asch 2014 [243]
Case reports – Kuge 2017 [245], Cwojdzinska 2009 [247]

and discharge. One study included 26 adolescents who received 13 weeks of inpatient treatment based on the Cognitive Behavioural Therapy- Enhanced (CBT-E) model followed by 7 weeks of Day Treatment Program (DTP) [249]. EDE scores decreased significantly pre-post for global score and all subscales other than Shape Concern. This study also reported on frequency of eating disorder symptoms. Binge eating was present in eight patients (30%) at admission and only two patients (7.7%) at discharge. Purging by vomiting was present at admission for 10 patients (28.5%) and at discharge for 4 patients (15.1%). Laxative misuse was present for 3 patients at admission and none at discharge.

One study reported on change in motivation as measured by the ANOSCQ in 35 patients [251]. These patients received 15.1 weeks of inpatient and day treatment. Overall scores increased a mean of 21.7 points, which signified moving from contemplation to preparation phases.

One study which included 71 patients who completed 7.9 weeks of combined inpatient and DTP (33 days inpatient and 22 days DTP) reported on "overall outcome" [200]. At the end of DTP 35.2% were deemed to have an excellent outcome, 26.8% were deemed good outcome, 14.1% deemed below average outcome and 23.9% were deemed to have a poor outcome.

Admission to weight restoration versus short admission for medical stabilization with either FBT or day treatment

Anorexia nervosa Two high quality studies examined the difference between patients randomized to receive a relatively short inpatient admission followed by either 20 sessions of FBT ($n = 82$) [252] or Day Treatment ($n = 172$) [253] compared to a lengthy inpatient stay to weight restoration (Table 53). In the Inpatient/FBT study [252]

Table 52 Inpatient and day treatment in combination for children and adolescents with anorexia nervosa

Certainty assessment							Impact	Certainty	Importance
№ of studies	Study design	Risk of bias	Inconsistency	Indirectness	Imprecision	Other considerations			
Weight Change (assessed with: Change in weight during treatment)									
5	Case Control and Case Series	very serious [a]	not serious	not serious	not serious	none	265 patients over 5 studies, all with AN. All studies treated patients as inpatients and then transferred to day treatment once medically stable. Details regarding the number of hours/days spent in day treatment not completely reported. Mean LOS were 3.9 months, 15.1 weeks and 7.9 weeks. Patients gained weight as described by BMI in 3 studies where BMI increase from 12.1 (SD1.1) to 18.6 (SD 0.42) in one study, 15.7 (SD1.2) to 18.0 (SD 1.0) in the second study and 15.19 (+/− 1.54) to 17.56 (+/− 1.07) in the third study. The second study also reported weight as %TGW which rose from 77.6% at admission to inpt to 88.5% at end of day treatment. In 2 studies weight change was described using BMI centiles and weight rose from a mean BMI centile of 2.7 (+/− 4.2) to 34.2 (+/− 15.7) in one study and 1.6 (+/− 5.1) to 49.4 (+/− 3.9) in the second study. 5/40 patients eligible for one study left treatment AMA and were not included in analysis.	⊕◯◯◯ VERY LOW	CRITICAL
Eating Disorder Inventory - 2 Score at discharge (assessed with: Rating Scale)									
1	Case Series	very serious [a,b]	not serious	not serious	not serious	none	35 patients completed inpt, day treatment and measures. Mean LOS 15.1 weeks. Change in ED1-2 total, drive for thinness and body dissatisfaction not significantly different between admission and discharge.	⊕◯◯◯ VERY LOW	IMPORTANT
Anorexia Nervosa Stages of Change Questionnaire (assessed with: Rating Scale)									
1	Case Series	very serious [a,c]	not serious	not serious	serious [d]	all plausible residual confounding would reduce the demonstrated effect	35 patients completed ANSOCQ at admission and d/c (ie after 15.1 weeks of inpatient + day treatment). Overall score increased a mean of 21.7 points which would signify moving from contemplation to preparation phases. Overall 29.4% (up from 0% at admission) of patients were classified as in "maintenance phase" and 26.5% (up from 15% at admission) in "action phase" at time of discharge.	⊕◯◯◯ VERY LOW	IMPORTANT
Overall Outcome (assessed with: Rating combining weight + compensatory symptoms)									
1	Case series	very serious [a,e]	not serious	not serious	not serious	all plausible residual confounding would reduce the demonstrated effect	One study which included 71 patients who completed 7.9 weeks of combined inpatient and DTP (33 days inpatient and 22 days DTP). At end of DTP 35.2% were deemed to have an excellent outcome (> 90% ideal BMI, maintaining weight and no use of compensatory symptoms in last week of program), 26.8% were deemed good outcome (85–90% ideal BMI, maintaining weight and no use of compensatory symptoms in last week of treatment), 14.1% deemed below average outcome (80–85% ideal BMI and maintaining weight OR > 85% ideal BMI, but losing 0.15–0.45 kg/week with no compensatory symptoms in the last week of treatment) and 23.9% were deemed to have a poor outcome (either < 80% ideal BMI OR < 85% ideal BMI and losing > 0.15 kg/week OR readmitted to inpatient unit OR use of compensatory symptoms in	⊕◯◯◯ VERY LOW	IMPORTANT

Table 52 Inpatient and day treatment in combination for children and adolescents with anorexia nervosa *(Continued)*

Certainty assessment							Impact	Certainty	Importance
№ of studies	Study design	Risk of bias	Inconsistency	Indirectness	Imprecision	Other considerations			
							the last week of treatment).		
Eating Disorder Symptomatology (assessed with: Pre-post EDE-Q)									
1	Case series	very serious [a]	not serious	not serious	serious [d]	none	One study, including $n = 26$ adolescents. Patients received 13 weeks of inpatient treatment based on CBT-E model followed by 7 weeks of DTP. EDE scores decreased significantly pre-post for global and all subscales other than Shape Concern. Global EDE at admission 3.7 (+/− 1.3) to d/c 2.0 (+/− 1.1), % of patients with Global EDE < 1 SD above the community mean at admission 2% (+/− 7.7) and at d/c 10% (+/− 38.5). Dietary restraint at admission 4.1 (+/− 1.2) and at d/c 1.1 (+/− 1.0), Eating Concern (3.3 (+/− 1.4) and at d/c 1.5 (+/− 1.4), Shape Concern (3.8 (+/− 1.8) and at d/c 3.2 (+/− 1.4), Weight Concern at admission 3.5 (+/− 1.9) and at d/c 2.3 (+/− 1.4).	⊕○○○ VERY LOW	IMPORTANT
Change in Frequency of Eating Disorder Symptoms (assessed with: Pre-post ED symptom frequency)									
1	Case series	very serious [a]	not serious	not serious	serious [d]	none	One study, including $n = 26$ adolescents. Patients received 13 weeks of inpatient treatment based on CBT-E model followed by 7 weeks of DTP. Binge eating was present in 8 patients (30%) at admission and only 2 patients (7.7%) at discharge. Median frequency of bingeing in previous 28 days was 17 (range 2–148) at admission and 8 (range 1–15) at discharge. Purging by vomiting was present at admission for 10 patients (28.5%) and at d/c for 4 patients (15.1%). Frequency of vomiting in previous 28 days was 25 (range 1–196) at admission and 10.5 (range 0–30) at dscharge. Laxative misuse was present for 3 patients at admission and none at discharge. Frequency of laxative abuse in previous 28 days was 1 (range 1–20) at admission and nil at d/c.	⊕○○○ VERY LOW	CRITICAL

Explanations
[a]Observational study with no comparison/control
[b]Self-rating scale (EDI-2)
[c]Self-rating scale (ANSOCQ)
[d]Lower end of confidence interval overlaps with score that would signify no change
[e]Information on compensatory symptoms was taken only from clinician notes
Bibliography:
Case control - El Ghoch 2015 [250], Strober 2006 [248]
Case series - Delle Grave 2014 [249], Hillen 2015 [251], Treat 2008 [200]

patients had all been unwell less than 3 years and in the inpatient/day treatment study [253] the patients were included only if it was their first admission. At the end of FBT or Day Treatment, there were no significant differences between those who were discharged after a short admission versus those who remained in hospital for weight restoration in terms of weight outcome, rate of readmissions over 12-month follow-up, or eating disorder symptoms [252, 253].

Day treatment

Multimodal day treatment

Anorexia nervosa Two case series and one case report describe the outcomes of patients treated in their multimodal day hospital programs [254–256] (Table 54). Admission to day treatment in these studies could occur from an inpatient setting or an outpatient setting based on clinical need. Weight related

Table 53 Inpatient medical stabilization followed by outpatient treatment versus inpatient weight restoration for children and adolescents with anorexia nervosa

Certainty assessment							Impact	Certainty	Importance
№ of studies	Study design	Risk of bias	Inconsistency	Indirectness	Imprecision	Other considerations			
Change in weight (assessed with: Pre/post measures of weight), Rate of Readmission, psychological symptoms (EDE and EDI)									
2	randomised trials	serious [a]	not serious	not serious	not serious	none	Two RCT examined the difference between patients randomized to receive a relatively short inpatient admission followed by either 20 sessions of FBT (*n* = 82) or DTP (*n* = 172). In the FBT F/U study patients had all been unwell less than 3 years and in the day treatment F/U study the patients we only included if it was their first admission. The first study randomized patients to be d/c once medically stable (mean LOS 21.73 +/− 5.92 days) vs to remain in hospital until 90%TGW (mean LOS 36.89 +/− 17.06). Both groups received 20 sessions of FBT following discharge. Patients discharged at point of medical stability (ie mean 84.40%TGW) had attained a mean of 95.20%TGW by the end of 20 sessions of FBT, whereas those who remained in hospital until they were 90%TGW (ie mean 92.00%TGW) were at a mean of 93.10%TGW by session 20. ES in this study was 1.28 at the end of hospitalization and 0.27 at end of session 20. There was a significant difference in weight at end of hospitalization, but not by end of session 20. The other study randomized patients to remain as inpatients for 3 weeks vs until attaining TGW (total mean treatment time 14.6 weeks). Those d/c at 3 weeks entered a DTP with similar programming (total mean treatment time 16.5 weeks). At end of treatment patients in inpatient only group had reached a mean of 89%TGW (+/− 3.8) and those in inpt + DTP had reached 88.1%TGW (+/− 4.7) - no significant difference in weight outcome in intention to treat analysis.	⊕⊕⊕○ MODERATE	CRITICAL
		serious [a]	not serious	not serious	not serious	none	Both RCTs examined Rate of readmission measured over the 12 months following admission in the FBT-f/u study (*n* = 82). Re admission rates were similar re gardless of allocation (ie 35% in med stability group vs 36.8% in the weight restoration group). However, given that the med stability group had a shorter	⊕⊕⊕○ MODERATE	IMPORTANT

Table 53 Inpatient medical stabilization followed by outpatient treatment versus inpatient weight restoration for children and adolescents with anorexia nervosa *(Continued)*

Certainty assessment							Impact	Certainty	Importance
№ of studies	Study design	Risk of bias	Inconsistency	Indirectness	Imprecision	Other considerations			
							initial admission, the total hospital days was 45.2 d in this group vs 65.5 in the weight restoration group. In inpatient weight restoration vs DTP F/U 8/87 patients were readmitted during their DTPtreatment due to medical instability and 25.3% (inpt WR) vs 15.1% (DTP), $p = 0.12$ required readmission to inpatient unit at 12 months F/U.		
		serious [a]	not serious	not serious	not serious	none	One study - EDI-2 scores pre treatment and post treatment similar between groups regardless of allocation (total $n = 143$).	⊕⊕⊕○ MODERATE	IMPORTANT
		serious [a]	not serious	not serious	not serious	none	One study - EDE global scores not significantly different between groups at baseline or at end of FBT, 6 month or 12 month F/U ($n = 69$).	⊕⊕⊕○ MODERATE	IMPORTANT

Explanations
[a]No blinding of participants possible
Bibliography:
RCT - Herpertz-Dahlmann 2014 [253], Madden 2015 [252]

outcomes were reported in various ways. Improvements in BMI from admission to discharge were described [255]. Two studies reported improvements in %TGW at admission and discharge [255, 256]. One study reported an increase in weight from 81.6 to 84.2%TGW [255]. The other study reported weight change separately for patients above and below 85%TGW at admission and found both cohorts gained weight [256]. Mean length of stay varied between 70 to 92 days. One case report described a weight change from 87 lbs to 101 lbs over the admission to the day program [254].

One study examined eating disorder psychological symptoms with 26 patients remaining in DTP for mean length of 10 weeks [255]. EDI scores for Drive for Thinness and Perfectionism improved significantly, whereas body dissatisfaction and maturity fears did not change significantly.

Two studies reported on percent of patients successfully completing the day treatment program [255, 256]. Definition of "successful completion" was based on a combination of symptom change, weight gain and progression in program (versus leaving against medical advice (AMA) or need for admission to an inpatient unit). Mean length of stay ranged from 11.6 to 15.3 weeks. Successful completion rates in these studies were 30 to 50%. One study examined whether completion rate varied between those that started at greater than or less that 85%TGW, and reported that there was no difference based on this factor [256].

Mixed diagnoses Several studies address mixed diagnoses of eating disorders within a multimodal day hospital program [257–261] (Table 55). Weight in all studies improved over the course of day treatment. Weight gain was correlated with a diagnosis of AN or EDNOS (versus BN), longer length of stay and lower weight at admission [261]. The length of stay in these studies varied between 15.3 weeks and 13.1 weeks.

Lazaro and colleagues [259] reported outcomes separately for those with AN and BN within their day treatment program. The sample size was 160 patients (116 AN patients and 44 BN patients). Mean length of stay was 15 weeks. For both groups, self-esteem improved in relation to others and in relation to weight and shape. No significant differences were found between the AN and BN groups [259].

Table 54 Multimodal day treatment be used in the treatment of children and adolescents with anorexia nervosa

Certainty assessment							Impact	Certainty	Importance
№ of studies	Study design	Risk of bias	Inconsistency	Indirectness	Imprecision	Other considerations			
Weight Gain From Admission to Discharge (assessed with: BMI/%TGW/Wt), EDI-3, EAT-26, Motivation, successful completion (%)									
2	Case Series	very serious [a]	serious [b]	not serious	serious [c]	all plausible residual confounding would reduce the demonstrated effect	Admission to DTP could occur from inpatient setting or outpatient setting based on clinical judgment of need for this level of care. Weight related outcomes reported in various ways. One study reported admission and discharge BMI with a change from 16.5 (SD 1.5) to 17.1 (SD 1.9). Two studies reported %TGW at admission and discharge. One reported an increase in weight from 81.6 to 84.2%TGW. The other study reported weight change separately for patients above and below 85%TGW at admission. For those < 85%TGW at admission, TGW rose from 81.5 to 88.3%, in those > 85%TGW at admission %TGW rose from 88.0 to 92.2%.. Mean LOS varied between 70 to 92 days.	⊕○○○ VERY LOW	CRITICAL
		very serious [a]	not serious	not serious	serious [c]	all plausible residual confounding would reduce the demonstrated effect	One study - 26 patients in study, remained in DTP for mean LOS of 10 weeks. Eighty-five % of patients were referred to DTP from out patient setting, remainder from in patient program. Only criterion from admission to DTP vs inpatient was medical stability. EDI-3 scores for Drive for Thinness and Perfectionism improved significantly with Drive for Thinness changing from 13.81 (SD 9.08) to 10.08 (SD 8.32) and Perfec tionism changing from 8.96 (6.79) to 8.19 (SD 6.87), signifying a small ef fect size (0.43 and 0.11 respectively). Body dissatisfaction and maturity fears did not change significantly during course of DTP.	⊕○○○ VERY LOW	IMPORTANT
		very serious	not serious	not serious	serious [c]	all plausible residual confounding would reduce the demonstrated effect	One study - 26 patients in study, remained in DTP for mean LOS of 10 weeks. EAT-26 scores decreased from 28.08 (SD 20.61) at admission to 22.19 (SD 19.34) at discharge which signifies a small effect size (ie 0.30).	⊕○○○ VERY LOW	IMPORTANT
		very serious [a]	not serious	not serious	serious [c]	all plausible residual confounding would reduce the demonstrated effect	One study - 26 patients in study, remained in DTP for mean LOS of 10 weeks. ANSOCQ score changed from 53.48 (SD 20.42) to 65.63 (SD 21.27) signifying no change in "stage" (patients remained in "preparation phase" throughout).	⊕○○○ VERY LOW	IMPORTANT
		very serious [a]	serious [b]	not serious	not serious	none	Two studies reported on "% completing" the DTP, including 53 patients with AN. Definition of "successful completion" was based on a combination of symptom change, weight gain and progression in program (vs leaving AMA or need for admission to inpatient unit). Mean LOS ranged	⊕○○○ VERY LOW	CRITICAL

Table 54 Multimodal day treatment be used in the treatment of children and adolescents with anorexia nervosa *(Continued)*

Certainty assessment							Impact	Certainty	Importance
№ of studies	Study design	Risk of bias	Inconsistency	Indirectness	Imprecision	Other considerations			
							from 11.6 to 15.3 weeks. "Successful Completion" rates in these studies were 30 to 50%. One study examined whether completion rate varied between those that started at greater than or less that 85%TGW, and reported that there was no difference based on this factor.		
Weight									
1	Case report	very serious [a]	serious [b]	not serious	serious [c]	all plausible residual confounding would reduce the demonstrated effect	The case report described a weight change from 87lbs to 101 lbs. over the DTP admission	⊕○○○ VERY LOW	CRITICAL

Explanations
[a] Observational study, no comparison/control
[b]Varying BMI/TGW at admission to various programs, programs provided differing levels/hours of support and results on this outcome varied
[c]Confidence intervals wider than actual effect in some studies
Bibliography:
Case series - Ngo 2014 [256], Goldstein 2011 [255]
Case reports – Garner 2002 [254]

Two studies treating mixed diagnoses of eating disorders for total of 61 patients looked at successful completion of the program [257, 258]. Success was defined using various criteria such as adequate weight gain, symptom reduction, and no AMA discharge or inpatient admission. Success rate was 49% [258] and 50% [257].

One study including 30 patients with mixed diagnoses examined motivational stage of change [260]. Length of stay was 10.5 weeks. Motivational Stage of Change was measured pre-post with the MSCARED [260]. Patients were noted to progress through the stages of change during treatment. The change in stage of change from intake to discharge was significantly correlated with the change in the Children's Eating Attitudes Test (ChEAT) score during the same time period [260].

Family-based day treatment

Anorexia nervosa/low weight eating disorders Nine studies for a total of 427 patients examined a family-based day treatment program [262–270] (Table 56). Studies varied with regards to the degree to which they included parents in treatment, number of hours/week of programming and length of stay. Criteria for admission to the day treatment program varied.

Five studies reported improvement in BMI [264, 265, 268–270]. Three studies reported on total weight gained in program [262, 263, 269]. Two studies reported on change in %TGW which rose from 83 to 93% in one study [266], and 83 to 98% in another study [269]. Length of stay in these studies varied from 28 days to 1.3 years.

One study reported on difference in weight outcomes between their Maudsley and non-Maudsley DTP, noting no difference between these two groups [264]. Another study reported on differences between patients who received "formal psychotherapy" (individual and/or family) outside of program thereby needing to leave program for approx 2 h/week and noted that patients who received external psychotherapy within the first 2 months of entering DTP gained significantly less weight [262]. One study examined predictors of weight restoration in DTP and reported that higher BMI at admission, greater gain in the first 4 weeks and lower caregiver empowerment at baseline were predictive of weight restoration at end of intensive treatment [269].

Six studies examined psychological symptoms with the EDE-Q [264, 266, 267, 269–271]. EDE-Q scores, global and all subscales decreased significantly in these studies. In a study reporting on a control group which was treated in the same program, but without the inclusion of Maudsley/family interventions, the EDE-Q scores decreased more in the Maudsley group than the non-Maudsley [264]. Of note the scores for Weight Concern and Restraint Concerns did not change significantly in the non-Maudsley group whereas they decreased significantly in the Maudsley group [264].

Table 55 Multimodal day treatment be used in the treatment of children and adolescents with eating disorders

Certainty assessment							Impact	Certainty	Importance
№ of studies	Study design	Risk of bias	Inconsistency	Indirectness	Imprecision	Other considerations			
Weight Change (assessed with: BMI/TGW), Change in self esteem, successful completion, change in motivation									
5	Case series	very serious [a]	not serious	not serious	serious [b]	none	Reasons for referral to DTP were based on severity of symptomatology, but could occur from inpatient or outpatient or initial assessment. Two studies reported all patients together, the other ($n = 160$) reported AN ($n = 116$) vs BN ($n = 44$). In one mixed study the mean BMI rose from 18.9 (SD 2.6) to 20.9 (SD 2.9) which related to a change in %TGW from 94% at admission to 102% at discharge. In the other mixed study the weight gain was reported as 0.95 kg over the 2.6 weeks LOS. It was noted that approx one-quarter of patients lost weight, one quarter gained 0–0.9 kg, on quarter gained 0.9–1.8 kg and one quarter gained > 1.8 kg. Weight gain was correlated with dx of AN or EDNOS vs BN, longer LOS and lower weight at admission. The last study reported that patients with AN started at a mean BMI of 18.3 (SD 1.2) and gained 0.9 points, whereas patients with BN started with a mean BMI of 20.3 (SD 3.3) and gained a mean of 0.3 points. The LOS in these studies was 15.3 weeks and 13.1 weeks respectively.	⊕○○○ VERY LOW	CRITICAL
		very serious [a]	not serious	not serious	serious [b]	all plausible residual confounding would reduce the demonstrated effect	One study - Total of 160 patients (ie 116 AN patients and 44 BN patients). Mean LOS was 15 weeks. For AN group the SEED in relation to others decreased from 16.5 (SD 9.7) to 15.0 (SD 10.7) ($p = 0.039$) and SEED related to weight and shape changed from 14.6 (SD 7.8) to 13.5 (SD 9.0) ($p = 0.046$). In the BN group SEED in relation to others changed from 17.3 (SD 7.8) to 13.2 (SD 8.5) ($p = 0.000$) and SEED related to weight and shape changed from 17.6 (SD 7.0) to 13.2 (SD 8.0) ($p = 0.001$). No significant difference in effect between AN and BN.	⊕○○○ VERY LOW	IMPORTANT
		very serious [a]	not serious	not serious	not serious	none	Two studies for total of 61 patients. Success defined using various criteria such as adequate weight gain, symptom reduction, and no AMA discharge or inpatient admission. "Success" rate was 49 and 50% in these 2 studies.	⊕○○○ VERY LOW	IMPORTANT
		very serious [a]	not serious	not serious	not serious	all plausible residual confounding would reduce the demonstrated effect	One study including 30 patients. LOS was 10.5 weeks. Motivational Stage of Change was measured pre-post with the MSCARED. Patients were noted to progress through 1.9 +/− 1.3 stages from beginning to end of treatment ($p < 0.0001$). The change in SOC from intake to discharge was significantly correlated	⊕○○○ VERY LOW	IMPORTANT

Table 55 Multimodal day treatment be used in the treatment of children and adolescents with eating disorders *(Continued)*

Certainty assessment							Impact	Certainty	Importance
№ of studies	Study design	Risk of bias	Inconsistency	Indirectness	Imprecision	Other considerations			
							with the change in the ChEAT score during the same time period ($p = 0.001$).		

Explanations
[a]Observational study with no comparison/control
[b]Confidence intervals wider than effect size
Bibliography:
Case series - Bustin 2013 [260], Lazaro 2011 [259], Dancyger 2002 [257], Dancyger 2003 [258], deGraft-Johnston 2013 [261]

One study consisting of 32 patients reported on body image disturbance [263]. Body image disturbance disappeared completely in 59%, decreased partially in 28% and remained unchanged in 13%. Prolonged duration of meals improved during treatment and "normalized" in 87.5% by end of treatment. Eighty-seven percent stopped ritualistic exercise habits by end of treatment.

One study including 60 patients, with median length of stay 8 months showed statistically significant change in EDI Drive for Thinness and body dissatisfaction [268]. Statistically significant change was reported on the EAT.

Mixed eating disorder diagnoses Five case series and one case report for total of 262 patients studied a family-based day treatment program with adolescents with mixed eating disorder diagnoses [272–277] (Table 57). Studies varied with regard to the form of parent involvement, hours/week in treatment and admission criteria. Four studies reported change in BMI from admission to discharge and found that BMI improved [272, 275–277] (Table 57). Three studies reported on change in %TGW and found significant improvements [272, 274, 276]. One study reported weight change as 12/19 patients reaching 100%TGW at 3 months and the other 7/19 reaching a mean %TGW of 94% [273]. The mean LOS varied between these studies from 3.2 weeks to 28.5 weeks. (Table 57).

In terms of psychological symptoms, one study with total of 51 patients looked at EDE-Q scores and found improvements [276]. Two studies for a total of 82 patients reported on change in EDI [273, 275]. EDI drive for thinness subscale decreased in one study [275], and in the second study EDI scores were reported to have improved significantly on all subscales other than maturity fears by 3 months [273]. One study examining ChEAT scores, involved 56 patients, however, only 30 patients had pre-post data to analyze. The mean length of stay was 10.3 weeks [272]. ChEAT scores improved.

One study with 51 patients [276] examined a family therapy with group DBT skills training in an intensive outpatient program. Fifteen out of 36 patients (30%) were considered not successful due to need for higher level of care, psychiatric hospitalization or left treatment against medical advice.

One study was found with eight patients and their parents [277] describing family-based treatment with CBT principles within a DTP. Statistically significant decreases were seen in all subscales of the EDE-Q and the Yale Brown Cornell Eating Disorder Scale (YBC-EDS) total score decreased significantly [277] (Table 57).

Avoidant/restrictive food intake disorder One study examined 32 patients with ARFID, compared to patients with AN ($n = 68$), BN ($n = 15$) and OSFED ($n = 15$) in the same DTP [278] (Table 58). This study reported that the reason for patients with ARFID to be admitted to their day treatment program was "acute onset of severe food restriction that results in significant weight loss or failure to gain weight." Length of stay for ARFID patients was significantly shorter than for those with AN, but not compared to those with BN or OSFED. Patients with ARFID gained weight from 86% median BMI to 95% median BMI which did not differ from the median weight gain for the AN or OSFED groups (Table 58). This study also reported that patients with ARFID had total ChEAT scores that were subclinical at admission and demonstrated minimal change in scores during treatment. There were no significant differences between the diagnostic groups at the end of treatment on ChEAT scores [278].

Family-based day treatment combined with dialectical Behavioural therapy

Bulimia nervosa One study including 35 adolescent females with BN examined DBT combined with FBT principles within a day hospital setting [279] (Table 59). Length of stay was 77.18 days. Binge-purge symptoms monitored via self-report on EDE-Q decreased significantly [279]. EDE-Q global, shape and weight concerns decreased significantly pre-post, whereas restraint and

Table 56 Family-based day treatment for children and adolescents with anorexia nervosa and low-weight eating disorders

Certainty assessment							Impact	Certainty	Importance
№ of studies	Study design	Risk of bias	Inconsistency	Indirectness	Imprecision	Other considerations			
Change in Weight (assessed with: Pre-post change in weight outcomes), Change in EDE-Q scores, change in symptoms									
9	Case Control and Case Series	very serious [a]	serious [b]	not serious	serious [c]	strong association all plausible residual confounding would reduce the demonstrated effect	Nine studies for a total of 427 patients. Studies varied with regards to degree/method of including parents in treatment, # of hours/week of programming and LOS. Criteria/reasons for admission to the DTP program varied, studies which reported referral source/reasons described that patients could be referred from either initially assessment, inpatient or outpatient based on the severity of their symptoms. Five studies reported on change in BMI which rose from 17.5 (SD 0.4) to 19.5 (SD 0.4), 16.4 to 19.6, 16.3 (+/−1.6) to 17.3 (+/− 1.3), 17.01 (range 12.3–22.1) to 20.05 (range 14.8–25.1), and 16.2 (+/− 1.98) to 19.4 (+/−2.87). Three studies reported on total weight gained in program (8.6 kg +/− 4.5 kg; 5.0 kg +/− 2.5; 7.3 kg +/− 3.1 and 17.58 kg). Two studies reported on change in %TGW which rose from 82.56 to 93.00% in one study and 82.3 to 97.99%. LOS in these studies varied from 27.6 (SD 12.13) days to 1.3 (SD 0.2) years. One study reported on difference in weight outcomes between their Maudsley and non-Maudsley DTP, noting no difference be tween these 2 groups. One other study reported on differ ences between patients who re ceived "formal psychotherapy" (individual and/or family) outside of program thereby needing to leave program for approx 2 h/ week and noted that patients who received psychotherapy within the first 2 months of en tering DTP gained significantly less weight (ie 5.0 +/− 2.5 kg vs 7.3 +/− 3.1 kg). One study exam ined predictors of weight restor ation in DTP and reported that Higher BMI at admission (range 12.3–22.1), greater gain in %TGW in first 4 weeks (range − 0.18 to 25.27% TGW) and lower care giver empowerment at baseline were predictive of weight restor ation at end of intensive treat ment (ie DTP + IOP).	⊕◯◯◯ VERY LOW	CRITICAL
		very serious [d]	not serious	not serious	not serious	all plausible residual confounding would reduce the demonstrated effect	Five studies receiving a family-based DTP treatment. LOS was 37.05 days, 28.41 days (SD 13.55) over 11.7 weeks (patients did not attend every day as they were transitioning back to school), 27.6 days (SD 12.13) and 11.56 days (SD 6.61), and one was a 3 month follow up. Weight at onset in 4 studies were similar although reported in different	⊕◯◯◯ VERY LOW	IMPORTANT

Table 56 Family-based day treatment for children and adolescents with anorexia nervosa and low-weight eating disorders *(Continued)*

Certainty assessment							Impact	Certainty	Importance
№ of studies	Study design	Risk of bias	Inconsistency	Indirectness	Imprecision	Other considerations			
							ways (ie 80.94%TGW in first study, BMI 16.3/79.9% in the second study, 82.56% in third study and BMI 16.4 in forth study). EDE scores, global and all subscales decreased significantly in all studies, although confidence intervals overlapped with size of effect. In the study reporting on a control group which was treated in the same program, but without the inclusion of Maudsley/family interventions, the EDE-Q scores decreased more in the Maudsley group than the non-Maudsley as the Maudsley group started with higher EDE-Q scores and at the end of the treatment period their scores were similar to the non-Maudsley. Of note the scores for Wt Concern and Restraint Concerns did not change significantly in the non-Maudsley group whereas they decreased significantly in the Maudsley group.		
		very serious [e]	not serious	not serious	not serious	all plausible residual confounding would reduce the demonstrated effect	One study consisted of 32 patients. LOS not reported in study. Body image disturbance disappeared completely in 59%, decreased partially in 28% and remained unchanged in 13%. Prolonged duration of meals improved during treatment and "normalized" in 87.5% by end of treatment. Eighty-seven percent stopped ritualistic exercise habits by end of treatment.	⨁◯◯◯ VERY LOW	IMPORTANT
		very serious [a]	not serious	not serious	serious [c]	all plausible residual confounding would reduce the demonstrated effect	One study including 60 patients, LOS median stay 8 months (SD 2.27). Statistically significant change was reported in EDI-3 Drive for Thinness (53.40 +/− 35 to 30.68 +/− 31.70) and Dissatisfaction (50.88 +/− 27.60 to 31.62 +/− 29.80), $p < 0.001$.	⨁◯◯◯ VERY LOW	IMPORTANT
		very serious [a]	not serious	not serious	serious [c]	all plausible residual confounding would reduce the demonstrated effect	One study including 60 patients, LOS median stay 8 months (SD 2.27). Statistically significant change was reported in EAT-26. Mean EAT-26 score was 26.70 (+/− 17.7) at admission and 7.97 (+/− 11.5) at discharge, $p < 0.001$.	⨁◯◯◯ VERY LOW	IMPORTANT

Explanations
[a]Many studies did not include a control or comparison group
[b]Admission weight, # hours/weeks of treatment, process of family involvement and LOS varied among studies, likely affecting outcome
[c]Confidence intervals wider than effect size in some studies
[d]Only one study included a control comparison, no blinding of participants possible
[e]No validated scale used, no comparison/control group
Bibliography:
Case control - Bean 2010 [264], Danziger 1989 [262]
Case series - Danziger 1988 [263], Gezelius 2016 [265], Martin-Wagar 2019 [269], Rienecke 2016 [266], Rienecke 2018 [267], Simic 2018 [270], Zanna 2017 [268]

Table 57 Family-based day treatment/intensive outpatient for adolescents with eating disorders

Certainty assessment							Impact	Certainty	Importance
№ of studies	Study design	Risk of bias	Inconsistency	Indirectness	Imprecision	Other considerations			
Improved Weight at Discharge (assessed with: %TGW/BMI), Change in EDE-Q (assessed with: Pre-post EDE-Q scores)									
5	Case Series	very serious [a]	serious [b]	not serious	serious [c]	none	Five studies for total of 254 patients. Studies varied with regard to the form of parent involvement, hours/ week in treatment and admission criteria. Referral to receive treatment in DTP or IOP was noted in the studies to be due to the presence of severe symptoms impairing the patients' functioning or physical health. In some cases the patients had to have already received another form of treatment (ie inpatient or outpatient), but in other cases patients could be referred directly for services in DTP/IOP. Weight related outcomes reported as change in BMI or % TGW. Four studies reported change in BMI from admission to discharge and found that weight rose from 17.4 (SD 2.0) to 18.3 (SD 1.8); 16.5 (SD 2.3) to 18.4 (SD 1.6);18.7 (SD 2.4) to 20.5 (SD 2.0) and by a mean of 0.91 +/−0.55 in the final study. Three studies reported on change in %TGW and found an increase in %TGW from 86 (SD 10) to 96 (SD 7) and 91.7 (SD 6.1) to 101.8% (SD 7.7) and 88 to 93.47%. One study reported weight change as 12/19 patients reaching 100%TGW at 3 months and the other 7/19 reaching a mean %TGW of 94% with mean %TGW at admission of 88%). The mean LOS varied between these studies from 3.2 weeks to 28.5 weeks.	⊕○○○ VERY LOW	CRITICAL
		very serious [a]	not serious	not serious	not serious	all plausible residual confounding would reduce the demonstrated effect	One study with total of 51 patients looking at EDE-Q. Fifty-three % of patients were referred directly from the inpatient unit in which case the treating inpatient clinician and insurance provider had to have determined that the patient/family required higher intensity treatment than outpatient could provide. Thirty-five % were referred due to inability to make progress in outpatient treatment. In 12% of cases, no referral source was recorded/available. Previous treatment and route of referral was not noted in other study. LOS was 7 weeks and mean of 40 +/− 17.2 days in each program. Global EDE-Q score decreased from 3.76 (SD 1.55) to 2.08 (SD 1.4) from admission to discharge ($p = 0.001$) in one study and from a mean of 3.83 +/− 0.95 to 1.50 (+/−1.03) in the other study ($p = 0.012$). Adolescent norm score	⊕○○○ VERY LOW	IMPORTANT

Table 57 Family-based day treatment/intensive outpatient for adolescents with eating disorders *(Continued)*

Certainty assessment							Impact	Certainty	Importance
№ of studies	Study design	Risk of bias	Inconsistency	Indirectness	Imprecision	Other considerations			
							reported in study was 1.6 (SD 1.4).		
		very serious [a]	not serious	not serious	serious [c]	all plausible residual confounding would reduce the demonstrated effect	Two studies for a total of 82 patients reported on change in EDI. Admission to the program was determined based on clinical assessment that the patients required a high level of treatment intensity based on symptomatology, in some cases patients had not received any prior treatment. LOS were 15 and 21.4 weeks. Change in EDI-2 was reported in one study and stated that EDI-DT decreased from 16.05 (SD 6.04) to 11.56 (SD 7.42) and EDI-BD decreased from 19.85 (SD 8.39) to 17.31 (SD 9.21), this study also reported that of those starting above the norm at beginning of study, 40% of patients improved on EDI-DT and 24.6% on EDI-BD). In the second study EDI-3 scores were reported to have improved significantly on all subscales other than maturity fears by 3 months. Scores for EDI-DT decreased from 49.24 (SD 12.61) to 42.06 (SD 11.52) and EDI-BD from 48.47 (SD 11.85) to 46.65 (SD 11.74).	⊕○○○ VERY LOW	IMPORTANT
		very serious [a]	not serious	not serious	serious [c]	all plausible residual confounding would reduce the demonstrated effect	One study involved 56 patients, only 30 patients had pre-post data to analyze, mean LOS of 10.3 weeks. ChEAT scores reported only in graph format, all subscales significantly improved, although upper and lower confidence intervals overlapped with median effect in all subscales.	⊕○○○ VERY LOW	IMPORTANT
		very serious [a]	not serious	not serious	not serious	none	Completion rate - One study with 51 patients. Patients were referred from both inpatient and outpatient sources based on severity of symptoms. 15/36 patients (30%) were considered not successful (ie premature d/c) due to need for higher level of care, psychiatric hospitalization or left treatment AMA. Mean LOS was 22.2 (SD 3.8) days.	⊕○○○ VERY LOW	CRITICAL
Change in EDE, YBC-EDS (assessed with: Pre/post YBC-EDS), Body Checking Questionnaire									
1	Case Report	very serious [a]	not serious	not serious	serious [c]	all plausible residual confounding would reduce the demonstrated effect	One study with 8 patients and their parents. LOS mean of 40 days +/−17.2. Intervention was	⊕○○○ VERY LOW	

Table 57 Family-based day treatment/intensive outpatient for adolescents with eating disorders *(Continued)*

Certainty assessment							Impact	Certainty	Importance
№ of studies	Study design	Risk of bias	Inconsistency	Indirectness	Imprecision	Other considerations			
							family-based with CBT principles. EDE-Q subscales --statistically significant decreases in all subscales (range $p = 0.012$ to 0.028).		
		very serious [a]	not serious	not serious	serious [c]	all plausible residual confounding would reduce the demonstrated effect	YBC-EDS total score decreased from mean 39.29 (+/−8.42) to 17.12 (+/−11.47) ($p = 0.028$), Concerns scores from mean of 15.57 to 9.43 ($p = 0.034$) and Rituals from mean of 14.71 to 7.71 ($p = 0.028$).	⨁◯◯◯ VERY LOW	
		very serious [a]	not serious	not serious	serious [c]	all plausible residual confounding would reduce the demonstrated effect	BCQ total scores decreased pre/post from 59.67 (+/−20.96) to 43.50 (+/−15.15) ($p = 0.075$). Scores also decreased for idiosyncratic checking and body dimensions subscales ($p = 0.027$ and 0.046)	⨁◯◯◯ VERY LOW	

Explanations
[a]Observational study with no control comparison
[b]Differences in admission BMI/%TGW, LOS, amount of hours/week of treatment which are likely to affect outcomes
[c]Confidence intervals wider than effect size in some studies
Bibliography:
Case Series - Girz 2013 [273], Henderson 2014 [275], Johnston 2015 [276], Grewal 2014 [274], Ornstein 2012 [272]
Case Report – Iniesta Sepulveda 2017 [277]

Table 58 Family-based day treatment for children and adolescents with ARFID

Certainty assessment							Impact	Certainty	Importance
№ of studies	Study design	Risk of bias	Inconsistency	Indirectness	Imprecision	Other considerations			
Change in Weight (assessed with: Pre/post % median BMI), Change in ED symptomatology (assessed with: Pre/post ChEAT scores)									
1	Case Control	serious [a]	not serious	not serious	serious [b]	none	One study of 32 patients with ARFID, compared to patients with AN ($n = 68$), BN ($n = 15$) and OSFED ($n = 15$) in the same DTP. Study reported that the reason for patients with ARFID to be admitted to their PHP was "acute onset of severe food restriction that results in significant weight loss or failure to gain weight." LOS for ARFID was significantly lower than AN (7.03 +/− 3.38 weeks vs 11.94 +/− 4.21 weeks), but not BN or OSFED. Patients with ARFID gained weight from 86.21%MBMI (+/− 9.96) to 95.45%MBMI (+/− 7.96) which did not differ from the median weight gain for the AN or OSFED groups.	⨁◯◯◯ VERY LOW	CRITICAL
		serious [a]	not serious	not serious	serious [b]	none	Patients with ARFID had Total ChEAT scores that were subclinical at admission and demonstrated minimal change in scores during treatment. There were no significant differences between the diagnostic groups at the end of treatment on ChEAT scores.	⨁◯◯◯ VERY LOW	NOT IMPORTANT

Explanations
[a]No control or comparison with no treatment, just patients in same program with other ED diagnoses
[b]Confidence intervals wide
Bibliography:
Case Control - Ornstein 2017 [278]

Table 59 Family-based combined with DBT-based day treatment for children and adolescents with bulimia nervosa

Certainty assessment							Impact	Certainty	Importance
№ of studies	Study design	Risk of bias	Inconsistency	Indirectness	Imprecision	Other considerations			
Weight Change (assessed with: Pre-post BMI), Change in frequency of bingeing and purging (assessed with: Pre-post frequency of binge/purge symptoms), Change in EDE-Q (assessed with: Pre-post EDE-Q)									
1	Case Series	very serious [a]	not serious	not serious	not serious	none	Study included 35 adolescent females. Criteria for referral/admission to the program was not reported. BMI did not change. At admission mean BMI was 26.3 (SD 2.34) and at discharge mean BMI was 24.9 (SD 2.87) (p 0.68). LOS 77.18 days.	⊕○○○ VERY LOW	IMPORTANT
		very serious [a]	not serious	not serious	serious [b]	none	Study included 35 adolescent females. LOS 77.18 days. B/P symptoms monitored via self-report on EDE-Q re ported as monthly frequency of these symptoms. At admission the mean fre quency of objective bingeing was 4.03 (SD 6.69) and at discharge it was 1.43 (SD 3.66) ($p = 0.04$). At admission the self-reported (ie EDE-Q) mean frequency of purging was 10.82 (SD 11.57) and at discharge it was 3.51 (SD 2.26) ($p = 0.005$).	⊕○○○ VERY LOW	CRITICAL
		very serious [a]	not serious	not serious	not serious	none	EDE-Q global, shape and weight concerns decreased significantly pre-post (p 0.001–0.002). Restraint and eating concerns scores were unchanged at end of treatment.	⊕○○○ VERY LOW	IMPORTANT

Explanations
[a]No comparison/control
[b]Wide confidence intervals, larger than actual effect
Bibliography:
Case Series - Murray 2015 [279]

eating concerns scores were unchanged at end of treatment [279].

CBT- based day treatment

Anorexia nervosa One case series including 42 patients with AN examined a CBT- based day treatment program [280] (Table 60). Length of stay in day treatment was a mean of 22.2 weeks. Patients gained weight, with a mean increase of 5.37 kg or BMI increase of 1.87 kg/m over the course of treatment (Table 60). It was noted the increase in weight was correlated with the number of months in program, as well as EDI scores and Motivational Stages of Change score. Of note only 38 completed 2 months, 25 completed 4 months and 9 completed 6 months of treatment.

Behaviour therapy based day treatment

Avoidant/restrictive food intake disorder Two case reports were found describing patients aged 4 years (fear of choking) [281] and 8 years (emetophobia) [282]. Length of stay in the day treatment program was 9 days and 7 days respectively. At the end of treatment, the patients had increased their intake (Table 61). The 4 year old was no longer supplement dependent and accepting 30 new foods. The 8 year old had increased her intake from having nothing by mouth to meeting her daily nutritional needs.

Resistance training as an adjunct in a day treatment program

Mixed diagnoses This randomized controlled study involved 36 patients with mixed diagnoses of eating disorders (18 intervention and 18 control) [283]. The study took place within a day treatment program and consisted of supervised exercise (50–60 min), for 3 days per week for 8 weeks. In order to be included in the study the patients must have had a BMI greater than 14 and could not be "excessive exercisers" (ie < 6 h per week). Intervention patients received resistance training plus 150 kcal extra to compensate for this activity. There was

Table 60 CBT-based day treatment for children and adolescents with anorexia nervosa

Certainty assessment							Impact	Certainty	Importance
№ of studies	Study design	Risk of bias	Inconsistency	Indirectness	Imprecision	Other considerations			
Change in Weight (assessed with: Pre/post measures of weight)									
1	Case Series	serious [a]	not serious	not serious	serious [b]	none	One study, including 42 patients. Unclear reasons for patients being referred to the program. Mean duration of illness prior to admission to this program was 2.40 years (SD = 2.02). LOS in Day Treatment was a mean of 22.2 weeks (range 0–52 weeks). Patients gained weight, with a mean increase of 5.37 kg or BMI increase of 1.87 kg/m over the course of treatment. It was noted the increase in weight was correlated with the number of months in program (0.23, $p < 0.01$), EDI-DT (− 4.90, $p < 0.001$), EDI-BD (− 3.56, $p < 0.001$) and Motivational Stages of Change (6.15, $p < 0.001$). Of note only 38 completed 2 months, 25 completed 4 months and 9 completed 6 months -- unclear how many were discharged due to improved clinical presentation vs deterioration or inability to meet program requirements.	⨁◯◯◯ VERY LOW	CRITICAL

Explanations
[a]Observational study with no comparison or control group
[b]Confidence intervals not reported
Bibliography:
Case Series - Green 2015 [280]

no difference in weight restoration between groups (Table 62).

Residential treatment

Four case series examined residential treatment and included 1068 patients with AN, BN and EDNOS, along with two additional case reports (Table 63). One case series examined patients with AN exclusively [287]. Reasons for admission to residential treatment were not noted and all studies took place in the United States. These studies measured change in weight in various ways. Four studies utilized BMI [284–287]. Admission mean BMI varied from 15.8 to 18.6. Discharge mean BMI varied from 17.8 to 21.3. Change in mean BMI from admission to discharge varied from 1.92 to 2.72. Two studies additionally reported on %TGW at admission and discharge. Admission mean %TGW were 83.4% [284] and 76.7% [287] and discharge mean %TGW were 94.7 and 86.6% respectively.

Table 61 Behaviour therapy based day treatment for children with ARFID

Certainty assessment							Impact	Certainty	Importance
№ of studies	Study design	Risk of bias	Inconsistency	Indirectness	Imprecision	Other considerations			
Change in eating behaviours/intake (assessed with: Pre/post measures of intake)									
2	Case Reports	very serious [a]	not serious	not serious	not serious	none	Two case reports, patients were 4 yrs. (fear of choking) and 8 yrs. (emetophobia). LOS in DTP were 9 days and 7 days respectively. At end of treatment the patients had increased their intake. The 4 yo was no longer supplement dependent and accepting 30 new foods. The 8 yo had increased her intake from NPO to meeting her daily nutritional needs.	⨁◯◯◯ VERY LOW	CRITICAL

Explanations
[a]Case studies only, no comparison/control
Bibliography:
Case Reports - Seiverling 2016 [281], Williams 2011 [282]

Table 62 Resistance training in combination with day treatment for adolescents with eating disorders

Certainty assessment							Impact	Certainty	Importance
№ of studies	Study design	Risk of bias	Inconsistency	Indirectness	Imprecision	Other considerations			
Body Mass Index at Discharge (assessed with: BMI calculated)									
1	randomised trials	serious [a]	not serious	not serious	not serious	none	36 patients participated (18 intervention and 18 control) another 8 patients were lost to follow-up. Study took place within a day treatment program and consisted of 3 day per week × 8 weeks of supervised exercise (50–60 min). In order to be included in the study the patients must have had a BMI > 14 kg/m and could NOT be "excessive exercisers" (ie < 6 h /week). Intervention patients re ceived resistance training + 150 kcal extra to compensate for this activity. There was no dif ference in weight restoration between groups. Mean BMI at initiation of study ranged was greater than 17 in both groups and patients had already been hospitalized for a mean of 50.8 and 61.5 days prior to enroll ment in the study. Exclusion factor - excessive exercise as part of illness.	⊕⊕⊕○ MODERATE	IMPORTANT

Explanations
[a]No concealment or blinding for patients or study team noted
Bibliography:
RCT - Fernandez-del-Valle 2016 [283]

One study reported on 361 patients that were purging at admission a mean of 3.25 times per day [284]. At discharge, they were purging a mean of 0.02 times per day. Differing diagnostic groups were not reported separately. Length of stay was an average of 52 days. Treatment was multimodal.

In terms of psychological symptoms, three studies looked at EDI scores and included 313 patients with AN, BN and EDNOS [285–287]. The treatment provided was multimodal. Length of stay varied between studies from 28.5 to 56.4 days. In general, EDI scores were improved when admission scores were compared with discharge scores. One study looked at the EDE-Q pre to post and included 105 patients with AN, BN and EDNOS [285]. The EDE-Q changed from 3.6 (SD = 1.58) to 1.95 (SD = 1.35).

One study including 65 patients with AN examined readiness for change. Treatment was multimodal [287]. Mean readiness for change (ANSOQC) at admission was 53.98 (SD 16.36) and at discharge was 67.28 (SD 20.06). This difference was statistically significant, but does not signify a change in actual stage of change. Participants were further divided into low readiness and high readiness. High readiness patients had a shift from 66.86 (SD 11.78) at admission to 76.80 (SD 15.71) at discharge, signifying a shift from Preparation to Action Phases. Low readiness patients shifted from 40.70 (SD 7.12) to 57.47 (SD 19.5), signifying a shift from Contemplative to Preparation Phases.

Two case reports both described patients with AN and Type 1 diabetes and reported weight gains and better glycemic control after residential treatment [288, 289]. Varying types of treatment were provided in multimodal format.

Recommendations

Family therapy

Family-based treatment

Family-based treatment (FBT) is strongly recommended for any child or adolescent with Anorexia Nervosa or Bulimia Nervosa, especially for those who have been ill less than 3 years. Strong recommendation

Qualifying statements:

There are implementation challenges with Family-Based Treatment (FBT) including requirements for specialized, well-trained staff, access and costs of training.

Table 63 Residential treatment for children and adolescents with eating disorders

Certainty assessment							Impact	Certainty	Importance
№ of studies	Study design	Risk of bias	Inconsistency	Indirectness	Imprecision	Other considerations			
Change in Mean Body Mass Index at Discharge (assessed with: Calculated BMI), change in purge frequency, EDI 3 Drive for thinness, EDE-Q, Readiness for Change									
4	Case Series	very serious [a]	serious [b]	not serious	serious [c,d]	none	Studies included patients with AN, BN and EDNOS for a total $n = 1068$. Reasons for admission to residential treatment were not noted and all studies took place in the US (ie decision for admission likely influenced by insurance coverage/ parental finances). One study noted that they included only data from the first admission for patients admitted more than once to residential treatment and that only patients who remained in treatment > 2 weeks were included. Another study noted that patients had a mean of 1.2 previous inpatient admissions prior to residential treatment. Otherwise there was a paucity of information describing previous treatments. They measured change in weight in various ways. Four studies utilized BMI. Admission mean BMI varied from 15.8 to 18.65. Discharge mean BMI varied from 17.8 to 21.3. Change in mean BMI from admission to discharge varied from 1.92 to 2.72. Two studies additionally reported on %TGW at admission and discharge. Admission mean %TGW were 83.4 and 76.7% and discharge mean %TGW were 94.7 and 86.6% respectively.	⊕○○○ VERY LOW	CRITICAL
		very serious [e]	serious [f]	not serious	serious [d]	all plausible residual confounding would reduce the demonstrated effect	One study reported on 361 patients that were purging at admission a mean of 3.25 times per day. At discharge they were purging a mean of 0.02 times per day. Differing diagnostic groups not reported separately. LOS 51.8 days +/− 25.8. Treatment was multimodal.	⊕○○○ VERY LOW	IMPORTANT
		very serious [g]	serious [b]	not serious	serious [c]	all plausible residual confounding would reduce the demonstrated effect	Three studies looked at EDI 3 scores and included 313 patients with AN, BN and EDNOS. Treatment provided was multimodal. Various subscales and EDI-3 Risk Composite as well as EDI-3 Global were reported in the some of the studies. EDI-3 Risk Composite was reported in 2 studies (total $n = 212$) mean decrease in EDI-3 RC varied from 14 to 31 (SD = 23.1 and 17.62 respectively). EDI-3 Global was reported in 1 study ($n = 101$) where it decreased a mean of 39.3 points (SD = 55.2). EDI-3 Drive for Thinness was reported in 3 studies ($n = 277$) where it decreased a mean of 3.53, 5.11 and 12.37 (SD 6.9, 7.81 and 6.42). EDI-3 was reported in 1 study ($n = 111$) and decreased 3.75 (SD = 2.21). EDI-3 Body Dissatisfaction was reported in 1 study	⊕○○○ VERY LOW	CRITICAL

Table 63 Residential treatment for children and adolescents with eating disorders *(Continued)*

Certainty assessment							Impact	Certainty	Importance
№ of studies	Study design	Risk of bias	Inconsistency	Indirectness	Imprecision	Other considerations			
							(*n* = 101) where it decreased 3.45 (SD = 10.88). LOS varied between studies from 28.5–56.4 days, one study did not report their LOS.		
		very serious [g]	not serious	not serious	not serious	all plausible residual confounding would reduce the demonstrated effect	One study looked at the EDE-Q Pre to Post and included 105 patients with AN, BN and EDNOS. Treatment was multimodal a nd mean LOS was 56 days. EDE-Q changed from 3.6 (SD = 1.58) to 1.95 (SD = 1.35), mean change – 1.56 (SD = 1.27) -- similar to reported norms in adolescent girls.	⊕◯◯◯ VERY LOW	CRITICAL
		very serious [c,g]	not serious	not serious	not serious	all plausible residual confounding would reduce the demonstrated effect	One study included 65 patients with AN and treatment was multimodal. Mean readiness for change (ANSOQC) at admission was 53.98 (SD 16.36) and at discharge was 67.28 (SD 20.06). This difference was statistically significant, but signifies no change in actual stage of change (ie Preparation Phase scores are 50–69). They were further divided into low readiness and high readiness. High readiness patients had a shift from 66.86 (SD 11.78) at admit to 76.80 (SD 15.71) at d/c, signifying a shift from Preparation to Action Phases. Low readiness patients shifted from 40.70 (SD 7.12) to 57.47 (SD 19.5), signifying shift from Contemplative to Preparation Phases. LOS was 28.5 days.	⊕◯◯◯ VERY LOW	IMPORTANT
Weight gain									
2	Case Reports	very serious [g]	not serious	not serious	not serious	none	The 2 case reports both described patients with Type 1 diabetes and reported weight gains of 2.2 and 4.3 kg during admission. Varying types of treatment provided in multimodal format. LOS varied among studies from 28 days to 56 days and in one study LOS was not reported.	⊕◯◯◯ VERY LOW	IMPORTANT

Explanations
[a]Observational study with no comparison
[b]Mixed diagnostic group (AN, BN and EDNOS)
[c]Large or overlapping confidence intervals wide in some studies included here
[d]Confidence intervals not reported or not reported in all studies
[e]Observational study with no comparison, self-reported # of purges/day
[f]Mixed diagnostic group (AN-B/P and BN) - results not differentiated
[g]Observational study with no comparison, self-rated scale
Bibliography:
Case Series - Fisher 2015 [284], Weltzin 2014 [285], Twohig 2016 [286], McHugh 2007 [287]
Case Reports – Pitel 1998 [288], Rodigue 1990 [289]

Parent-Focused Family Therapy – where the patient is seen separately from the family – may be just as effective as traditional FBT where the family is seen together. Adaptations to FBT such as shorter or longer treatment, removal of the family meal, guided self-help, parent to parent consult, short term intensive formats, and delivery of FBT by telehealth, require more study. Structural and Systemic Family therapy might be helpful for children and adolescents with Anorexia Nervosa, but the evidence generally does not indicate superiority to FBT, especially when costs are taken into consideration.

Key Evidence:

Anorexia Nervosa

One meta-analysis [21] and three high quality RCTs [6, 22, 23] have demonstrated that greater weight gain and higher remission rates are achieved in FBT compared to individual treatment, particularly when focusing on one year follow-up. Eight large case series also show improvement in weight following treatment [26–32, 40].

Bulimia Nervosa

Three high quality RCTs for Bulimia Nervosa have been completed and compared FBT to various control conditions [48–50]. When FBT was compared to Cognitive Behavioral Therapy (CBT), remission rates were significantly higher in the FBT group (39% versus 20%) [50]. Remission rates were also significantly better in the FBT group, when FBT was compared to supportive psychotherapy (39% versus 18%)[48]. However, when family therapy (with some elements consistent with FBT) was compared to guided self-help CBT, there were no significant differences in remission (10% versus 14%) [49]. A case series and case report also support the use of FBT for Bulimia Nervosa [34, 51].

Multi-family therapy

Multi-family therapy (MFT) may be a reasonable treatment option for children and adolescents with Anorexia Nervosa. Weak recommendation

Qualifying statements:

Multi-Family Therapy (MFT) provides workshops for multiple families at once and generally is delivered alongside single-family therapy following FBT principles, although some studies just report on the delivery of the multi-family workshops alone. It may be challenging for programs to run MFT as it requires several staff present for several full days and requires several families interested at the same time to begin the treatment. The delivery of MFT for children and adolescents with Bulimia Nervosa may be beneficial but requires more study. Members of the guideline committee indicated that the value of parents having support from each other cannot be understated. The panel voiced that peer support is often a missing component of treatment and hospital administration can place barriers to the implementation of this option.

Key evidence:

One large high quality RCT found that MFT (multi-family workshops plus single FBT) conferred additional benefits compared to FBT alone in terms of remission rates in adolescents with Anorexia Nervosa (75% in MFT versus 60% in FBT) [76]. Several case series have also demonstrated a benefit of MFT [77–80]. There is one small case series examining MFT for adolescents with Bulimia Nervosa which found improvements in eating disorder symptoms [81].

Additional promising therapies

Other outpatient family therapies exist that have some data showing their promise but where more research is required before definitive recommendations can be made. These are treatment options in which research efforts should be prioritized.

They are:

- FBT for children with atypical Anorexia Nervosa.
- FBT for children with Avoidant/Restrictive Food Intake Disorder (ARFID).
- FBT for children across the gender spectrum, including individuals who are gender variant or gender non-conforming.
- Adjuncts to FBT, such as cognitive remediation therapy, art therapy and cognitive behavioural therapy for children and adolescents with Anorexia Nervosa.
- Emotion focused family therapy (EFFT) for Bulimia Nervosa and Anorexia Nervosa, as stand- alone treatment, or as an adjunct to FBT.

Individual or group outpatient psychotherapies

Cognitive Behavioural therapy

Cognitive behavioural therapy may be a reasonable treatment option for children and adolescents with Anorexia Nervosa or Bulimia Nervosa. Weak recommendation

Qualifying statements:

Across the studies, Cognitive Behavioural Therapy was not offered in a uniform manner. Motivational interviewing as a component of treatment or prior to initiating treatment, may also be helpful although strong scientific evidence is lacking due to a paucity of studies.

Key evidence:

Anorexia nervosa

Eight case reports [97–104] and one large case series [96] indicate that CBT results in weight gain and improvement in eating disorder psychological symptoms for children and adolescents with Anorexia

Nervosa. A small RCT ($n = 22$) did not show any difference between CBT and Behavioural Family Therapy in terms of these outcomes for children with Anorexia Nervosa, however, both improved [24]. Efficacy has also been shown when CBT is delivered in a group setting for Anorexia Nervosa [105, 106].

Bulimia nervosa

For Bulimia Nervosa, three high quality RCTs exist examining CBT. One RCT compared CBT to psychodynamic therapy in primarily adolescents, but also some young adults. This trial did not find any difference in terms of remission from Bulimia Nervosa. There were small advantages in terms of greater reduction in binge/purge frequency in the CBT group [107]. There are also two high quality RCTs comparing CBT to family-based approaches for Bulimia Nervosa [49, 50]. There are conflicting results between these two studies, with the study by Le Grange and colleagues [50] indicating significantly greater remission rates in the FBT group compared to the CBT group, whereas the study by Schmidt and colleagues [49] showed no significant difference between the groups with only a small proportion remitted in each group. Two large case series indicate significant decreases in binge/purge frequency pre to post treatment [108, 109]. Several case reports indicating improvement in binge/purge symptoms exist [110–114].

Adolescent focused psychotherapy

Adolescent focused psychotherapy may be a reasonable treatment option for children and adolescents with Anorexia Nervosa. Weak recommendation

Qualifying statements:

Adolescent Focused Psychotherapy (AFP) could be delivered in situations in which FBT has been attempted, but been ineffective, or if FBT is contraindicated, not possible, or not available.

A manual is not yet available to clinicians, which makes training and dissemination difficult.

It is a challenge to study this type of treatment due to its lengthy nature and lack of clarity around essential elements. Adolescent Focused Psychotherapy includes elements of: an emphasis on therapeutic relationship with a goal to improve symptoms, psychoeducation, the role of the eating disorder as a coping mechanism, along with the development of more positive coping mechanisms. Panel members agreed that treatment of this nature is commonly delivered and can be quite beneficial to some patients. This treatment for Anorexia Nervosa may be beneficial, however other treatments have some advantages in terms of cost and more rapid improvement in symptoms.

Key evidence:

Anorexia Nervosa

Adolescent Focused Psychotherapy (AFP; based on psychodynamic principles) has some evidence to support its use [22, 23, 128], as does individual psychodynamic treatment [129], and group analytic psychotherapy [130]. Remission rates were not significantly different between AFP and FBT in two RCTs involving a total sample of 158 adolescents [22, 23]. Rates of 20% (12/60) remitted in AFP compared to 34% (21/60) in FBT were found in the study by Lock and colleagues [23], whereas 41% in the AFP group met the weight goal of the 50th percentile in the study by Robin and colleagues [22] compared to 53% in the FBT group. Differences between FBT and AFP become more apparent at one year follow up with FBT having an advantage [23].

Additional promising psychotherapies

Other promising outpatient psychotherapies exist that require more research before definitive recommendations can be made.

These include:

- Cognitive Behavioural Therapy for Avoidant/ Restrictive Food Intake Disorder.
- Dialectical Behavioural Therapy for eating disorders.

Other therapies - adjunctive yoga

Yoga, in addition to standard treatments, may be a reasonable option for medically stable youth with Anorexia Nervosa, Bulimia Nervosa, and Other Specified Feeding and Eating Disorders. Weak recommendation

Qualifying statements:

There is no evidence to guide the specific regimen (e.g. duration, frequency) of yoga. Yoga should only be undertaken with support by the physician involved in the individual's care. Hot yoga or other strenuous forms of Yoga are not recommended when medical concerns exist. If Yoga interferes with recovery, or worsens symptoms, it should be discontinued.

Key Evidence:

One high quality study suggests some benefits in terms of the psychological symptoms of eating disorders, as well as depressive and anxious symptoms in the context of an eating disorder [136].

Medications

The clinical trials environment to test medications for the treatment of eating disorders is fraught with ethical and methodological complexity. Obtaining the required informed consent to bring a child or adolescent into a study requires disclosure of the study intent, hypotheses, and potential for side effects attributable to the medication. In some cases, these effects (e.g. weight gain) are connected specifically to outcomes patients may strongly fear. In addition, parents are often reluctant to give their children psychotropic medication. This often results in studies that have prolonged enrollment phases, that struggle or fail to meet recruitment goals, and suffer from high rates of patient drop out. As a consequence, study quality is poor and prone to bias.

Atypical antipsychotics

Olanzapine or aripiprazole may be reasonable treatment options for certain populations of children and adolescents with Anorexia Nervosa if monitored carefully. Weak recommendation

Qualifying statements:

In specific contexts, consideration of olanzapine and aripiprazole use may be undertaken for the adjunct treatment of low weight children and adolescents with Anorexia Nervosa. Although the evidence-base supporting these specific medications is scant and of poor quality, expert opinion suggests potential benefit in carefully selected treatment contexts. Given their propensity for side effects, these medications should only be considered with appropriate consultation and monitoring by trained specialists in Child and Adolescent Psychiatry or Pediatrics who have expertise in the treatment of children and adolescents with eating disorders. When utilized, these medications should be initiated at a very low dose (0.625–1.25 mg for olanzapine, or 0.5–1.0 mg for aripiprazole) and titrated very carefully. Target doses in research trials are often modest. Informed consent from the young person, or their substitute decision maker including risk of side effects must be obtained and appropriate monitoring undertaken while these medications are in use.

Key evidence:

Olanzapine

Olanzapine has been the most commonly studied psychotropic medication for children and adolescents with Anorexia Nervosa. At present, only one small double-blind placebo-controlled trial in this population has been published [137], and no beneficial effect in favour of olanzapine was found in the 15 subjects who completed the trial. Several open trials and case series have examined the use of olanzapine in children and adolescents with Anorexia Nervosa [138–142]. While some have demonstrated benefit (e.g. weight gain), reported adverse effects associated with the medication as well as patient attrition were common.

Aripiprazole

Three small poor-quality studies found aripiprazole showed some modest benefit in adolescents with Anorexia Nervosa [165–167].

Additional promising medications

The use of other medications for the purposes of eating disorder treatment require more research before definitive recommendations can be made. These medications should be a priority for research. These include:

- Selective Serotonin Reuptake Inhibitors (fluoxetine for Bulimia Nervosa).
- Risperidone and Quetiapine for use in Anorexia Nervosa.
- Atypical Antipsychotics for use in Avoidant/Restrictive Food Intake Disorder.
- Mirtazapine use for patients with Anorexia Nervosa.

Medications that are not recommended

The medications below have no evidence to support their use in the treatment of primary eating disorder symptoms, or are harmful.

- Selective Norepinephrine Reuptake Inhibitors – no evidence.
- Mood Stabilizers - no evidence.
- Buproprion - not recommended for use in eating disorders, due to the elevated risks of seizures in this population.

Level of care – inpatient/day treatment/residential care

In contrast to the above sections that examine specific treatment modalities, this section focuses on the level – or setting - where care takes place. Research on level of care is generally sparse. Moreover, the setting where care takes place is often conflated with the treatment activities themselves making it difficult to attribute which mechanism(s) contributed to outcomes. Some tools already exist to guide the practitioner on which level of care might be indicated (e.g. residential, inpatient, day treatment, or outpatient care) based on a variety of clinical factors [290].

Level of care

It is strongly recommended that the least intensive treatment environment be provided (e.g. family-based treatment or day treatment versus lengthy hospitalizations) especially for those children and adolescents with Anorexia Nervosa requiring a first admission to hospital and/or with a duration of illness less than 3 years. Strong recommendation

Qualifying statements:

Definitive clinical research does not currently exist that identifies the specific characteristics of what comprises "least intensive environment" or an agreed upon hierarchy of least to most intensive environments. However, the evidence-base does provide signals of reasonable options and areas that should be prioritized for further study. In addition, definitive clinical research does not currently exist that identifies the specific elements required to optimize inpatient, specialist outpatient, and community outpatient programs.

Key evidence:

Studies comparing different levels of care and length of stay

One trial of 167 adolescents randomized to inpatient care, a specialist outpatient program, or a generalist community outpatient program found significant improvements across all three groups with no differences between the groups [291]. In order to examine length of inpatient treatment related to outcome, two high quality studies examined the difference between patients randomized to receive a relatively short inpatient admission followed by either 20 sessions of FBT ($n = 82$) [252] or day treatment ($n = 172$) [253] compared to a lengthy inpatient stay to weight restoration. In the inpatient/FBT study [252] patients had all been unwell less than 3 years, and in the inpatient/day treatment study [253] the patients were included only if it was their first admission. At the end of FBT or day treatment, there were no significant differences between those who were discharged after a short admission versus those who remained in hospital for weight restoration in terms of: weight outcome, rate of readmissions over 12-month follow-up, or eating disorder symptoms.

Studies examining inpatient treatment only

Multiple low-quality studies have been published examining the outcomes for children and adolescents with eating disorders [187, 188, 193, 194, 197, 213, 216, 222, 224, 227, 232–234, 251, 292]. The most consistent finding is that inpatient treatment leads to weight restoration regardless of the treatment framework used. There are no studies directly comparing treatment modalities. Outcomes related to the cognitive symptoms of the eating disorder were mixed in these inpatient studies. Some low quality studies have examined various adjuncts to inpatient treatment including non-select versus selective menus, meal support, multi-family versus multi-parent group therapy, cognitive remediation therapy, and bright light therapy. Non-select menus conferred a benefit related to rate of weight restoration and meal support appeared to decrease the need for nasogastric tube feeds. Other outcomes were less evident and potentially eclipsed by the effect of the inpatient treatment milieu.

Studies examining day treatment programming only

Several low-quality studies report a benefit of day hospital programming in terms of weight restoration and reduction in eating disorder symptoms [255, 256, 258, 259, 262, 266, 272–276, 280]. Of these studies 14 described using a family-based approach [262, 264–270, 272–277], eight a multimodal approach [254–261] and one a CBT framework [280] in their programs. All studies reported an increase in mean weight during day treatment, and most studies reported improvement in eating disorder symptoms. One study compared cohorts in their program with and without family involvement [264], and found that weight outcomes did not vary with family involvement, but there was a greater improvement observed in overall symptomatology, and in particular weight concerns and dietary restraint with family involvement. Only three small studies have examined the use of day treatment settings for patients with Avoidant/Restrictive Food Intake Disorder [278, 281, 282] and one small study examined this setting for Bulimia Nervosa [279]. One high quality study observed no harm with the addition of a standardized resistance training program to day treatment care as usual for patients with mixed eating disorder diagnoses [283].

Studies examining residential programming only

Six low quality studies examined outcomes for patients with eating disorders treated in a residential setting [284–289]. Studies included patients with Anorexia Nervosa, Bulimia Nervosa and Eating Disorder Not Otherwise Specified for a total of 1070 patients studied. Reasons for admission to residential treatment were not noted, there is a paucity of information reported on treatments received prior to admission to residential facilities, and all studies took place in the United States. Length of stay in these studies varied from 28 days to 56 days. All six studies reported that underweight patients gained weight during treatment. One study reported that episodes of purging were significantly reduced [284]. Three studies reported that eating disorder symptoms decreased significantly during treatment in the residential setting [285–287].

General care considerations when choosing level or setting of treatment

The following are reasonable care considerations as it relates to the choice of environment in which treatment is available for children and adolescents with eating disorders.

Care within an inpatient treatment environment

- Inpatient treatment may promote weight restoration regardless of model of care provided, but requires more study to determine the critical treatment elements related to weight restoration.

- Cognitive Behavioural Therapy (CBT) and family-based inpatient treatment may lead to improvement in eating disorder symptoms.
- Inpatient treatment combined with day treatment follow-up may be helpful in weight restoration, symptom change and motivation for children and adolescents with Anorexia Nervosa.
- Adjuncts to inpatient treatment, such as non-selective menus, meal support, cognitive remediation and bright light therapy may be helpful for certain children and adolescents with eating disorders.
- Inpatient treatment alone or in combination with day treatment for Bulimia Nervosa and Avoidant/Restrictive Food Intake Disorder requires more study.
- Peer support during inpatient treatment by other parents would be an asset.

Preparing for discharge from inpatient care

- Any transition in care is a period of high risk for deterioration and adverse events. Bridging these transitions with added supports is needed to prevent young people from suffering from adverse outcomes due to disruptions in continuity of care.
- Parental support is needed in order to prepare parents for discharge and the treatment that follows.
- Patient and parent preferences should be considered when planning for discharge.
- Issues of consent and capacity should also be considered when making decisions around admission and discharge.

Care within a day treatment environment

- Day treatment may promote weight restoration in Anorexia Nervosa regardless of model of care provided, but requires more study to determine the critical treatment elements related to weight restoration.
- Multimodal, CBT and family-based day treatment may lead to improvement in eating disorder symptoms.
- Day treatment for Avoidant/Restrictive Food Intake Disorder may be helpful in weight restoration and improved outcome.
- Resistance training may be offered to children and adolescents who do not have a history of compulsive exercise while participating in day treatment, but it remains unclear whether this intervention imparts any benefit.
- Day treatment varies significantly from study to study, so comparison is difficult. The common element appears to be a group-based treatment program with meal support.
- Equity and access to day treatment are issues to be considered. Families must live close to such a program in order to be able to attend, or must abandon their home/career to move close to a day treatment program in order for their child to attend.

Care within a residential treatment program

- Although literature was lacking to support a formal recommendation for residential treatment, many of the panel members opined that residential treatment is an essential component of treatment for some individuals with eating disorders who need lengthier treatment in a setting away from home. Based on expert opinion and those with lived experience, it was agreed that individuals who have had repeat admissions to the hospital and those with complex comorbid conditions, might benefit from residential treatment.

Discussion

These are the first Canadian Practice Guidelines to evaluate the evidence on psychotherapeutic and psychopharmacological treatments focused specifically on children and adolescents with eating disorders. Strong recommendations were supported in favour of Family-Based Treatment, and more generally in terms of least intensive treatment environment. Weak recommendations in favour of Multi-Family Therapy, Cognitive Behavioural Therapy, Adolescent Focused Psychotherapy, adjunctive Yoga, and atypical antipsychotics were confirmed. Several gaps for future work were identified including enhanced research efforts on new adjunctive treatments in order to address severe eating disorders and complex co-morbidities. Underlying the specific treatments emerged some general values and philosophies to be upheld, particularly apparent during the panel meeting. These philosophies included mutual trust and respect in the provider/patient/family relationship.

In addition, parent and patient representatives mentioned the critical importance of peer support (patient and parent), particularly in times of transition between different levels of care and from the pediatric to adult system of care. The importance of a coordinated continuum of care from outpatient to residential care was emphasized by the panel. The lack of services was also emphasized. Several individuals mentioned the lack of residential care across the country and the great need that exists for certain individuals with eating disorders for intensive inpatient and residential services. This need is particularly apparent for those who are medically stable, but have psychiatric co-morbidities and need longer term treatment in a highly structured environment. The comorbidity with substance abuse was mentioned as an area where there is a complete lack of services in Canada. Patient and parent choice/preferences of treatment were also mentioned as essential to consider when thinking of the treatments and levels of care available.

The strengths of this guideline are numerous. We used rigorous methodology for our literature review and synthesis as well as for our guideline development. Our literature synthesis methods included a thorough review of all literature (including gray literature and papers of any language). We translated 25 papers for full text review. In terms of guideline development, conflict of interest statements were reviewed by an impartial chair in order to address any biases. We had a face-to-face meeting to discuss our recommendations, followed by an anonymous voting procedure. Furthermore, our panel included the voices of various stakeholder groups including researchers, clinicians, policy makers, parents and those with lived experience.

Limitations

These guidelines serve as a starting point for Canadian Practice Guidelines for treating children and adolescents with eating disorders, and as such, they have several limitations. Our guidelines did not aim to review treatments within the scope of medical stabilization, or in terms of treatments for the physical complications of eating disorders in children and adolescents. A companion Canadian Guideline focused on these topics for children and adolescents is needed. The reader is encouraged to examine the Academy for Eating Disorders Guidelines on eating disorders, and the Clinical Practice Guidelines *for the* BC eating disorders continuum of services which includes a Short Term Allocation Tool for Eating Disorders (STATED) [290], specifically outlining medical criteria for hospital admission, and level of care recommendations for the full age spectrum. None of the outpatient treatments mentioned in our current guideline should be delivered with a medically unstable child needing hospital admission for medical reasons. Similarly, if outpatient treatments are attempted, and an individual deteriorates during these treatments, or fails to progress, stepping up to either day treatment, or inpatient care may be needed. Furthermore, if outpatient treatments are not available, then lengthier inpatient stays may be necessary.

We did not examine qualitative literature in our search. The scope of our guideline was so broad already, that these studies could not be incorporated. These studies should be included in future iterations of these guidelines. Qualitative meta-syntheses on the topic of treatment for and recovery from AN in particular, highlight the importance of therapeutic alliance, treatment targets, building identity and self-acceptance [293, 294]. These qualitative works, can shed light on the concept of recovery which can have several different definitions, not just focused on symptomatic change, but quality of life, and functionality of work and relationships. For the purposes of this guideline, we focused on studies reporting on symptomatic change, however, future iterations should include other outcomes as viewed as essential to those affected by these illnesses and their families. Caregiver outcomes would also be important to include in future guidelines. We also would recommend including transition age youth as an important population with unique needs. A more in-depth examination of transitions in the health care system in general would be beneficial.

Most of the published studies to date on pharmacotherapy of eating disorders in children and adolescents have focused on the role of antipsychotic medication in AN. Despite progress in recent years, the total number of subjects studied remains small, and there is a paucity of randomized controlled trials. Further, it has become increasingly clear that there are substantive challenges involved with the completion of such studies. As a result, there is still insufficient evidence to recommend medication as a first line consideration in children and adolescents with eating disorders. Due to the significant challenges in recruitment and retention in clinical trials to date, large multi-site collaborative trials are necessary to move the field forward in determining which young patients with eating disorders might benefit most from psychotropic medication and in what fashion. In addition, we did not systematically review the literature for certain classes of medications including benzodiazepines, or stimulants. We came across a couple of case reports through searching in the other areas [295, 296], however, searches on these drugs should be included in future iterations of this guideline.

Our search strategy also had limitations. Although our search was very thorough, we were unable to retrieve several citations as full text articles. Some of these were difficult to locate as they were dissertations, conference proceedings, books, or simply did not exist. We attempted to examine sex differences, but the numbers of male subjects were so small that no conclusions could be drawn. Furthermore, although we searched the literature thoroughly for art and music therapies, we could not find any articles on these topics. In addition, two papers in the family-based therapy section were identified through external review, indicating that these papers were not found through the initial search.

Despite these limitations, these guidelines represent a significant step forward in developing a collaborative process for identifying effective treatments for children and adolescents with eating disorders and will be reviewed every 5 years.

Future directions

Several gaps were noted by the guideline panel and these should be a focus for future study. These gaps included treatments for complex presentations of eating disorders, including complex co-morbidity such as borderline personality disorder, obsessive compulsive disorder, and substance use disorder. Determining which treatment benefits which individual in advance should be a priority for further study. There were also difficulties in making recommendations around medication use. Studies in the area of psychopharmacology are fraught with challenges in terms of a lack of recruitment and retention. Small and poorly designed studies, make it difficult to arise at recommendations. Perhaps multi-site trials, or innovative designs are needed to further promote and enhance the evidence base where psychopharmacology is concerned. The panel noted difficulty in making recommendations on inpatient and residential levels of care, but noted that these are sorely needed services, and should be expanded in Canada, along with a more rigorous investigation of effectiveness. Developing treatments, including new and adjunctive psychotherapeutic approaches for families unable to engage in Family-Based Treatment is essential. In addition, particular populations may have unique needs that have not yet been explored, such as predominantly male populations, and those with non-binary gender identities. Furthermore, creative ways of accessing evidence-based treatment need to be explored including the use of technology to treat patients and families at a distance.

Conclusions

Our Canadian Practice Guidelines for the treatment of children and adolescents with eating disorders recommend the provision of: 1) FBT for those with AN or BN (strong recommendation), 2) MFT for those with AN (weak recommendation), 3) CBT for those with AN or BN (weak recommendation), 4) AFP for those with AN (weak recommendation), and, 5) adjunctive Yoga for those with AN, BN and OSFED (weak recommendation). All of these treatments can only be delivered in a medically stable young person, and more intensive treatment should be considered if treatments are deeming to lack efficacy. In terms of medication, a weak recommendation was confirmed for olanzapine and aripiprazole for those with AN. A strong recommendation was agreed upon for providing care in a least intensive environment. Patient and parental preferences should be considered. Research efforts should be devoted to developing treatments for severe eating disorders with complex co-morbidity.

Abbreviations

%TGW: Percent treatment goal weight; ADHD: Attention deficit hyperactivity disorder; AFP: Adolescent focused psychotherapy; AGREE II: Appraisal of guidelines, research, and evaluation; AN: Anorexia nervosa; ANSOCQ: Anorexia nervosa stage of change questionnaire; ARFID: Avoidant/restrictive food intake disorder; BED: Binge eating disorder; BLT: Bright light therapy; BMI: Body mass index; BN: Bulimia nervosa; CBT: Cognitive behavioural therapy; CBT-E: Cognitive behavioural therapy - enhanced; ChEAT: Children's eating attitudes test; CRT: Cognitive remediation therapy; DBT: Dialectical behavioural therapy; DTP: Day treatment program; EAT: Eating attitudes test; EDE: Eating disorder examination; EDE-Q: Eating disorder examination - questionnaire; EDI: Eating disorders inventory; EDNOS: Eating disorder not otherwise specified; EFFT: Emotion focused family therapy; FBT: Family-based treatment; GDP: Guideline development panel; GRADE: Grading of recommendations assessment, development, and evaluation system; GUIDE-M: Guideline implementability for decision excellence model; LOS: Length of stay; MFT: Multi-family therapy; MPT: Multi-parent group therapy; MSCARED: Motivational stages of change for adolescents recovering from an eating disorder; NGY: Nasogastric tube; NJ: Nasojejunum; OCD: Obsessive compulsive disorder; OSFED: Other specified feeding and eating disorder; PRISMA: Preferred reporting items for systematic reviews and meta-analyses; SNRIs: Selective norepinephrine reuptake inhibitors; SSRIs: Selective serotonin reuptake inhibitors; TAU: Treatment as usual; YBC-EDS: Yale brown Cornell eating disorder scale

Acknowledgements

We would like to acknowledge the external reviewers of our guideline: Debra Katzman, Daniel Le Grange, James Lock, and Eric Vickar. Thank you for your expert input. We also acknowledge the following individuals for their contributions to this project – Zechen Ma, Kelsea McCready, Sadaf Sami, and Tracy Woodford. Thank you as well to all the patients and families with whom we work on a daily basis.

Authors' contributions

JC conceived the idea for this project with input from MN, WS, MB, MK, GM, CW, SF, NB, and CM. JC was primarily responsible for the overall project design, oversight of the project and drafting of the manuscript. Several authors participated in screening abstracts and full text articles including: JC, LI, MN, WS, MK, CW, NS, and AR. Panel members who contributed to the drafting and finalization of the recommendations included: WP, CM, JC, AB, CS, RL, TL, EW, CF, KB, JG, JG, AL, AL, JS, SG, MJ, GD, and DP. All authors read and edited the manuscript, and approved the final manuscript.

Competing interests

The authors declare that they have no competing interests.

Author details

[1]McMaster University, Hamilton, Canada. [2]University of Ottawa, Ottawa, Canada. [3]University of Toronto, Toronto, Canada. [4]National Initiative for Eating Disorders, Toronto, Canada. [5]Canadian Mental Health Association – Waterloo, Wellington, Dufferin, Kitchener, Canada. [6]The Univeristy of British Columbia, Vancouver, Canada. [7]Patient advocate, Woodstock, Canada. [8]Parent advocate, Woodstock, Canada. [9]Ontario Ministry of Health and Long-Term Care, Toronto, Canada. [10]St. Joseph's Care Group – Thunder Bay, Thunder Bay, Canada. [11]Dalhousie University, Halifax, Canada. [12]Laurentian

University, Sudbury, Canada. [13]McMaster Children's Hospital, Hamilton, Canada. [14]University of Calgary, Calgary, Canada.

References

1. Hoek HW, van Hoeken D. Review of the prevalence and incidence of eating disorders. Int J Eat Disord. 2003;34(4):383–96.
2. Arcelus J, et al. Mortality rates in patients with anorexia nervosa and other eating disorders. A meta-analysis of 36 studies. Arch Gen Psychiatry. 2011; 68(7):724–31.
3. Ward A, et al. Follow-up mortality study of compulsorily treated patients with anorexia nervosa. Int J Eat Disord. 2015;48(7):860–5.
4. Sullivan PF. Mortality in anorexia nervosa. Am J Psychiatry. 1995;152(7):1073–4.
5. Herzog DB, Nussbaum KM, Marmor AK. Comorbidity and outcome in eating disorders. Psychiatr Clin North Am. 1996;19(4):843–59.
6. Russell GF, et al. An evaluation of family therapy in anorexia nervosa and bulimia nervosa. Arch Gen Psychiatry. 1987;44(12):1047–56.
7. Treasure J, Russell G. The case for early intervention in anorexia nervosa: theoretical exploration of maintaining factors. Br J Psychiatry. 2011;199(1):5–7.
8. Lock J, et al. Practice parameter for the assessment and treatment of children and adolescents with eating disorders. J Am Acad Child Adolesc Psychiatry. 2015;54(5):412–25.
9. National Institute of Health and Care Excellence. Eating disorders: recognition and treatment. United Kingdom: the National Institute of Health and Care Excellence; 2017.
10. Guyatt GH, et al. GRADE guidelines: a new series of articles in the Journal of Clinical Epidemiology. J Clin Epidemiol. 2011;64(4):380–2.
11. Guyatt GH, et al. GRADE: an emerging consensus on rating quality of evidence and strength of recommendations. BMJ. 2008;336(7650):924–6.
12. Jaeschke R, et al. Use of GRADE grid to reach decisions on clinical practice guidelines when consensus is elusive. BMJ. 2008;337:a744.
13. Brouwers MC, et al. AGREE II: advancing guideline development, reporting and evaluation in health care. CMAJ. 2010;182(18):E839–42.
14. Higgins JPT, Thomas J, Chandler J, Cumpston M, Li T, Page MJ, Welch VA, editors. Cochrane Handbook for Systematic Reviews of Interventions. 2nd ed. Chichester: Wiley; 2019.
15. Guyatt G, Rennie D. Users' guides to the medical literature: a manual for evidence-based clinical practice. Chicago: American Medical Association; 2002.
16. Brouwers MC, et al. Validation of the guideline implementability for decision excellence model (Guide-M). BMJ Qual Saf. 2013;22(Suppl 1):A1–A94.
17. Eccles MP, et al. Developing clinical practice guidelines: target audiences, identifying topics for guidelines, guideline group composition and functioning and conflicts of interest. Implement Sci. 2012;7:60.
18. Kunz R, et al. Guideline group composition and group processes: article 3 in Integrating and coordinating efforts in COPD guideline development. An official ATS/ERS workshop report. Proc Am Thorac Soc. 2012;9(5):229–33.
19. Qaseem A, et al. Guidelines international network: toward international standards for clinical practice guidelines. Ann Intern Med. 2012;156(7):525–31.
20. Yousuf MI. Using experts' opinion through the Delphi technique. Pract Assess Res Eval. 2007;12(4):1–8.
21. Couturier J, Kimber M, Szatmari P. Efficacy of family-based treatment for adolescents with eating disorders: a systematic review and meta-analysis. Int J Eat Disord. 2013;46(1):3–11.
22. Robin AL, et al. A controlled comparison of family versus individual therapy for adolescents with anorexia nervosa. J Am Acad Child Adolesc Psychiatry. 1999;38(12):1482–9.
23. Lock J, et al. Randomized clinical trial comparing family-based treatment with adolescent-focused individual therapy for adolescents with anorexia nervosa. Arch Gen Psychiatry. 2010;67(10):1025–32.
24. Ball J, Mitchell P. A randomized controlled study of cognitive behavior therapy and behavioral family therapy for anorexia nervosa patients. Eat Disord. 2004;12(4):303–14.
25. Gusella JL, Campbell AG, Lalji K. A shift to placing parents in charge: does it improve weight gain in youth with anorexia? Paediatr Child Health. 2017; 22(5):269–72.
26. Paulson-Karlsson G, Engstrom I, Nevonen L. A pilot study of a family-based treatment for adolescent anorexia nervosa: 18- and 36-month follow-ups. Eat Disord. 2009;17(1):72–88.
27. Lock J, et al. Is family therapy useful for treating children with anorexia nervosa? Results of a case series. J Am Acad Child Adolesc Psychiatry. 2006; 45(11):1323–8.
28. Le Grange D, Binford R, Loeb KL. Manualized family-based treatment for anorexia nervosa: a case series. J Am Acad Child Adolesc Psychiatry. 2005; 44(1):41–6.
29. Loeb KL, et al. Open trial of family-based treatment for full and partial anorexia nervosa in adolescence: evidence of successful dissemination. J Am Acad Child Adolesc Psychiatry. 2007;46(7):792–800.
30. Goldstein M, et al. The effectiveness of family-based treatment for full and partial adolescent anorexia nervosa in an independent private practice setting: clinical outcomes. Int J Eat Disord. 2016;49(11):1023–6.
31. Couturier J, Isserlin L, Lock J. Family-based treatment for adolescents with anorexia nervosa: a dissemination study. Eat Disord. 2010;18(3):199–209.
32. Herscovici C, Bay L. Favorable outcome for anorexia nervosa patients treated in Argentina with a family approach. Eat Disord. 1996;4(1):59–66.
33. Le Grange D. Family therapy for adolescent anorexia nervosa. J Clin Psychol. 1999;55(6):727–39.
34. Le Grange D, Lock J, Dymek M. Family-based therapy for adolescents with bulimia nervosa. Am J Psychother. 2003;57(2):237–51.
35. Loeb KL, et al. Family-based treatment of a 17-year-old twin presenting with emerging anorexia nervosa: a case study using the "Maudsley method". J Clin Child Adolesc Psychol. 2009;38(1):176–83.
36. Sim LA, et al. Family-based therapy for adolescents with anorexia nervosa. Mayo Clin Proc. 2004;79(10):1305–8.
37. Krautter T, Lock J. Treatment of adolescent anorexia nervosa using manualized family-based treatment. Clin Case Stud. 2004;3(2):107–23.
38. Aspen V, Boutelle K. Family-based treatment without a family: case report of an adolescent with anorexia nervosa. Eat Weight Disord. 2014; 19(1):119–23.
39. Matthews A, Peterson CM. Intensive family-based therapy during an acute medical admission for anorexia nervosa: a case report. Clin Case Stud. 2016; 15(4):313–25.
40. Turkiewicz G, et al. Feasibility, acceptability, and effectiveness of family-based treatment for adolescent anorexia nervosa: an observational study conducted in Brazil. Braz J Psychiatry. 2010;32(2):169–72.
41. O'Neil J, Terry R, Connelly S. Family-based approach to anorexia nervosa. Osteopath Fam Physician. 2012;4:168–71.
42. Duvvuri V, et al. Differential weight restoration on olanzapine versus fluoxetine in identical twins with anorexia nervosa. Int J Eat Disord. 2012; 45(2):294–7.
43. Goldstein M, Madden S, Peters L. The use of effective treatments: the case of an adolescent girl with anorexia nervosa in the context of a conversion disorder. Clin Child Psychol Psychiatry. 2013;18(2):214–23.
44. Le Grange D, Schwartz S. Family therapy for identical twins with anorexia nervosa. Eat Weight Disord. 2003;8(1):84–7.
45. Eisler I, et al. Family therapy for adolescent anorexia nervosa: the results of a controlled comparison of two family interventions. J Child Psychol Psychiatry. 2000;41(6):727–36.
46. Le Grange D, et al. Randomized clinical trial of parent-focused treatment and family-based treatment for adolescent anorexia nervosa. J Am Acad Child Adolesc Psychiatry. 2016;55(8):683–92.
47. Le Grange D, et al. Evaluation of family treatments in adolescent anorexia nervosa: a pilot study. Int J Eat Disord. 1992;12(4):347–57.
48. Le Grange D, et al. A randomized controlled comparison of family-based treatment and supportive psychotherapy for adolescent bulimia nervosa. Arch Gen Psychiatry. 2007;64(9):1049–56.
49. Schmidt U, et al. A randomized controlled trial of family therapy and cognitive behavior therapy guided self-care for adolescents with bulimia nervosa and related disorders. Am J Psychiatry. 2007;164(4):591–8.
50. Le Grange D, et al. Randomized clinical trial of family-based treatment and cognitive-behavioral therapy for adolescent bulimia nervosa. J Am Acad Child Adolesc Psychiatry. 2015;54(11):886–94 e2.
51. Dodge E, et al. Family therapy for bulimia nervosa in adolescents: an exploratory study. J Fam Ther. 1995;17:59–77.
52. Hughes EK, et al. A case series of family-based treatment for adolescents with atypical anorexia nervosa. Int J Eat Disord. 2017;50(4):424–32.
53. Spettigue W, et al. Treatment of children and adolescents with avoidant/restrictive food intake disorder: a case series examining the feasibility of family therapy and adjunctive treatments. J Eat Disord. 2018;6(20):1–11.

54. Murray SB, Thornton C, Wallis A. Selective eating in a 9-year-old boy: family therapy as a first-line treatment. Clin Child Psychol Psychiatry. 2013;18(2): 270–5.
55. Strandjord SE, Ng H, Rome ES. Effects of treating gender dysphoria and anorexia nervosa in a transgender adolescent: lessons learned. Int J Eat Disord. 2015;48(7):942–5.
56. Lock J, et al. A comparison of short- and long-term family therapy for adolescent anorexia nervosa. J Am Acad Child Adolesc Psychiatry. 2005; 44(7):632–9.
57. Herscovici CR, Kovalskys I, Orellana L. An exploratory evaluation of the family meal intervention for adolescent anorexia nervosa. Fam Process. 2017;56(2):364–75.
58. Lock J, et al. Parental guided self-help family based treatment for adolescents with anorexia nervosa: A feasibility study. Int J Eat Disord. 2017; 50(9):1104–8.
59. Rhodes P, et al. Can parent-to-parent consultation improve the effectiveness of the maudsley model of family-based treatment for anorexia nervosa? A randomized control trial. J Fam Ther. 2008;30:96–108.
60. Lock J, et al. Can adaptive treatment improve outcomes in family-based therapy for adolescents with anorexia nervosa? Feasibility and treatment effects of a multi-site treatment study. Behav Res Ther. 2015;73:90–5.
61. Rockwell RE, Boutelle K, Trunko ME, Joy Jacobs M, Kaye WH. An innovative short-term, intensive, family-based. treatment for adolescent anorexia nervosa: case series. Eur Eat Disord Rev. 2011;19(4):362–7.
62. Marzola E, Knatz S, Murray SB, Rockwell R, Boutelle K, Eisler I, Kaye WH. Short-term intensive family. therapy for adolescent eating disorders: 30-month outcome. Eur Eat Disord Rev. 2015;23(3):210–8.
63. Goldfield GS, Boachie A. Delivery of family therapy in the treatment of anorexia nervosa using telehealth. Telemed J E Health. 2003;9(1):111–4.
64. Anderson KE, et al. Utilizing telehealth to deliver family-based treatment for adolescent anorexia nervosa. Int J Eat Disord. 2017;50(10):1235–8.
65. Lock J, et al. Feasibility study combining art therapy or cognitive remediation therapy with family-based treatment for adolescent anorexia nervosa. Eur Eat Disord Rev. 2018;26(1):62–8.
66. Ganci M, Pradel M, Hughes EK. Feasibility of a parent education and skills workshop for improving response to family-based treatment of adolescent anorexia nervosa. Int J Eat Disord. 2018;51(4):358–62.
67. Accurso EC, et al. Adaptation and implementation of family-based treatment enhanced with dialectical behavior therapy skills for anorexia nervosa in community-based specialist clinics. Eat Disord. 2018;26(2):149–63.
68. Peterson C, et al. FBT with adjunctive parent emotion coaching in an adolescent male with anorexia nervosa. Clin Case Stud. 2016;15(5):409–23.
69. Wagner I, et al. Attachment-based family therapy as an adjunct to family-based treatment for adolescent anorexia nervosa. Aust N Z J Fam Ther. 2016;37:207–27.
70. Hildebrandt T, et al. Exposure-based family therapy (FBT-E): An open case series of a new treatment for anorexia nervosa. Cogn Behav Pract. 2014;21: 470–84.
71. Timko CA, et al. An open trial of Acceptance-based Separated Family Treatment (ASFT) for adolescents with anorexia nervosa. Behav Res Ther. 2015;69:63–74.
72. Hurst K, Zimmer-Gembeck M. Family-based treatment with cognitive behavioural therapy for anorexia. Clin Psychol. 2019;23:61–70.
73. Merwin RM, Zucker NL, Timko CA. A pilot study of an acceptance-based separated family treatment for adolescent anorexia nervosa. Cogn Behav Pract. 2013;20(4):485–500.
74. Hurst K, Zimmer-Gembeck M. Focus on perfectionism in female adolescent anorexia nervosa. Int J Eat Disord. 2015;48(7):936–41.
75. Hurst K, Read S, Holtham T. Bulimia nervosa in adolescents: a new therapeutic frontier. J Fam Ther. 2017;39(4):563–79.
76. Eisler I, et al. A pragmatic randomised multi-centre trial of multifamily and single family therapy for adolescent anorexia nervosa. BMC Psychiatry. 2016; 16(1):422.
77. Gabel K, et al. The effect of multiple family therapy on weight gain in adolescents with anorexia nervosa: pilot data. J Can Acad Child Adolesc Psychiatry. 2014;23(3):196–9.
78. Hollesen A, Clausen L, Rokkedal K. Multiple family therapy for adolescents with anorexia nervosa: a pilot study of eating disorder symptoms and interpersonal functioning. J Fam Ther. 2013;35:53–67.
79. Salaminiou E, et al. Intensive multi-family therapy for adolescent anorexia nervosa: an open study of 30 families. J Fam Ther. 2017;39:498–513.
80. Gelin Z, et al. The effects of a multiple family therapy on adolescents with eating disorders: an outcome study. Fam Process. 2015;54(1):160–72.
81. Stewart C, et al. Multi-family therapy for bulimia nervosa in adolescence. Eat Disord. 2015;23(4):345–55.
82. Agras WS, et al. Comparison of 2 family therapies for adolescent anorexia nervosa: a randomized parallel trial. JAMA Psychiatry. 2014;71(11):1279–86.
83. Carr A, McDonnell D, Afnan S. Anorexia nervosa: the treatment of a male case with combined behavioural and family therapy. J Fam Ther. 1989;11: 335–51.
84. Merl H. Systemic family therapy in a case of anorexia nervosa in a boy--a case report within the scope of final interventions. Psychother Psychosom Med Psychol. 1989;39(12):444–51.
85. De Benedetta G, et al. Cancer and anorexia nervosa in the adolescence: a family-based systemic intervention. Int J Family Med. 2011;2011:1–8.
86. Minuchin S, et al. A conceptual model of psychosomatic illness in children. Family organization and family therapy. Arch Gen Psychiatry. 1975;32(8): 1031–8.
87. Wallin U, Kronvall P. Anorexia nervosa in teenagers: change in family function after family therapy, at 2-year follow-up. Nord J Psychiatry. 2002; 56(5):363–9.
88. Combrinck-Graham L. Structural family therapy in psychosomatic illness. Treatment of anorexia nervosa and asthma. Clin Pediatr (Phila). 1974;13(10): 827–33.
89. Liebman R, Minuchin S, Baker L. The role of the family in the treatment of anorexia nervosa. J Am Acad Child Psychiatry. 1974;13(2):264–74.
90. Godart N, et al. A randomized controlled trial of adjunctive family therapy and treatment as usual following inpatient treatment for anorexia nervosa adolescents. PLoS One. 2012;7(1):e28249.
91. Debow SL. Identical twins concordant for anorexia nervosa. A preliminary case report. Can Psychiatr Assoc J. 1975;20(3):215–7.
92. Lane D, Kern R. Multidimensional treatment of a 14-year-old anorexia nervosa patient. J Child Adolesc Psychother. 1987;4(3):211–5.
93. O'Halloran S. Family involvement in the treatment of anorexia nervosa: A solution-focused approach. Fam J. 1999;7(4):384–8.
94. Geist R, et al. Comparison of family therapy and family group psychoeducation in adolescents with anorexia nervosa. Can J Psychiatr. 2000;45(2):173–8.
95. Johnson S, Maddeaux C, Blouin J. Emotionally focused family therapy for bulimia: Changing attachment patterns. Psychotherapy. 1998;35(2):238–47.
96. Dalle Grave R, et al. Enhanced cognitive behaviour therapy for adolescents with anorexia nervosa: an alternative to family therapy? Behav Res Ther. 2013;51(1):R9–R12.
97. Cowdrey FA, Davis J. Response to enhanced cognitive behavioural therapy in an adolescent with anorexia nervosa. Behav Cogn Psychother. 2016;44(6): 717–22.
98. Cooper PJ, Fairburn CG. Cognitive behaviour therapy for anorexia nervosa: some preliminary findings. J Psychosom Res. 1984;28(6):493–9.
99. Martin-Murcia F, Diaz A, Gonzalez L. A case study of anorexia nervosa and obsessive personality disorder using third-generation behavioral therapies. Clin Case Stud. 2011;10(3):198–209.
100. Heffner M, Sperry J, Eifert G, Detweiler M. Acceptance and commitment therapy in the treatment of an adolescent female with anorexia nervosa: a case example. Cogn Behav Pract. 2002;9:232–6.
101. Scrignar C. Food as the reinforcer in the outpatient treatment of anorexia nervosa. J Behav Ther Exp Psychiat. 1971;2:31–6.
102. Fundudis T. Anorexia nervosa in a pre-adolescent girl: a multimodal behaviour therapy approach. J Child Psychol Psychiatry. 1986;27(2): 261–73.
103. Ollendick T. Behavioral treatment of anorexia nervosa: a five year study. Behav Modif. 1979;3(1):124–35.
104. Wildes JE, Marcus MD. Development of emotion acceptance behavior therapy for anorexia nervosa: a case series. Int J Eat Disord. 2011;44(5):421–7.
105. Pegado P, et al. Development, applicability, and effects of a pilot program of group cognitive-behavioral therapy in Brazilian adolescents with anorexia nervosa. Arch Clin Psychiatry. 2018;45(3):57–60.
106. Ohmann S, et al. Emotional aspects of anorexia nervosa: results of prospective naturalistic cognitive behavioral group therapy. Neuropsychiatr. 2013;27(3):119–28.
107. Stefini A, et al. Cognitive-behavioral and psychodynamic therapy in female adolescents with bulimia nervosa: a randomized controlled trial. J Am Acad Child Adolesc Psychiatry. 2017;56(4):329–35.

108. Dalle Grave R, et al. Transdiagnostic cognitive behaivour therapy for adolescents with an eating disorder who are not underweight. Behav Res Ther. 2015;73:79–82.
109. Lock J. Adjusting cognitive behavior therapy for adolescents with bulimia nervosa: results of case series. Am J Psychother. 2005;59(3):267–81.
110. Schapman-Williams AM, Lock J, Couturier J. Cognitive-behavioral therapy for adolescents with binge eating syndromes: a case series. Int J Eat Disord. 2006;39(3):252–5.
111. Cooper M, et al. Cognitive therapy for bulimia nervosa: an A-B replication series. Clin Psychol Psychother. 2007;14:402–11.
112. Anbar RD, Savedoff AD. Treatment of binge eating with automatic word processing and self-hypnosis: a case report. Am J Clin Hypn. 2005;48(2–3): 191–8.
113. Schapman-Williams AM, Lock J. Using cognitive-behavioral therapy to treat adolescent-onset bulimia nervosa: a case study. Clin Case Stud. 2007;6(6): 508–24.
114. Sysko R, Hildebrandt T. Enhanced cognitive behavioural therapy for an adolescent with purging disorder: a case report. Eur Eat Disord Rev. 2011; 19(1):37–45.
115. Seigel L. Classical and operant procedures in the treatment of a case of food aversion in a young child. J Clin Child Psychol. 1982;11(2):167–72.
116. Chatoor I, Conley C, Dickson L. Food refusal after an incident of choking: a posttraumatic eating disorder. J Am Acad Child Adolesc Psychiatry. 1988; 27(1):105–10.
117. Culbert TP, et al. Hypnobehavioral approaches for school-age children with dysphagia and food aversion: a case series. J Dev Behav Pediatr. 1996;17(5): 335–41.
118. Chorpita BF, Vitali AE, Barlow DH. Behavioral treatment of choking phobia in an adolescent: an experimental analysis. J Behav Ther Exp Psychiatry. 1997; 28(4):307–15.
119. Nock MK. A multiple-baseline evaluation of the treatment of food phobia in a young boy. J Behav Ther Exp Psychiatry. 2002;33(3–4):217–25.
120. Bailly D, et al. Choking phobia in childhood: a differential diagnosis with anorexia nervosa. Arch Pediatr. 2003;10(4):337–9.
121. Ciyiltepe M, Turkbay T. Phagophobia: a case report. Turk J Pediatr. 2006; 48(1):80–4.
122. Okada A, et al. A study of psycho-pathology and treatment of children with phagophobia. Acta Med Okayama. 2007;61(5):261–9.
123. de Roos C, de Jongh A. EMDR treatment of children and adolescents with a choking phobia. J EMDR Pract Res. 2008;2(1):201–11.
124. Fischer A, Luiselli J, Dove M. Effects of clinic and in-home treatment on consumption and feeding-associtied anxiety in an adolescent with avoidant/restrictive food intake disorder. Clin Pract Pediatr Psychol. 2015;3(2): 154–66.
125. Murphy J, Zlomke K. A behavioral parent-training intervention for a child with avoidant/restrictive food intake disorder. Clin Pract Pediatr Psychol. 2016;4(1):23–34.
126. Reid DB. A case study of hypnosis for phagophobia: it's no choking matter. Am J Clin Hypn. 2016;58(4):357–67.
127. Bloomfield B, et al. Treatment of food selectivity in a child with avoidant/ restrictive food intake disorder through parent teleconsultation. Bahav Anal Prac. 2018;12:33.
128. Fitzpatrick K, et al. Adolescent focused psychotherapy for adolescents with anorexia nervosa. J Contemp Psychother. 2010;40:31–9.
129. Pharis M, Penn M. A model for outpatient treatment of young adolescents with anorexia nervosa. Child Adolesc Soc Work. 1984;1:34–48.
130. Prestano C, et al. Group analytic therapy for eating disorders: preliminary results in a single-group study. Eur Eat Disord Rev. 2008;16(4):302–10.
131. Fischer S, Peterson C. Dialectical behavior therapy for adolescent binge eating, purging, suicidal behavior, and non-suicidal self-injury: a pilot study. Psychotherapy (Chic). 2015;52(1):78–92.
132. Safer D, Lock J, Couturier J. Dialectical behavior therapy modified for adolescent binge eating disorder: a case report. Cogn Behav Pract. 2007;14:157–67.
133. Salbach-Andrae H, et al. Dialectical behavior therapy of anorexia and bulimia nervosa among adolescents: a case series. Cogn Behav Pract. 2008; 15(4):415–25.
134. Dahlgren CL, et al. Neuropsychological functioning in adolescents with anorexia nervosa before and after cognitive remediation therapy: a feasibility trial. Int J Eat Disord. 2013;46(6):576–81.
135. van Noort BM, et al. Cognitive remediation therapy for children with anorexia nervosa. Z Kinder Jugendpsychiatr Psychother. 2015;43(5):351–5.
136. Carei TR, et al. Randomized controlled clinical trial of yoga in the treatment of eating disorders. J Adolesc Health. 2010;46(4):346–51.
137. Kafantaris V, et al. A placebo-controlled pilot study of adjunctive olanzapine for adolescents with anorexia nervosa. J Child Adolesc Psychopharmacol. 2011;21(3):207–12.
138. Spettigue W, et al. Evaluation of the effectiveness and safety of olanzapine as an adjunctive treatment for anorexia nervosa in adolescents: an open-label trial. J Can Acad Child Adolesc Psychiatry. 2018;27(3):197–208.
139. Norris ML, et al. Olanzapine use for the adjunctive treatment of adolescents with anorexia nervosa. J Child Adolesc Psychopharmacol. 2011;21(3):213–20.
140. Hillebrand JJ, et al. Olanzapine reduces physical activity in rats exposed to activity-based anorexia: possible implications for treatment of anorexia nervosa? Biol Psychiatry. 2005;58(8):651–7.
141. Swenne I, Rosling A. No unexpected adverse events and biochemical side effects of olanzapine as adjunct treatment in adolescent girls with eating disorders. J Child Adolesc Psychopharmacol. 2011;21(3):221–7.
142. Leggero C, et al. Low-dose olanzapine monotherapy in girls with anorexia nervosa, restricting subtype: focus on hyperactivity. J Child Adolesc Psychopharmacol. 2010;20(2):127–33.
143. Pisano S, et al. Second generation antipsychotics in adolescent anorexia nervosa: a new hypothesis of eligibility criteria. J Child Adolesc Psychopharmacol. 2014;24(5):293–5.
144. Dennis K, Le Grange D, Bremer J. Olanzapine use in adolescent anorexia nervosa. Eat Weight Disord. 2006;11(2):e53–6.
145. Boachie A, Goldfield GS, Spettigue W. Olanzapine use as an adjunctive treatment for hospitalized children with anorexia nervosa: case reports. Int J Eat Disord. 2003;33(1):98–103.
146. Mehler C, et al. Olanzapine in children and adolescents with chronic anorexia nervosa. A study of five cases. Eur Child Adolesc Psychiatry. 2001; 10(2):151–7.
147. La Via MC, Gray N, Kaye WH. Case reports of olanzapine treatment of anorexia nervosa. Int J Eat Disord. 2000;27(3):363–6.
148. Dadic-Hero E, et al. Olanzapine treatment in anorexia nervosa: case report. Psychiatr Danub. 2009;21(1):122–5.
149. Hein IM, Huyser C. Olanzapine in the treatment of adolescents with anorexia nervosa. Tijdschr Psychiatr. 2010;52(6):417–21.
150. Tateno M, et al. Successful olanzapine treatment of anorexia nervosa in a girl with pervasive developmental disorder not otherwise specified. Psychiatry Clin Neurosci. 2008;62(6):752.
151. Ercan ES, et al. Olanzapine treatment of an adolescent girl with anorexia nervosa. Hum Psychopharmacol. 2003;18(5):401–3.
152. Dodig-Curkovic K, et al. The case report of treatment strategy for anorexia nervosa with psychotic elements in adolescent. Coll Antropol. 2010;34(3): 1093–9.
153. Ayyildiz H, et al. Olanzapine-induced atypical neuroleptic malignant syndrome in an adolescent man with anorexia nervosa. Eat Weight Disord. 2016;21(2):309–11.
154. Ritchie B, Norris ML. QTc prolongation associated with atypical antipsychotic use in the treatment of adolescent-onset anorexia nervosa. J Can Acad Child Adolesc Psychiatry. 2009;18(1):60–3.
155. Norris ML, et al. Factors influencing research drug trials in adolescents with anorexia nervosa. Eat Disord. 2010;18(3):210–7.
156. Bozabali O, Baykara B, Baykara A. Olanzapine use in five different psychiatric disorders in children and adolescents. Bull Clin Psychopharmacol. 2002; 12(4):179–85.
157. Brewerton TD, D'Agostino M. Adjunctive use of olanzapine in the treatment of avoidant restrictive food intake disorder in children and adolescents in an eating disorders program. J Child Adolesc Psychopharmacol. 2017;27(10): 920–2.
158. Hagman J, et al. A double-blind, placebo-controlled study of risperidone for the treatment of adolescents and young adults with anorexia nervosa: a pilot study. J Am Acad Child Adolesc Psychiatry. 2011;50(9):915–24.
159. Fisman S, et al. Case study: anorexia nervosa and autistic disorder in an adolescent girl. J Am Acad Child Adolesc Psychiatry. 1996;35(7):937–40.
160. Kracke EJ, Tosh AK. Treatment of anorexia nervosa with long-term risperidone in an outpatient setting: case study. Springerplus. 2014;3:706.
161. Umehara H, Iga J, Ohmori T. Successful treatment of anorexia nervosa in a 10-year-old boy with risperidone long-acting injection. Clin Psychopharmacol Neurosci. 2014;12(1):65–6.
162. Newman-Toker J. Risperidone in anorexia nervosa. J Am Acad Child Adolesc Psychiatry. 2000;39(8):941–2.

163. Pennell A, et al. Severe avoidant/restrictive food intake disorder and coexisting stimulant treated attention deficit hyperactivity disorder. Int J Eat Disord. 2016;49(11):1036–9.
164. Mehler-Wex C, et al. Atypical antipsychotics in severe anorexia nervosa in children and adolescents--Review and case reports. Eur Eat Disord Rev. 2008;16(2):100–8.
165. Frank GK, et al. The partial dopamine D2 receptor agonist aripiprazole is associated with weight gain in adolescent anorexia nervosa. Int J Eat Disord. 2017;50(4):447–50.
166. Frank GK. Aripiprazole, a partial dopamine agonist to improve adolescent anorexia nervosa-a case series. Int J Eat Disord. 2016;49(5):529–33.
167. Trunko ME, et al. Aripiprazole in anorexia nervosa and low-weight bulimia nervosa: case reports. Int J Eat Disord. 2011;44(3):269–75.
168. Colak Sivri R, Hizarcioglu Gulsen H, Yilmaz A. Phagophobia successfully treated with low-dose aripiprazole in an adolescent: a case report. Clin Neuropharmacol. 2018;41(4):148–50.
169. Holtkamp K, et al. A retrospective study of SSRI treatment in adolescent anorexia nervosa: insufficient evidence for efficacy. J Psychiatr Res. 2005; 39(3):303–10.
170. Frank GK, Kaye WH, Marcus MD. Sertraline in underweight binge eating/ purging-type eating disorders: five case reports. Int J Eat Disord. 2001;29(4): 495–8.
171. Lyles B, Sarkis E, Kemph JP. Fluoxetine and anorexia. J Am Acad Child Adolesc Psychiatry. 1990;29(6):984–5.
172. Gee RL, Telew N. Obsessive-compulsive disorder and anorexia nervosa in a high school athlete: a case report. J Athl Train. 1999;34(4):375–8.
173. Kotler LA, et al. An open trial of fluoxetine for adolescents with bulimia nervosa. J Child Adolesc Psychopharmacol. 2003;13(3):329–35.
174. Tor PC, Lee EL. Treatment emergent mania responding to valproate in a Chinese female adolescent population with eating disorders: a case series. Eur Eat Disord Rev. 2008;16(6):421–6.
175. Wolter H, et al. Diagnostic crossover from obesity to atypical anorexia nervosa - a case report. Obes Facts. 2009;2(1):52–3.
176. Banerjee SP, Bhandari RP, Rosenberg DR. Use of low-dose selective serotonin reuptake inhibitors for severe, refractory choking phobia in childhood. J Dev Behav Pediatr. 2005;26(2):123–7.
177. Hosoglu E, Akca OF. Escitalopram in the treatment of a 3-year-old child with posttraumatic feeding disorder. J Child Adolesc Psychopharmacol. 2018; 28(2):153–4.
178. Celik G, et al. Fluoxetine in posttraumatic eating disorder in two-year-old twins. J Child Adolesc Psychopharmacol. 2007;17(2):233–6.
179. Hrdlicka M, et al. Mirtazapine in the treatment of adolescent anorexia nervosa. Case-control study. Eur Child Adolesc Psychiatry. 2008;17(3):187–9.
180. Jaafar NR, et al. Mirtazapine for anorexia nervosa with depression. Aust N Z J Psychiatry. 2007;41(9):768–9.
181. Naguy A, Al-Mutairi A. An adolescent male with anorexia nervosa favorably responded to mirtazapine. Am J Ther. 2018;25(6):e675–6.
182. Gray E, et al. Mirtazapine and weight gain in avoidant and restrictive food intake disorder. J Am Acad Child Adolesc Psychiatry. 2018;57(4):288–9.
183. Tanidir C, Herguner S. Mirtazapine for choking phobia: report of a pediatric case. J Child Adolesc Psychopharmacol. 2015;25(8):659–60.
184. Anis N, Isomaa R, Kaltiala-Heino R. Adolescent psychiatric inpatients with first hospitalization due to anorexia nervosa: can rehospitalization be predcited by clinical features. Psychiatr Fenn. 2016;47:76–94.
185. Ayton A, Keen C, Lask B. Pros and cons of using the mental health act for severe eating disorders in adolescents. Eur Eat Disord Rev. 2009;17(1):14–23.
186. Castro-Fornieles J, et al. Predictors of weight maintenance after hospital discharge in adolescent anorexia nervosa. Int J Eat Disord. 2007;40(2):129–35.
187. Fennig S, et al. Inpatient treatment has no impact on the core thoughts and perceptions in adolescents with anorexia nervosa. Early Interv Psychiatry. 2017;11(3):200–7.
188. Goddard E, et al. A multi-centre cohort study of short term outcomes of hospital treatment for anorexia nervosa in the UK. BMC Psychiatry. 2013;13:287.
189. Heinberg LJ, et al. Clinical course and short-term outcome of hospitalized adolescents with eating disorders: the success of combining adolescents and adults on an eating disorders unit. Eat Weight Disord. 2003;8(4):326–31.
190. Kalisvaart JL, Hergenroeder AC. Hospitalization of patients with eating disorders on adolescent medical units is threatened by current reimbursement systems. Int J Adolesc Med Health. 2007;19(2):155–65.
191. Leon GR, et al. Sexual, body-image, and personality attitudes in anorexia nervosa. J Abnorm Child Psychol. 1985;13(2):245–57.
192. Lievers LS, Curt F, Wallier J, Perdereau F, Rein Z, Jeammet P, Godart N. Predictive factors of length of inpatient treatment in anorexia nervosa. Eur Child Adolesc Psychiatry. 2009;18(2):75–84.
193. Mekori E, et al. Predictors of short-term outcome variables in hospitalised female adolescents with eating disorders. Int J Psychiatry Clin Pract. 2017; 21(1):41–9.
194. Morris J, Simpson AV, Voy SJ. Length of stay of inpatients with eating disorders. Clin Psychol Psychother. 2015;22(1):45–53.
195. Nova E, Lopez-Vidriero I, Varela P, Casas J, Marcos A. Evolution of serum biochemical indicators in anorexia nervosa patients: a 1-year follow-up study. J Hum Nutr Diet. 2007;21:23–30.
196. Roux H, et al. Predictive factors of dropout from inpatient treatment for anorexia nervosa. BMC Psychiatry. 2016;16(1):339.
197. Schlegl S, et al. Inpatient treatment for adolescents with anorexia nervosa: clinical significance and predictors of treatment outcome. Eur Eat Disord Rev. 2016;24(3):214–22.
198. Shugar G, Krueger S. Aggressive family communication, weight-gain, and improved eating attitudes during systemic family-therapy for anorexia-nervosa. Int J Eat Disord. 1995;17(1):23–31.
199. Tasaka K, et al. Long-term follow up of hospitalized pediatric anorexia nervosa restricting type. Pediatr Int. 2017;59(4):482–9.
200. Treat TA, et al. Treatment of anorexia nervosa in a specialty care continuum. Int J Eat Disord. 2008;41(6):564–72.
201. Vall E, Wade TD. Predictors and moderators of outcomes and readmission for adolescent inpatients with anorexia nervosa: a pilot study. Clin Psychol. 2017;21(2):143–52.
202. Bourion-Bedes S, et al. Prognostic value of early therapeutic alliance in weight recovery: a prospective cohort of 108 adolescents with anorexia nervosa. J Adolesc Health. 2013;52(3):344–50.
203. Rothschild-Yakar L, Lacoua L, Stein D. Changes in patient measures as predictors of therapists' ratings of treatment collaboration and change in eating disorder subgroups. Assessment. 2013;20(6):752–63.
204. Toms DA, Crisp AH. Weight phobia in an adolescent male with stunted development. J Psychosom Res. 1972;16(4):289–95.
205. Strik Lievers L, Curt F, Wallier J, Perdereau F, Rein Z, Jeammet P, Godart N. Predictive factors of length of inpatient treatment in anorexia nervosa. Eur Child Adolesc Psychiatry. 2009;18(2):75–84.
206. Avnon A, et al. Inpatient weight curve trajectory as a prognostic factor among adolescents with anorexia nervosa: a preliminary report. Eat Weight Disord. 2018;23(5):645–51.
207. Hetman I, et al. Percentage from target weight (PFTW) predicts re-hospitalization in adolescent anorexia nervosa. Isr J Psychiatry Relat Sci. 2017;54(3):28–34.
208. Singer L, et al. Cognitive-behavioural treatment of health-impairing food phobias in children. J Am Acad Child Adolesc Psychiatry. 1992;31(5):847–52.
209. Pitt PD, Middleman AB. A focus on behavior management of avoidant/ restrictive food intake disorder (ARFID): a case series. Clin Pediatr (Phila). 2018;57(4):478–80.
210. Rhodes P, Prunty M, Madden S. Life-Threatening Food Refusal in Two Nine-Year-Old Girls: Re-Thinking the Maudsley Model. Clin Child Psychol Psychiatry. 2009;14(1):63–70.
211. Halvorsen I, et al. Naturalistic outcome of family-based inpatient treatment for adolescents with anorexia nervosa. Eur Eat Disord Rev. 2018;26(2):141–5.
212. Paul P, Mehta S, Coffey BJ. Anorexia nervosa in a 14-year-old second-generation hispanic adolescent boy. J Child Adolesc Psychopharmacol. 2013;23(4):295–9.
213. Salbach-Andrae H, et al. Short-term outcome of anorexia nervosa in adolescents after inpatient treatment: a prospective study. Eur Child Adolesc Psychiatry. 2009;18(11):701–4.
214. Leitenberg H, Agras WS, Thomson LE. A sequential analysis of the effect of selective positive reinforcement in modifying anorexia nervosa. Behav Res Ther. 1968;6(2):211–8.
215. Blinder BJ, Freeman DM, Stunkard AJ. Behavior therapy of anorexia nervosa: effectiveness of activity as a reinforcer of weight gain. Am J Psychiatry. 1970;126(8):1093–8.
216. Garfinkel PE, Kline SA, Stancer HC. Treatment of anorexia nervosa using operant conditioning techniques. J Nerv Ment Dis. 1973;157(6):428–33.
217. Halmi KA, Powers P, Cunningham S. Treatment of anorexia nervosa with behavior modification. Effectiveness of formula feeding and isolation. Arch Gen Psychiatry. 1975;32(1):93–6.

218. Pertschuk M, Edwards N, Pomerleau O. A multiple-baseline approach to behavioural intervention in anorexia nervosa. Behav Ther. 1978;9:368–76.
219. Poole AD, Sanson-Fisher RW, Young P. A behavioural programme for the management of anorexia nervosa. Aust N Z J Psychiatry. 1978;12(1):49–53.
220. Clark DB, Munford PR. Behavioral consultation to pediatrics. Child Behavior Therapy. 1981;2(3):25–33.
221. Cinciripini PM, et al. A behavioral program for the management of anorexia and bulimia. J Nerv Ment Dis. 1983;171(3):186–9.
222. Collins M, Hodas GR, Liebman R. Interdisciplinary model for the inpatient treatment of adolescents with anorexia nervosa. J Adolesc Health Care. 1983;4(1):3–8.
223. Boey KW. The restoration of body weight in anorexia nervosa through operant conditioning: a case report. Singap Med J. 1985;26(2):187–91.
224. Steinhausen HC. Evaluation of inpatient treatment of adolescent anorexic patients. J Psychiatr Res. 1985;19(2–3):371–5.
225. Alessi NE, et al. Prepubertal anorexia nervosa and major depressive disorder. J Am Acad Child Adolesc Psychiatry. 1989;28(3):380–4.
226. Nygaard JA. Anorexia nervosa. Treatment and triggering factors. Acta Psychiatr Scand Suppl. 1990;361:44–9.
227. Solanto MV, et al. Rate of weight gain of inpatients with anorexia nervosa under two behavioral contracts. Pediatrics. 1994;93(6 Pt 1):989–91.
228. Blanchet-Collet C, et al. Anorexia nervosa hyperactivity-induced ischemic colitis (ANHIC): a new cause of anaemia. Eat Weight Disord Stud Anorexia Bulimia Obes. 2016;21(3):507–10.
229. Wockel L, et al. Serotonin-induced decrease of intracellular Ca(2+) release in platelets of bulimic patients normalizes during treatment. J Neural Transm (Vienna). 2009;116(1):89–95.
230. Groen JJ, Feldman-Toledano Z. Educative treatment of patients and parentsin anorexia nervosa. Br J Psychiatry. 1966;112(488):671–81.
231. Kronenberg J, et al. The treatment of anorexia-nervosa in a general-hospital - a case vignette of a multidisciplinary general hospital-based approach. J Adolesc. 1994;17(2):163–71.
232. Maxmen JS, Siberfarb PM, Ferrell RB. Anorexia nervosa. Practical initial management in a general hospital. JAMA. 1974;229(7):801–3.
233. Jenkins ME. An outcome study of anorexia nervosa in an adolescent unit. J Adolesc. 1987;10(1):71–81.
234. Lock J, Litt I. What predicts maintenance of weight for adolescents medically hospitalized for anorexia nervosa? Eat Disord. 2003;11(1):1–7.
235. Meilleur D, et al. Sociodemographic, clinical, psychological and behavioral characteristics of children 8–12 years old hospitalized for an eating disorder. J Adolesc Health. 2012;50(2):S42.
236. Depestele L, et al. An adjunctive multi-family group intervention with or without patient participation during an inpatient treatment for adolescents with an eating disorder: a pilot study. Eur Eat Disord Rev. 2017;25(6):570–8.
237. Salbach H, et al. Family-oriented group therapy in the treatment of female patients with anorexia and bulimia nervosa--a pilot study. Z Kinder Jugendpsychiatr Psychother. 2006;34(4):267–74.
238. Couturier J, Mahmood A. Meal support therapy reduces the use of nasogastric feeding for adolescents hospitalized with anorexia nervosa. Eat Disord. 2009;17(4):327–32.
239. Kells M, et al. Examining supervised meals in patients with restrictive eating disorders. Appl Nurs Res. 2013;26(2):76–9.
240. Kells M, et al. Meal supervision during medical hospitalization for eating disorders. Clin Nurs Res. 2017;26(4):525–37.
241. Leacy KA, Cane JN. Effect of non-select menus on weight and eating concern in adolescents hospitalized with anorexia nervosa. Eat Disord. 2012; 20(2):159–67.
242. Janas-Kozik M, et al. Bright light treatment of depressive symptoms in patients with restrictive type of anorexia nervosa. J Affect Disord. 2011; 130(3):462–5.
243. Asch M, et al. Cognitive remediation therapy for children and adolescents with anorexia nervosa in France: an exploratory study. Encephale. 2014; 40(3):240–6.
244. Herbrich L, et al. Follow-up assessment of cognitive remediation therapy in adolescent anorexia nervosa: a pilot study. Eur Eat Disord Rev. 2017;25(2):104–13.
245. Kuge R, et al. Group cognitive remediation therapy for younger adolescents with anorexia nervosa: a feasibility study in a Japanese sample. BMC Res Notes. 2017;10(1):317.
246. Harrison A, et al. Cognitive remediation therapy for adolescent inpatients with severe and complex anorexia nervosa: a treatment trial. Eur Eat Disord Rev. 2018;26(3):230–40.
247. Cwojdzinska A, Markowska-Regulska K, Rybakowski F. Cognitive remediation therapy in adolescent anorexia nervosa--case report. Psychiatr Pol. 2009; 43(1):115–24.
248. Strober M, et al. Are there gender differences in core symptoms, temperament, and short-term prospective outcome in anorexia nervosa? Int J Eat Disord. 2006;39(7):570–5.
249. Dalle Grave R, et al. Inpatient cognitive behavior therapy for adolecents with anorexia nervosa: immediate and long-term effects. Front Psychiatry. 2014;5:14.
250. El Ghoch M, et al. Regional fat distribution in adolescent and adult females with anorexia nervosa: a longitudinal study. Clin Nutr. 2015; 34:1224–32.
251. Hillen S, et al. Motivation to change and perceptions of the admission process with respect to outcome in adolescent anorexia nervosa. BMC Psychiatry. 2015;15:140.
252. Madden S, et al. A randomized controlled trial of in-patient treatment for anorexia nervosa in medically unstable adolescents. Psychol Med. 2015; 45(2):415–27.
253. Herpertz-Dahlmann B, et al. Day-patient treatment after short inpatient care versus continued inpatient treatment in adolescents with anorexia nervosa (ANDI): a multicentre, randomised, open-label, non-inferiority trial. Lancet. 2014;383(9924):1222–9.
254. Garner D, Magana C. Anorexia nervosa, in clinical behavior therapy: adults and children, M. Hersen, Editor. New York: Wiley; 2002.
255. Goldstein M, et al. The effectiveness of a day program for the treatment of adolescent anorexia nervosa. Int J Eat Disord. 2011;44(1):29–38.
256. Ngo M, Isserlin L. Body weight as a prognostic factor for day hospital success in adolescents with anorexia nervosa. Eat Disord. 2014;22(1):62–71.
257. Dancyger I, et al. Cultural factors in orthodox Jewish adolescents treated in a day program for eating disorders. Int J Adolesc Med Health. 2002;14(4):317–28.
258. Dancyger I, et al. Adolescents and eating disorders: an examination of a day treatment program. Eat Weight Disord. 2003;8(3):242–8.
259. Lazaro L, et al. Effectiveness of self-esteem and social skills group therapy in adolescent eating disorder patients attending a day hospital treatment programme. Eur Eat Disord Rev. 2011;19(5):398–406.
260. Bustin LA, et al. Motivational stage of change in young patients undergoing day treatment for eating disorders. Int J Adolesc Med Health. 2013;25(2):151–6.
261. de Graft-Johnson A, et al. Weight gain in an eating disorders day program. Int J Adolesc Med Health. 2013;25(2):177–80.
262. Danziger Y, et al. Is psychotherapy mandatory during the acute refeeding period in the treatment of anorexia nervosa? J Adolesc Health Care. 1989; 10(4):328–31.
263. Danziger Y, et al. Parental involvement in treatment of patients with anorexia nervosa in a pediatric day-care unit. Pediatrics. 1988;81(1):159–62.
264. Bean P, et al. Clinical observations of the impact of maudsley therapy in improving eating disorder symptoms, weight, and depression in adolescents receiving treatment for anorexia nervosa. J Groups Addict Recover. 2010;5(1):70–82.
265. Gezelius C, et al. Adolescent patients with eating disorders and their parents: a study of self-image and outcome at an intensive outpatient program. Eat Weight Disord. 2016;21(4):607–16.
266. Rienecke RD, Richmond R, Lebow J. Therapeutic alliance, expressed emotion, and treatment outcome for anorexia nervosa in a family-based partial hospitalization program. Eat Behav. 2016;22:124–8.
267. Rienecke RD, Richmond RL. Three-month follow-up in a family-based partial hospitalization program. Eat Disord. 2018;26(3):278–89.
268. Zanna V, et al. Day-hospital multifocal integrated treatment for anorexia nervosa in adolescents: a one-year follow-up. J Child Fam Stud. 2017;26(5): 1460–71.
269. Martin-Wagar CA, Holmes S, Bhatnagar KAC. Predictors of weight restoration in a day-treatment program that supports family-based treatment for adolescents with anorexia nervosa. Eat Disord. 2019; 27(4):400–17.
270. Simic M, et al. Intensive treatment program (ITP): A case series service evaluation of the effectiveness of day patient treatment for adolescents with a restrictive eating disorder. Int J Eat Disord. 2018;51(11):1261–9.
271. Hoste R. Incorporating family-based therapy principles into a partial hospitalization programme for adolescents with anorexia nervosa: challenges and considerations. J Fam Ther. 2015;37:41–60.

272. Ornstein RM, Lane-Loney SE, Hollenbeak CS. Clinical outcomes of a novel, family-centered partial hospitalization program for young patients with eating disorders. Eat Weight Disord. 2012;17(3):e170–7.
273. Girz L, et al. Adapting family-based therapy to a day hospital programme for adolescents with eating disorders: preliminary outcomes and trajectories of change. J Fam Ther. 2013;35:102–20.
274. Grewal S, et al. Factors associated with successful completion in an adolescent-only day hospital program for eating disorders. Eat Disord. 2014;22(2):152–62.
275. Henderson K, et al. A family-based eating disorder day treatment program for youth: examining the clinical and statistical significance of short-term treatment outcomes. Eat Disord. 2014;22(1):1–18.
276. Johnston JA, et al. A pilot study of maudsley family therapy with group dialectical behavior therapy skills training in an intensive outpatient program for adolescent eating disorders. J Clin Psychol. 2015;71(6):527–43.
277. Iniesta Sepulveda M, et al. Intensive family exposure-based cognitive-behavioral treatment for adolescents with anorexia nervosa. Psicothema. 2017;29(4):433–9.
278. Ornstein RM, et al. Treatment of avoidant/restrictive food intake disorder in a cohort of young patients in a partial hospitalization program for eating disorders. Int J Eat Disord. 2017;50(9):1067–74.
279. Murray SB, et al. Integrating family-based treatment and dialectical behavior therapy for adolescent bulimia nervosa: preliminary outcomes of an open pilot trial. Eat Disord. 2015;23(4):336–44.
280. Green J, et al. Day program for young people with anorexia nervosa. Australas Psychiatry. 2015;23(3):249–53.
281. Seiverling L, et al. The effects of a brief behavioral intervention on food refusal in a child with a fear of choking. Clin Case Stud. 2016;15(2):117–25.
282. Williams K, et al. Brief, intensive behavioural treatment of food refusal secondary to emetophobia. Clin Case Stud. 2011;10(4):304–11.
283. Fernandez-del-Valle M, et al. Muscle function and body composition profile in adolescents with restrictive anorexia nervosa: does resistance training help? Disabil Rehabil. 2016;38(4):346–53.
284. Fisher M, et al. Demographics and outcomes of adolescents with eating disorders treated in residential care. J Adolesc Health. 2015;56(2):S87.
285. Weltzin T, et al. Long-term effects of a multidisciplinary residential treatment model on improvements of symptoms and weight in adolescents with eating disorders. J Groups Addict Recover. 2014;9:71–85.
286. Twohig MP, et al. Effectiveness and clinical response rates of a residential eating disorders facility. Eat Disord. 2016;24(3):224–39.
287. McHugh MD. Readiness for change and short-term outcomes of female adolescents in residential treatment for anorexia nervosa. Int J Eat Disord. 2007;40(7):602–12.
288. Pitel AU, et al. Diagnosis and treatment of an adolescent with comorbid type 1 diabetes mellitus and anorexia nervosa. Clin Pediatr (Phila). 1998; 37(8):491–6.
289. Rodrigue J, et al. Multi-modal treatment of an adolescent with anorexia nervosa and insulin-dependent diabetes mellitus: a case report. Fam Syst Med. 1990;8(4):349–58.
290. van der Leer, G., et al., Clinical practice guidelines for the BC eating disorders continuum of services. 2012: www.healthservices.gov.bc.ca.
291. Gowers SG, et al. A randomised controlled multicentre trial of treatments for adolescent anorexia nervosa including assessment of cost-effectiveness and patient acceptability - the TOuCAN trial. Health Technol Assess. 2010; 14(15):1–98.
292. Dalle Grave R, et al. Inpatient cognitive behavior therapy for adolescents with anorexia nervosa: immediate and longer-term effects. Front Psychiatry. 2014;5:14.
293. Sibeoni J, et al. Metasynthesis of the Views about Treatment of Anorexia Nervosa in Adolescents: Perspectives of Adolescents, Parents, and Professionals. PLoS One. 2017;12(1):e0169493.
294. Stockford C, et al. Women's recovery from anorexia nervosa: a systematic review and meta-synthesis of qualitative research. Eat Disord. 2019;27(4):343–68.
295. Dukarm CP. Bulimia nervosa and attention deficit hyperactivity disorder: a possible role for stimulant medication. J Women's Health (Larchmt). 2005; 14(4):345–50.
296. Kardas M, et al. Lorazepam in the treatment of posttraumatic feeding disorder. J Child Adolesc Psychopharmacol. 2014;24(5):296–7.

3

"Our daily life was mainly comprised of eating and sitting:" a qualitative analysis of adolescents' experiences of inpatient eating disorder treatment in China

Yi Wu and Amy Harrison*

Abstract

Background: Some individuals with Eating Disorders (EDs) require hospitalization to stabilize and improve life-threatening physical complications. The experiences of those receiving inpatient treatment for EDs are well-documented in western samples, but less is known about the experiences of those in China, the world's most populous country in which the incidence of EDs may be increasing.

Methods: This qualitative study aimed to use Interpretative Phenomenological Analysis to understand the experiences of four adolescents receiving inpatient treatment for EDs in China. Individual, semi-structured interviews were conducted.

Results: Four themes emerged from the data: perceptions of the treatment received, peer influences during admission, the impact of treatment on wellbeing and participants' sense of self.

Conclusions: This is the first published study on the experience of Chinese participants with EDs. Their experiences share commonalities with those reported by participants in Western studies and also illuminate differences in how EDs are understood and managed in inpatient settings in China. Cross-cultural collaborations will be important to share knowledge and practice.

Keywords: Anorexia nervosa, Eating disorders, China, Inpatient treatment, Patient experience

Plain English summary

Eating disorders are being reported more frequently in China, and while past research has largely explored the treatment experiences of those in Europe, the USA and Australia, little is known about Chinese participants' experiences of treatment for an eating disorder. In this study, four adolescents receiving inpatient treatment for an eating disorder were interviewed and the experiences they shared are illustrated through four 'themes' which represent participants' perceptions of the treatment they received, how their peers impacted them during their hospital admission, the degree to which treatment impacted their own wellbeing and the impact of treatment of their sense of self. Knowing more about how treatment is delivered in different countries will enable practitioners to collaborate around good practice for treating eating disorders.

* Correspondence: a.harrison@ucl.ac.uk
Department of Psychology and Human Development, Institute of Education, University College London, 25 Woburn Square, London WC1H 0AA, UK

Background

Eating disorders (EDs), including anorexia nervosa (AN) and bulimia nervosa (BN) are psychiatric disorders with severe physical complications. Their typical onset is during adolescence and EDs have the highest death rate of any psychiatric illness [1]. Behaviors include food restriction, bingeing, self-induced vomiting and excessive exercise [2]. Life-time risk is increasing [3] and in the United Kingdom (UK), adolescents with EDs occupy the largest number of child and adolescent psychiatric beds [4]. Due to effects of starvation on the body, including cardiovascular risks, many people require hospitalization, which for the 20% who have the more severe and enduring form of illness, can be extensive and repeated [5].

Previous work has investigated the lived experiences of this group of individuals requiring hospitalization using qualitative methodologies. Studies from the UK [6–13], The Netherlands [14], Norway [15] and Australia [16] all report themes of control versus collaboration, removal from normality, the negative and positive impacts of peer relationships, transition and recovery, disconnection from the outside world, the role of meals and eating, battling the ED and taking responsibility. In these countries, in-patient treatment tends to involve physical rehabilitation alongside psychotherapies including cognitive behavioral therapy (CBT) and family therapy [17] and individuals may be admitted voluntary or detained and treated using legal frameworks like the UK's Mental Health Act [18]. One key limitation of the current literature is that research on the experience of inpatient treatment is restricted to these western countries, perhaps because erroneously, it was once thought that EDs were culturally bound [19]. Therefore, little is known about experiences of inpatient treatment for EDs in countries such as China, which, hosting the world's largest population, has a developing literature on the prominence of eating difficulties [20–27]. Indeed, although under-researched relative to western countries, EDs are becoming formidable public health challenges in China [28], showing significant increases in prevalence, with similar rates to the west [28–30], with which China shares thinness as a desirable trait [31]. Therefore, this study aimed to use Interpretive Phenomenological Analysis (IPA; [32]) to understand the experiences of four adolescents receiving inpatient treatment for EDs in mainland China.

Methods

Design

This qualitative inquiry employed a within-participants design.

Participants

A purposive, volunteer sample of four Chinese adolescent girls (aged 16–19) admitted to a university hospital in Beijing for treatment of anorexia nervosa (AN) was recruited to take part in the study. The study was publicized through an online forum for families affected by EDs in the region. The researcher was given permission by the forum moderator to advertise the study in this space. Participants aged 16 to 20 of any gender were eligible to take part if they were receiving inpatient treatment for an ED and could consent to agree to speak about their experiences. Participants' identities are protected through the use of pseudonyms.

Measures

A semi-structured interview was selected due to its flexibility [33] and ability to permit unforeseen ideas to emerge [34] and was developed and piloted beforehand. The interview schedule consisted of a series of open-ended questions informed via a systematic review of the literature on the inpatient experience, discussions with service users and experts in the field. The semi-structured interview is provided in Appendix.

Procedure

Participants were provided with an information sheet, and, having consented to participation, were interviewed individually, using video conferencing and the interview was audio recorded. Participants were informed that they had the right to withdraw at any point with no impact on their hospital treatment. Interviews lasted around 30 min. At the end, participants received a full debrief which involved discussing the project in more depth with participants, answering any outstanding questions that participants might have and providing a space to discuss and provide support around any issues or challenges that had arisen for them during the interviews. Interviews were conducted in Chinese, transcribed verbatim and then professionally translated into English. A sample back translation was conducted by an expert native speaker to ensure accuracy of meaning. The study received ethical approval from the University College London Research Ethics Committee (Ref 17.406) and was conducted in keeping with the principles of the Declaration of Helsinki and in agreement with the hospital where the participants were being treated.

Data analysis

An inductive approach [35] was used to permit the generation of themes from the data. Interpretative Phenomenological Analysis (IPA; [32, 36]), an ideographic approach used widely in health and clinical psychology research (e.g. [37]) and in similar studies exploring the experience of inpatient treatment for EDs [6] was employed. IPA was selected due to its focus on understanding in-depth psychological perspectives and lived experience in small samples [36]. IPA takes both phenomenology and social constructionism into consideration, sitting between the critical realist and social constructionist perspectives [38]. IPA assumes all individuals are self-interpretative and underlines how individuals reflect upon and make sense of their experiences [39] and is associated with the hermeneutic (i.e. to interpret) tradition [40], adopting a 'double hermeneutic,' such that researchers are required to interpret the participants' interpretations of their experience while being affected by their preoccupied experience and/or understanding [32]. An analytic process involving three steps [41] was followed. First, interviews were analyzed individually to permit immersion in the detail of the data. Meanwhile, all audio-recordings and transcripts were revised several times, and the intonation and expression were carefully noted down to increase precision and clarity. This was particularly important given that interviews were conducted in Chinese and then translated into English. Where direct translation was not possible, comments were provided to aid the understanding of the second author, a non-Chinese speaker. Second, emergent themes were identified and clustered as per Smith et al. [41] which involved abstraction (naming the clusters of inter-correlated emergent themes), subsumption (making specific emergent themes which can fully represent other related themes as super-ordinate themes), polarization (detecting oppositional ideals), contextualization (recognizing contextual/narrative components within analyses), numeration (counting how frequent a theme was supported), and function (examining themes' functions). Third, master themes, which represented shared superior patterns, were developed by bringing all identified themes from individual cases into collective consideration. This process was conducted independently by two coders (YW and AH) who met regularly to discuss and agree on the emerging and final thematic map.

Results

The final sample consisted of four female participants all diagnosed on admission by a Consultant Psychiatrist with the binge-purge subtype of AN according to the DSM 5 [2]. They were aged 16 to 19. For three participants (75%), this was their second admission and for one participant (25%), this was their first admission. Participants had been unwell for a mean of 3.7 years (SD = 2.2). Four master themes emerged from the data: participants' understanding of the nature of the treatment received, peer influences during the admission, the impact of treatment on wellbeing and participants' sense of self. The section below explores each master theme and its subordinate themes in turn, using quotations taken from the transcripts to explain the themes/subthemes further.

Master Theme 1: *Nature of the Treatment Received*

The first master theme reflected participants' ideas about the nature of the treatment received (Fig. 1).

Subordinate Theme 1: Discrepancies between the dominant focus of physical improvement at the expense of the psychological support desired by participants

The first subordinate theme reflects the discrepancy participants experienced between what they felt was the focus of the intervention they received and what they felt they needed. Participants all perceived that inpatient treatment mainly focused on modifying their eating behaviors and improving their physiological condition (i.e. nutrition improvement and weight gain) and that negligible attention was allocated to psychological improvement, which they felt was equally, if not more, important:

> *"I felt they could have tried to provide more psychological interventions... I did not think they provided that much psychological intervention...". (Bik)*

> *"I felt that the nutrition intervention was the dominant intervention, and psychological intervention was the sub-intervention". (Daiyu)*

> *"Psychological help they provided was too little. They could not help soothe you psychologically or reduce your anxiety...they normally just asked about whether you felt any physical discomfort these days...they would prescribe medications to you...and some issues like changing your meal plan. And something like bathing or other very tiny little things. Psychological help was extremely rare". (Ah Lam)*

Chun summarized her daily life as follows:

> *"Our daily life was mainly composed of eating and sitting...". (Chun)*

This combination of a lack of psychological care alongside weight restoration was experienced as problematic and traumatic by participants.

Subordinate Theme 2: Inadequate professional psychological support

The subordinate theme of there being inadequate psychological intervention from qualified professionals and little contact with the ED expert in the team further highlighted the contrast they experienced between what they reported to be an absence of psychological treatment alongside the treatment for the physiological complications of their illness:

> *"During the whole period of receiving inpatient care, I only saw her (the ED expert team member) twice or three times, maximum. Once you started to live inside, she might talk to you once. And after a while, let's say a month later, she would talk to you for the second time. And just before discharging you, she would talk to you again". (Ah Lam)*

> *"The chief doctor...actually I did not have that many chances to talk to her". (Bik)*

Participants reported being matched with junior doctors, who were directly responsible for them and met people more frequently. However, participants perceived

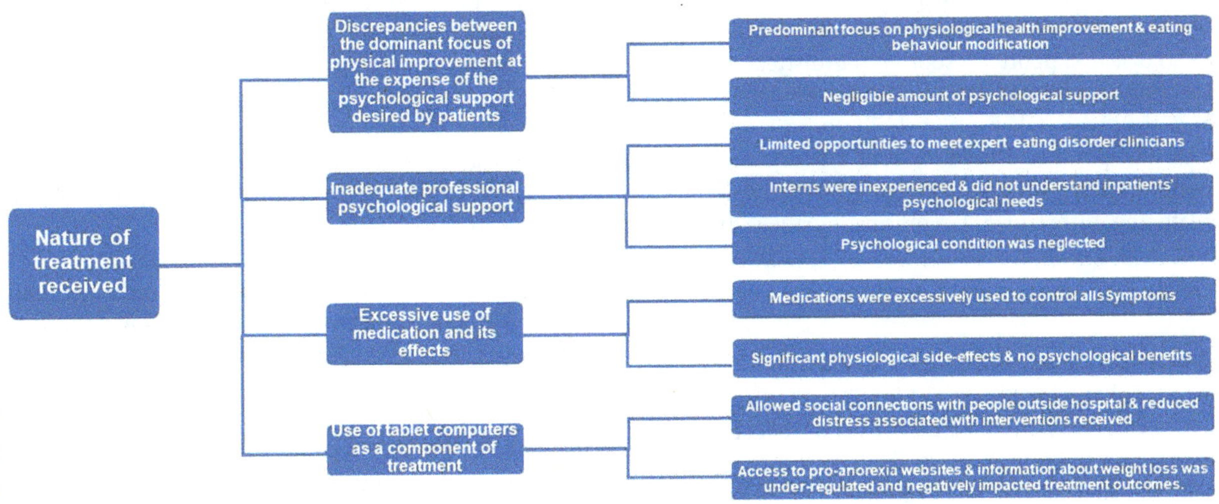

Fig. 1 The master theme the *"Nature of treament received"* is presented in the furthest left-hand box, and subordinate themes are presented in the middle boxes. Supplementary explanations are provided in the furthest right-hand boxes provide further explanation. The connecting lines indicate the hierarchical organisation of the themes

these doctors as inexperienced and felt they struggled to meet their psychological needs:

> *"The doctors were quite perfunctory...these doctors were mainly interns and some of them were really being silly—they always misunderstood what you were talking about...they might be not that experienced and probably answered your questions with something irrelevant". (Daiyu)*

Subordinate Theme 3: Excessive use of medication and its effects

A further subordinate theme reflected participants' experiences of their illness being primarily treated using medications. They expressed concerns regarding overuse of medication:

> *"If you cannot not sleep well, they give you sleeping pills...if you want to eat (binge), they would give you pills to suppress appetite. And if you want to exercise, they give you pills to sedate you. Everything in the ward is solved by taking medication". (Ah Lam)*

Participants reported negative physiological outcomes from medication (e.g. over-reliance on medication, tolerance and withdrawal) and perceived that this treatment offered little psychological benefits:

> *"They prescribed Lorazepam to control my anxiety... while I was taking it, it was not effective at all. But when I stopped taking it, I could not bear my condition..., my anxiety was extreme, I could not sit still and felt anxious all the time. And finally...I just re-took it and increased the dose". (Ah Lam)*

> *"My body became reliant on these medications... [when I stopped taking Olanzapine] I could not fall asleep and became very anxious". (Chun)*

Subordinate Theme 4: Use of tablet computers as a component of treatment

The final subordinate theme was the use of tablet computers on the ward which participants were encouraged to use as part of treatment. For some, being permitted to use tablet computers was viewed as a positive component of treatment, as it lessened boredom and facilitated connections with others which distracted participants from their distress:

> *"There were definitely more positive influences such as using the iPad which could help reduce anxiety and you could facetime your parents". (Ah Lam)*

However, participants also noted that unmonitored access to tablet computers seemed at odds with the overall treatment approach, as they had access to nutritional and weight-loss information:

> *"Others used their iPad to calculate the calories in their meals. I saw others going online to look at diets so that they could lose weight after discharge". (Chun)*

What seemed to be implicit in these narratives was that participants perceived their psychological distress not to matter in the treatment approach, as they saw it to focus mainly on nutritional restoration. They desired psychological support to 'soothe' the distress related to re-feeding and wanted a relationship with staff members where they were taken seriously by those treating them which may point to a need for staff training and support around working with this patient group who have life-threatening forms of ED requiring inpatient treatment which will evoke anxiety in the staff members trying to help.

Master Theme 2: Peer Influence

The second master theme reflected participants' experiences of peers during admission and reflected group dynamics on the ward (Fig. 2).

For all participants, the experience of being treated alongside peers with the same illness created a 'bubble' which they existed in during hospitalization:

> *"Being with other girls inside [the hospital] was like living in a micro-society". (Daiyu)*

Like many young people in English speaking countries, being on the ward was the participants' first time living apart from their families. The group dynamics that seemed to involved elements of cooperation and conflict, with participants reporting on both positive and negative aspects of social interactions with their peers. Both authors were curious about whether some of these dynamics might reflect what it might be like for young people who were likely to be only children (due to the one child policy in China) to live with others of a similar age/generation perhaps for the first time.

Subordinate Theme 1: Positive Peer Influences

Participants discussed how being amongst peers with a similar illness provided a platform to freely talk about EDs without worrying about being stigmatized:

> *"I had been keeping this secret (my ED) for an extremely long time without finding somebody to talk to. I think I have found someone to talk to here". (Daiyu)*

The presence of peers also prevented some ED behaviors, as concerned peers reported concerning behaviors to the nurses:

> *"And about vomiting... lots of people would definitely go to the nurses and report this issue. This stopped me from vomiting so much". (Ah Lam)*

Subordinate Theme 2: Negative Peer Influences

There were also a number of negative peer influences, including a shared focus on food and weight:

> *"We spent a significant amount of time together talking about weight gain and calorie intake and the like. I felt this did impact me more or less since. I felt my body had gained lots of weight and ...focusing on talking about weight, I felt psychologically uncomfortable and planned to lose weight". (Bik)*

Participants discussed making comparisons with each other and reported spending significant amounts of time comparing food intake and who gained weight faster (or slower). This seemed to intensify fears around nutritional intake and weight gain:

> *"I feel I was living in a space full of comparison, everything would be compared between us. They (peers) compared things like whose was larger or smaller, who ate more or less, who gained weight faster or slower". (Chun)*

Peers negatively impacted one another through discussions around ED behaviors and weight:

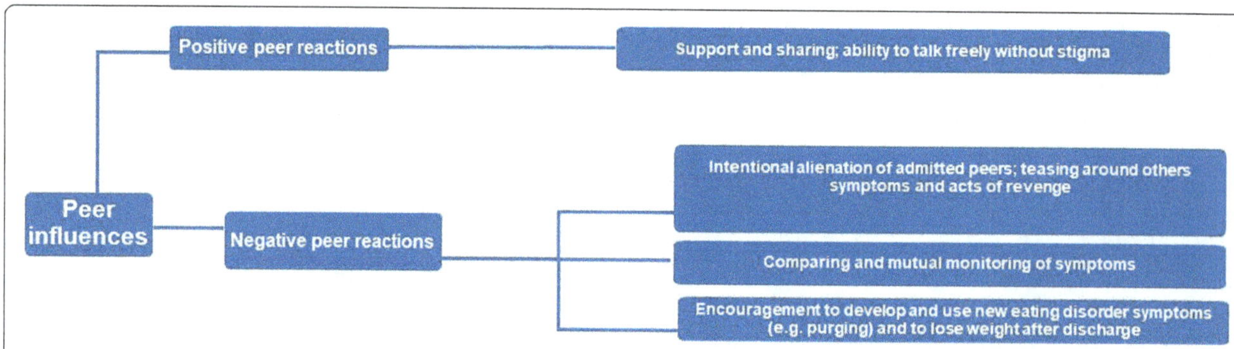

Fig. 2 The master theme *"Peer Influence"* is presented in the furthest left-hand box, and subordinate themes are presented in the middle boxes. Supplementary explanations are provided in the furthest right-hand boxes provide further explanations. The connecting lines indicate the hierarchical organisation of the themes

"Patients were discussing how to not gain weight and saying how anxious they were". (Ah Lam)

"I felt there were more negative influences since I cared so much about the weight and they (peers) talked too much about the issues surrounding weight". (Bik)

"I will be sometimes negatively influenced by them (those who don't want to recover)". (Daiyu)

Participants also discussed how to cope with weight gain in hospital by encouraging weight loss after discharge:

"Being told (be peers) to lose weight after getting discharged can reduce that person's anxiety a lot". (Ah Lam)

Participants reported learning new ED behaviors while in hospital and being encouraged to use them by other experienced people:

"Some people would tell the others how they binged outside and taught the others who did not know how to purge before where to suppress and to release the pressure". (Ah Lam)

"She taught me so many different ways to manually induce vomiting". (Chun)

Participants discussed bullying, teasing and alienation perpetrated by peers on the ward:

"Some of them would intentionally create alienation between patients".

"I realized that there was nobody who did not say bad things about the others (including care workers, nurses, patients and doctors)... And this made me feel living inside was extremely painful. I understood that I had negatively influenced the others (because of my physical symptoms), which had made me feel guilty already; they were still talking like that (telling each other I was disgusting), which made me even more stressed". (Ah Lam)

Sometimes these negative peer interactions resulted in acts of revenge from other experiencing people:

"She hid half of the steam bun in her clothes... we (myself and another patient) decided to report this to the nurses. ... just before she left (the hospital), she taunted me while the other patients were all there". (Chun)

These experiences seemed indicative of difficulties managing group dynamics and peer abuse on the ward which then allowed for new ED behaviors to be discussed and acquired, and for comparisons to be made amongst the group which may have maintained the ED or contributed to possible relapse on discharge.

Master Theme 3: *Impact of Treatment on Wellbeing*

The third master theme reflects an analysis of participant experiences related to the impacts of treatment on their wellbeing. This differs to the first master theme, in that rather than reporting participants' perceptions of the treatment they received, this theme relates to what participants believed were the benefits of inpatient treatment for their ED (Fig. 3).

Subordinate Theme 1: Physiological and behavioral improvements

The first subordinate theme related to the physiological and behavioral improvements participants reported, like improvements in physical wellbeing (weight restoration) and a reduction in disruptive behaviors (bingeing and purging). Some participants discussed how inpatient treatment had saved their life:

"It has already saved my life more than once or twice. Probably without receiving inpatient care I would have already died". (Ah Lam)

"I have gained lots of weight during the period of receiving inpatient care...". (Bik)

"Now I am eating normally and can stop bingeing and purging.... The only positive impact was on physical health, and the other impacts were all negative". (Ah Lam)

Subordinate Theme 2: Limited psychological or cognitive benefits

The second subordinate theme reflects a lack of improvement in psychological or cognitive functioning. Their experiences highlight that in spite of the physical improvement achieved through their hospitalization, they continued to experience heightened fear of gaining weight and other ED cognitions:

"I did not find that the staff helped me with my anxieties about my weight... I was not helped psychologically, it was all about the physical improvements". (Chun)

Subordinate Theme 3: Short-term impacts of treatment

The third subordinate theme reflects frustrations with the longevity of behavioral improvements. Participants reported that while positive health outcomes were

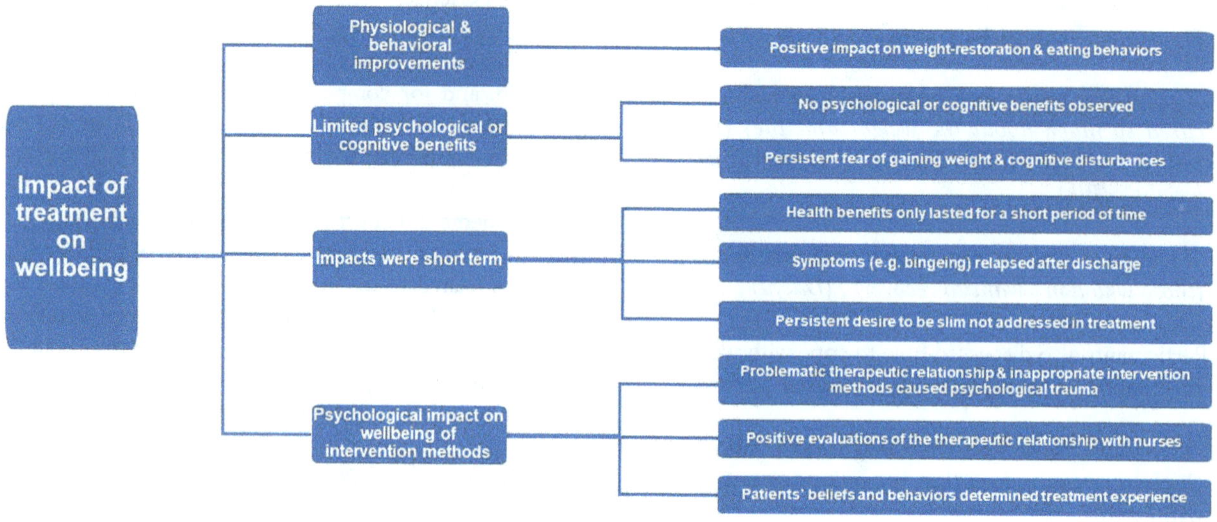

Fig. 3 The master theme– *The Impact of Treatment on Wellbeing*–is presented in the furthest left-hand box, and subordinate themes are presented in the middle boxes. Supplementary explanations are provided in the furthest right-hand boxes provide further explanations. The connecting lines indicate the hierarchical organisation of the themes

achieved, these were short-lived; meanwhile, more adverse long-term health outcomes were reported:

> *"I think it did help in terms of short-term outcomes...but I did not see any long-term effects. After I got discharged from the hospital, the bingeing got even worse". (Bik)*

> *"These influences (the positive outcomes) only lasted for a short period of time". (Daiyu)*

Participants said that behavioral improvements did not continue into the longer term. They felt that this was because their psychological wellbeing had been neglected:

> *"I think it [bingeing and purging becoming even worse after discharge] might be because I have gained lots of weight during the period of receiving inpatient care, but I could not psychologically accept it...thus...I started to fast badly, and after a while, my bingeing emerged and my urge to eat got even stronger". (Bik)*

Further, participants expressed ideas that longer-term change may not have been achieved because their overvaluation of slimness wasn't addressed in treatment:

> *"I still want to lose weight and keep slim. So I will not change my behaviors". (Daiyu)*

Subordinate Theme 4: Psychological impact of intervention methods on wellbeing

The fourth subordinate theme reflected negative experiences of inpatient treatment which had a psychological impact. Participants perceived their inpatient treatment experience as traumatic and perhaps shameful:

> *"The hospital is called mental health center, but it is just an asylum. So living inside can definitely induce psychological distress and discomfort". (Ah Lam)*

> *"The experience still brings me some psychological traumas. Sometimes, I dream about the events that happened during inpatient care. Anyway, they were nightmares". (Bik)*

One aspects of participants' negative experiences of treatment was a challenging therapeutic relationship between patients and nurses. For example, two participants reporting a damaging relationship with traumatic experiences and frightening memories:

> *"Whenever they (the nurses who were extremely fierce) would be on duty tomorrow I could not sleep well in the night before, because of fear". (Bik)*

> *"The way the nurses treated us was not respectful at all...the nurses yelled at us...they did not treat you with dignity". (Ah Lam)*

> *"The most unacceptable intervention method for me was to be tied-up. The patients...every time while I saw this (others being 'tied-up' – mechanical restraint), I felt so sad...those being tied up would scream and cry their lungs out". (Ah Lam)*

Other participants experienced the patient-nurse relationship as less traumatic and dangerous, and held contrary views, suggesting that this strong approach was needed. These participants explained that they dealt with the patient-nurse relationship through being extremely co-operative and obedient and reflected that this provoked positive interactions between themselves and the nurses:

"At least they (nurses and care-workers) did this (being harsh, forcing us to eat, 'protecting' us – (here the participants is referring to the use of mechanical restraint)) for our health, and they were just following the doctors' instructions...". (Chun)

"It was possibly because I was being really cooperative, the nurses treated me well". (Daiyu)

Master Theme 4: *Sense of self*

This master theme related to how inpatient treatment had influenced participants' sense of self (Fig. 4).

Subordinate theme 1: Self-perception

The first subordinate theme, self-perception, relates to participants' self-evaluation having undergone inpatient treatment. This appeared to be strongly dominated by their experiences of being 'psychiatric patients.' Some participants reported negative self-evaluations:

"I have been taking too many psychiatric drugs and this has made me think I am a psychopath". (Ah Lam)

However, other participants felt they needed medicine because they were ill and that this fact shouldn't impact their self-evaluation:

"I don't think taking medication means I am psychopathic.... I feel taking medication is normal while being ill". (Daiyu)

Nonetheless, all participants worried that this new experience which had contributed to their self-perception in some way might be perceived negatively by others:

"Whenever I hear somebody else mentioning words like 'mental institution' I become very sensitive... And I cannot stop worrying about whether others will know I had an experience of being hospitalized". (Ah Lam)

This comment suggests that Ah Lam's experience of their identity following the inpatient admission reflects more than an experience of being a 'psychiatric patient' and relates to the process of recruitment into the identity of a 'disordered person.' This highlights the power imbalance within the context of a setting like an inpatient unit.

"I am worrying about how teachers and peers will evaluate me". (Chun)

These statements may also reflect the sense of shame and stigma that many participants felt around their diagnosis and the treatment their symptoms had required.

Subordinate Theme 2: Confidence in 'normal' living and eating

The second subordinate theme reflects how inpatient treatment had led to experiencing people incorporating a sense of normal versus abnormal eating behavior into their sense of self. They discussed their renewed confidence to be able to eat like others in their communities with the help of their meal plan:

"I can generally understand the amount of food normal people consume every day". (Bik)

"I am determined to eat meals normally by following the guidance set up by the hospital...while I was unable to control my disordered eating before, I can use this as a way to find a new balance and be more like normal people around food". (Daiyu)

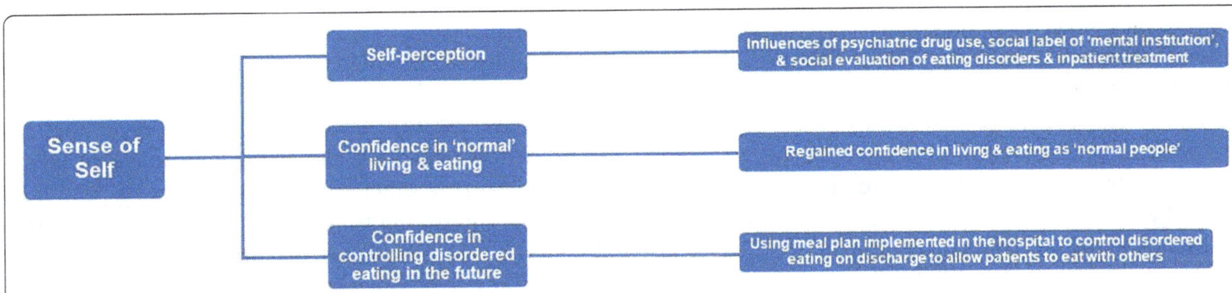

Fig. 4 The master theme– Participants' *Sense of Self*– is presented in the furthest left-hand box, and subordinate themes are presented in the middle boxes. Supplementary explanations are provided in the furthest right-hand boxes provide further explanations. The connecting lines indicate the hierarchical organisation of the themes

"Though ...I ate a lot and felt uncomfortable [during the admission], I was eating like a normal person. You would enjoy the food there [in hospital] and realized that you hadn't been eating normal meals for years". (Daiyu)

There was a sense that through treatment participants had become more able to 'eat normally' alongside others in their society:

"I can live like a normal person". (Chun)

Subordinate Theme 3: Confidence in controlling disordered eating in the future

Finally, participants discussed how they planned to use what they had learnt in the hospital to manage their symptoms in the community in future:

"I feel much more in charge of my eating behaviors and I think I can control my binges". (Chun)

"My meal plan gives me confidence that I can continue to get better outside of the hospital". (Bik)

Discussion

The aim of this study was to use Interpretive Phenomenological Analysis [32] to understand the experiences of four adolescents receiving inpatient treatment for EDs in mainland China. Four master themes emerged from the data: the first reflecting what participants perceived to be the nature of the treatment they received as inpatient; the second reflecting participants' ideas around the positive and negative impacts of peers during their inpatient admission; the third relating to the experienced impacts of treatment on wellbeing and the fourth relating to the impact of inpatient treatment on participants' sense of self.

The overall experience of these participants was mixed. They perceived inpatient treatment to offer and deliver welcome, positive, short-term improvements in their physical wellbeing, largely achieved through medication (infrequent) interactions with ED specialists and the presence of (some) supportive and understanding peers. For some, a strict, controlled ward environment was warranted as a means of saving lives. At the end of treatment, they felt like they could live and eat more 'normally' alongside others in their community. Conversely, participants felt that a combination of factors resulted in their psychological needs not being well met. These included the inexperience of the 'intern doctors' with whom they had more regular contact, 'strict, cold, punitive' nurses who often resorted to mechanical restraint, difficult interactions with (some) peers who encouraged competition and ED behaviors, over-reliance on medication and under-use of psychological therapies (which participants said they wanted). This seemed to reflect difficulties in understanding and managing difficult ED behaviors and the anxiety of the staff in working with this group of individuals. Because treatment benefits were largely limited to the restoration of physical health at any cost, credited with saving participants' lives, they felt they were vulnerable to relapse after discharge. A clear message from these experiencing people was the need for a more psychologically driven treatment as a means of supporting longer-term recovery. Finding balance between physical interventions and psychological treatments is a discussion held in treatment settings in other countries like the UK [17]. Participants' experiences of mechanical and chemical restraint may reflect the greater issue of the need for alternative ways of engaging the person in the process of change within an inpatient context. This highlights the need for improved training and support for staff in the uptake of interventions that support rather than potentially traumatize the experiencing person. Furthermore, this raises the question of fiscal support in the training and supervision of staff in the treatment of EDs, including in inpatient contexts. Adequate financial support for ED treatment is a challenge shared with many countries. It could be that these negative experiences could be improved through supporting staff with training so that they could have alternative, less-traumatic ways of supporting individuals.

Like Smith et al.'s [16], Coltan and Pistrang's [6] and Offord et al.'s [10] UK studies, the positive impact of sharing experiences with understanding peers was similarly important to the UK and Chinese participants. The theme reflecting the contribution of the inpatient experience to participants' sense of self in this study is corroborated by Smith et al.'s master theme reflecting the sense of self-discovery obtained through the inpatient experience. An interesting parallel between this study and Smith et al.'s [16] was that while both samples discussed the importance of supportive staff relationships; in this sample there were mixed experiences of what this actually looked like in practice, with some participants experiencing staff as cold, punitive and overly strict which they felt was unhelpful. Interpersonal relationships in treatment were also highlighted as being salient to participants in other UK studies such as Fox and Diab [7]. It was interesting to note the bullying and alienation reported by the Chinese participants. These strong negative narratives provoked an interesting discussion between the two authors (one from the UK and the other Chinese) about cultural differences regarding the expression of negative emotions and attitudes which were strongly evident in the experiencing people's narratives and perhaps reflects a directness less present in the UK than China. Interestingly a difference between Fox and Diab's [7] work and this study is that none of the Chinese participants discussed staff members' views on their recovery, whereas participants in the UK context reported being attuned to staff members' pessimism about the likelihood of recovery.

In common with another study from the UK [9], Chinese participants also reported a culture of restriction, which they described as excessive 'strictness' and perceived the inpatient unit as an alternate reality, similar to the 'bubble' described in Seed et al.'s [12] UK sample. Haynes et al.'s [8] sample and the Chinese participants both reported using relational strategies to cope with the 'bubble' of hospitalization, such as being overly compliant and cooperative, secretive behaviors around eating and competing with other experiencing people. This compliance seemed to be associated with a loss of voice and a parallel between the use of ED behaviors which may have been employed to gain a sense of control over oneself and the punitive measures like mechanical restraint, albeit intended to save lives, which seemed to also be an attempt to control the experiencing person.

For some of the Chinese participants, hospitalization offered a means of acquiring new ED behaviors and they used their peers' knowledge to develop new behaviors, for example, around purging. This unhealthy modelling is an experience reported in other inpatient settings [42, 43]. It could be suggested that difficulties in asserting boundaries between oneself and others' behaviors might be understood to some degree by discussions around identity and it was interesting to us (both authors) that the Chinese participants did not discuss the impact of treatment on their identity and its development. As authors, we reflected on how this identity during treatment is a common narrative in the UK context (AH, second author), whereas individual identity may be less evident in the Chinese context (YW, first author).

It was interesting to note that a positive outcome for the Chinese participants was feeling more able to eat with others and live a 'normal' life (in their own words) and this experience is similar to that of the Dutch adolescents in Van Ommen et al.'s [14] study. Like the Dutch participants who used individual action plans, the Chinese participants reported how helpful the meal plans were to enable them to achieve 'a normal life'. Like Kezelman et al. [16] the Chinese participants reported strong ambivalence around re-feeding and weight gain and expressed needing more support with the anxiety this caused. In common with Pemberton and Fox's [11] theme entitled 'looking for ideal care,' derived from their interviews with participants in the UK, the master theme reflecting perceptions of treatment received by the Chinese participants also suggests that this participant group may have had an ideal treatment plan in mind. While the master theme in this study reflecting the impact of treatment suggests that physical rehabilitation was achieved, and indeed some participants even felt that their lives had been saved, they were unhappy that their psychological needs had been under-addressed as for them, this was a vital part of ideal care. On the other hand, it was difficult to know whether participants had an idealized view of care, or the degree to which their expectations of ideal care were realistic. Nonetheless, it is important to hear participants' desire for a tailored treatment focused on both physical and psychological recovery. National Institute for Care Excellence (NICE) guidelines [17] recommend a range of evidence-based treatments for EDs such as CBT [44], Family Based Treatment [45] and the Maudsley Model of Anorexia Treatment for Adults [46] although none of the Chinese participants discussed having received interventions beyond re-feeding and medication. While this reflects an opportunity to share good practice with international colleagues, it should be noted that the evidence base for these treatments and the context for the NICE Guidelines comes largely from UK, USA, and Australian studies and more research is needed on their efficacy in, for example, China.

Taken together, despite some important differences like participants' reports regarding the use of mechanical restraint and sedation to manage ED behaviors and negligible psychological intervention, which these experiencing individuals experienced as traumatic, the experiences of the Chinese participants in treatment for EDs are rather similar to those of participants studied in other countries (largely the UK, USA, Australia and the Netherlands).

There are some limitations which need to be considered when interpreting these findings. The generalizability of the findings is limited by the inclusion of young females with the binge-purge subtype of AN and further work is needed to explore whether these participants' of inpatient care are shared by those with other forms of EDs. The study participants were adolescents and developmentally, are highly susceptible to peer influence [47] and social evaluation [48]. Therefore their perceptions relating to these facets might be over-reported or biased. Further work should explore the reliability of these themes across the lifespan. Although the sample size is small, it provides adequate narratives for the idiographic nature of IPA [36]. The translation of the interviews from Chinese into English may have resulted in issues with vocabulary selection. However, there were some benefits noted from conducting the interviews in Chinese. The shared native language of the interviewer and participants reduced participant burden and may have improved the recording of the initial meaning of participants' narratives. The interviews were conducted at one time-point in the participants' recovery and future work could explore how their perceptions of inpatient treatment change after a longer period of time. Indeed, further work is needed to explore in more depth the damaging aspects of treatment discussed by participants and how these might impact them in the longer term. As representatives from the medical team at the hospital were not interviewed, it is not possible to know whether participants' experiences of inpatient treatment corroborate the treatment plan offered. Further work could build on this limitation by interviewing staff and family members to as have Davidson et al., 2019 [49] and Bravender et al., 2017 [50]. This would increase the reliability of the findings and better understand the training needs and anxieties of the staff working with this complex illness. The semi-structured interview tended to confine the construction of participant narratives to questions related to their experiences. Therefore, opportunities to generate data that richly described their identity negotiations was limited in the data collection phases. Future qualitative research is needed to scaffold participant narratives between experience to questions of identity to further analyze some of the effects of inpatient treatments on a person's identity formation. As our research question was focused on the Chinese patients' experiences of treatment, the data analysis did not analyse transcript data for the implicit identity negotiations that might be happening in the reported extracts and this would be an important construct to explore in future work with this group. Nonetheless, this work which was the first study to explore the experience of inpatient treatment for an ED in China highlights the usefulness of investigating health issues cross-culturally, as a means of improving global wellbeing based on a deeper understanding of illnesses. It would also be of interest to explore how the experiences of shame and stigma present in some of these experiencing people's narratives might be understood in these individuals' cultural context and how this experience might be similar or different to other cultural contexts. Shame, for example, has been discussed by Norwegians experiencing an ED [51].

There are a number of implications arising from this study. The data highlight both similarities and differences between China and other contexts in the treatment of EDs in an inpatient context. Experienced caregivers from the ED field could work to share ideas with international teams around other strategies which can be used to challenge ED behaviors and work collaboratively with those needing/requiring/wanting care. This is particularly important given that data suggest EDs are on the rise in China [28] and collaboration and knowledge-sharing are important tools in fighting global illness. The participants in this study were able to speak with family members through tablet computers, and to further develop these links, the team could be supported to involve families in treatment through information sharing and skills training as this is a low-cost, task sharing approach that has been useful in helping people to remain in the community for longer [52]. Given that the idealization of the thin ideal is also important in China, and this this was salient in the participants' narratives, international collaborations to influence policy and practice around images on social media, pro-AN websites and ED prevention are warranted. Further exploration of experiences of recovering from an ED which are shared across cultures and/or specific to particular cultures and contexts are needed in the context of the globalized world.

Conclusions

This qualitative study which is the first study to explore the experiences of inpatient care for an ED in four adolescent females in mainland China found four key themes reflecting both positive and negative experiences of the nature of the treatment received and peer influences, short-term, physical and behavioral improvements and a desire for more psychological treatment, as well as changes to participants' sense of self, such as perceived stigma associated with medication and mental health service use and improved confidence in the ability to manage ED symptoms in future. Further research into ways of increasing experiencing people's satisfaction is warranted.

Reflective section

YW: I have previously fought EDs for several years and suffering such an unforgettable experience intensely motivated me to investigate EDs and to further explore more efficient treatments. Reviewing the research literature, I recognized the impact of inpatient treatment can be controversial. Meanwhile, since I had never received any inpatient treatment, I was extremely interested in understanding inpatient treatment for EDs, particularly regarding what it could actually bring to the participants. I was deeply touched by my participants; they had demonstrated their strong willingness to contribute to the field of study, in order to prevent more people from developing EDs or to evaluate the weaknesses and strengths of inpatient treatment. I was shocked and impressed by the findings. First, the negative effects brought by taking medication significantly outweighed the positive ones, which made me question the most appropriate ways of using medication. Second, the unintentional physical and emotional harm, along with the use of physical restraint, experienced by participants on the ward struck me as extremely inhumane and unethical; though they were people with EDs, they were fundamentally humans deserving of respect. Similar to findings from Western cultures, it seemed hard to reduce or eliminate psychological and cognitive symptoms. What was surprising was that the people receiving treatment on the ward were not always supportive, but teased each other and promoted health-damaging/pro anorexia behaviors. Through regular supervision meetings, I was able to explore my beliefs and be mindful of how they might impact the interpretation of participants' narratives. It was an extraordinarily valuable experience to conduct this research as a former patient with EDs and a future psychologist.

AH: having worked in the UK in the field of EDs for around 11 years, largely with people with severe and enduring forms of ED on inpatient units, and as a white woman born in the UK with Polish heritage and a clinician researcher, I was really interested to understand how people in another country very different from my own experience of inpatient treatment for EDs. It was interesting to explore the similarities and differences between the UK and Chinese contexts through participants' testimonies. I was mindful of my western ethnocentric context when conducting the study and analyzing the data, wanting to acknowledge it yet trying to see participants' experiences through their own eyes. It struck me that there were many similarities between my experiences of being on inpatient units in the UK and the participants in China: participants were ambivalent about change; they desired psychological change yet found it hard to tolerate the physical improvements their bodies needed in order for them to think and feel differently. There were also some differences which for me were distressing: participants reported being mechanically restrained and sedated which made me feel uncomfortable and sad, and through discussions with clinical colleagues I became more mindful of how this was an approach to treatment we have taken in Europe in the past. It was interesting and surprising to hear participants reporting being teased by discharged patients about eating, something I haven't encountered in the UK. It was a really important learning experience to work with Yi to understand how EDs are understood and treated in her country and this made me reflect more on the diverse patient groups we work with in the UK and how it is vital to be mindful of the ways in which different communities might understand mental illness and treatment.

Appendix

Semi-Structured Interview Guide

1. From your point of view, in what ways has inpatient treatment contributed to your recovery? What was it like being on the ward? What were some of the best and worst things about being in hospital? Was there anything that was particularly helpful or problematic for you?

2. Could you please describe your perception/understanding of the intervention you have received during the period of inpatient care? How has the inpatient admission helped? Please think about this in terms of the bigger picture - your psychological and physiological wellbeing, as well as your quality of life. Could you please provide some examples? The examples could be in general or more specific.

3. How do you perceive the presence of peers who were being hospitalized with you and interacting with you during the period of receiving inpatient care? Any specific examples?

4. Could you discuss the staff you interacted with on the ward during your admission? How did you perceive and experience the support they provided? Can you give any examples to support this?

If you received any medication or other psychological treatment during your admission, how did you experience this? In what ways.

Abbreviations

AN: Anorexia nervosa; BN: Bulimia nervosa; CBT: Cognitive Behavioral Therapy; EDs: Eating disorders; UK: United Kingdom

Acknowledgements

Thank you to all participants who supported this research study.

Authors' contributions

All authors contributed to the conception and design of the work; YW acquired the data; YW and AH analysed and interpreted the data; AH drafted the work and worked with YW to provide critical revisions and produce the final manuscript. All authors approve the final version of this manuscript.

Authors' information

YW completed her MSc Psychology degree at University College London and is currently undertaking a PhD at Maastricht University in the Netherlands. AH is and a Lecturer in Psychology and Clinical Psychologist at University College London and a member of the Academy for Eating Disorders.

Competing interests

The authors declare that they have no competing interests.

References

1. Schmidt U, Adan R, Böhm I, Campbell IC, Dingemans A, Ehrlich S, Elzakkers I, Favaro A, Giel K, Harrison A, Himmerich H. Eating disorders: the big issue. Lancet Psychiat. 2016;3(4):313–5.
2. American Psychiatric Association. Diagnostic and statistical manual of mental disorders (DSM-5). Washington, DC: American Psychiatric Publishing; 2013.
3. Stice E, Becker CB, Yokum S. Eating disorder prevention: current evidence-base and future directions. Int J Eat Disord. 2013;46(5):478–85.
4. O'herlihy A, Worrall A, Lelliott P, Jaffa T, Hill P, Banerjee S. Distribution and characteristics of in-patient child and adolescent mental health services in England and Wales. Brit J Psychiat. 2003;183(6):547–51.
5. Arcelus J, Mitchell AJ, Wales J, Nielsen S. Mortality rates in patients with anorexia nervosa and other eating disorders: a meta-analysis of 36 studies. Arch General Psychiat. 2011;68(7):724–31.
6. Colton A, Pistrang N. Adolescents' experiences of inpatient treatment for anorexia nervosa. Eur Eat Disord Rev. 2004;12(5):307–16.
7. Fox JR, Diab P. An exploration of the perceptions and experiences of living with chronic anorexia nervosa while an inpatient on an eating disorders unit: an interpretative phenomenological analysis (IPA) study. J Health Psychol. 2015;20(1):27–36.
8. Haynes C, Eivors A, Crossley J. 'Living in an alternative reality': adolescents' experiences of psychiatric inpatient care. Child Adol Mental H-UK. 2011;16(3):150–7.
9. Long S, Wallis D, Leung N, Meyer C. "All eyes are on you": anorexia nervosa patient perspectives of in-patient mealtimes. J Health Psychol. 2012;17(3):419–28.
10. Offord A, Turner H, Cooper M. Adolescent inpatient treatment for anorexia nervosa: a qualitative study exploring young adults' retrospective views of treatment and discharge. Eur Eat Disord Rev. 2006;14(6):377–87.
11. Pemberton K, Fox JR. The experience and management of emotions on an inpatient setting for people with anorexia nervosa: a qualitative study. Clin Psychol Psychot. 2013;20(3):226–38.
12. Seed T, Fox J, Berry K. Experiences of detention under the mental health act for adults with anorexia nervosa. Clin Psychol Psychot. 2016;23(4):352–62.
13. Smith V, Chouliara Z, Morris PG, Collin P, Power K, Yellowlees A, Grierson D, Papageorgiou E, Cook M. The experience of specialist inpatient treatment for anorexia nervosa: a qualitative study from adult patients' perspectives. J Health Psychol. 2016;21(1):16–27.
14. Van Ommen J, Meerwijk EL, Kars M, Van Elburg A, Van Meijel B. Effective nursing care of adolescents diagnosed with anorexia nervosa: the patients' perspective. J Clin Nurs. 2009;18(20):2801–8.
15. Duesund L, Skårderud F. Use the body and forget the body: treating anorexia nervosa with adapted physical activity. Clin Child Psychol Psychiat. 2003;8(1):53–72.
16. Kezelman S, Rhodes P, Hunt C, Anderson G, Clarke S, Crosby RD, Touyz S. Adolescent patients' perspectives on rapid-refeeding: a prospective qualitative study of an inpatient population. Adv Eat Disord. 2016;4(3):277–92.
17. National Institute for Health and Care Excellence. Eating disorders: recognition and treatment, NG69. London: National Institute for Health and Care Excellence; 2017.
18. Department of Health. Mental health act. London: HMSO; 2007.
19. Prince R. The concept of culture-bound syndromes: anorexia nervosa and brain-fag. Soc Sci Med. 1985;21(2):197–203.
20. Chang YJ, Lin W, Wong Y. Survey on eating disorder–related thoughts, behaviors, and their relationship with food intake and nutritional status in female high school students in Taiwan. J Am Coll of Nutr. 2011;30(1):39–48.
21. Jackson T, Chen H. Risk factors for disordered eating during early and middle adolescence: a two year longitudinal study of mainland Chinese boys and girls. J Abnorm Child Psychol. 2014;42(5):791–802.
22. Lee S, Lee AM. Disordered eating in three communities of China: a comparative study of female high school students in Hong Kong, Shenzhen, and rural Hunan. Int J Eat Disord. 2000;27(3):317–27.
23. Liang XM, Guo LT, Liu KZ. A cross-sectional investigation on eating disorders in 1486 female students from universities, senior high schools and junior high schools in Chengdu. Zhonghua Liu Xing Bing Xue Za Zhi. 2008;29(4):321–4.
24. Liao Y, Liu T, Cheng Y, Wang J, Deng Y, Hao W, Chen X, Xu Y, Wang X, Tang J. Changes in eating attitudes, eating disorders and body weight in Chinese medical university students. Int J Soc Psychiatr. 2013;59(6):578–85.
25. Lu X, Zhang N. A survey of eating behaviors among 703 female university and middle school students in Nanjing. Chinese School H. 2008;29:637–8.
26. Tam CK, Ng CF, Yu CM, Young BW. Disordered eating attitudes and behaviours among adolescents in Hong Kong: prevalence and correlates. J Paediatr Child H. 2007;43(12):811–7.
27. Tsai MR, Chang YJ, Lien PJ, Wong YC. Survey on eating disorders related thoughts, behaviors and dietary intake in female junior high school students in Taiwan. Asia Pacific J Clin Nutr. 2011;20(2):196–205.
28. Tong J, Miao S, Wang J, Yang F, Lai H, Zhang C, Zhang Y, Hsu LG. A two-stage epidemiologic study on prevalence of eating disorders in female university students in Wuhan, China. Soc Psych Psych Epid. 2014;49(3):499–505.
29. Fu D. Eating disorder of female university students in Beijing and its relation with personality. Chinese J Clin Psychol. 2008;16(1):31.
30. Fan Y, Li Y, Liu A, Hu X, Ma G, Xu G. Associations between body mass index, weight control concerns and behaviors, and eating disorder symptoms among non-clinical Chinese adolescents. BMC Public Health. 2010;10(1):314.
31. Witcomb GL, Arcelus J, Chen J. Can cognitive dissonance methods developed in the west for combatting the 'thin ideal'help slow the rapidly increasing prevalence of eating disorders in non-Western cultures. Shanghai Arch Psychiat. 2013;25(6):332.
32. Smith JA, Flowers P, Osborn M. Interpretative phenomenological analysis and the psychology of health and illness. Mater Discourses H illness. 1997;11:68–91.
33. Holloway I, Galvin K. Qualitative research in nursing and healthcare. London: Wiley; 2016.
34. Edwards R, Holland J. What is qualitative interviewing? London: Bloomsbury; 2013.
35. Creswell JW, Hanson WE, Clark Plano VL, Morales A. Qualitative research designs: selection and implementation. Couns Psychol. 2007;35(2):236–64.
36. Smith JA, Flowers P, Larkin M. Interpretative phenomenological analysis: theory method and research. London: Sage; 2009.
37. Pearce A, Clare L, Pistrang N. Managing sense of self: coping in the early stages of Alzheimer's disease. Dementia. 2002;1(2):173–92.
38. Cosgrove L. Crying out loud: understanding women's emotional distress as both lived experience and social construction. Fem Psychol. 2000;10(2):247–67.
39. Chapman E, Smith JA. Interpretative phenomenological analysis and the new genetics. J H Psychol. 2002;7(2):125–30.
40. Palmer RE. Hermeneutics. Michigan: Northwestern University Press; 1969.
41. Spencer L, Ritchie J, Lewis J, Dillon L. Quality in qualitative evaluation: a framework for assessing research evidence. London: Government chief social Researcher's office; 2003.
42. Espíndola CR, Blay SL. Anorexia nervosa's meaning to patients: a qualitative synthesis. Psychopathology. 2009;42(2):69–80.
43. Vandereycken W. Can eating disorders become 'contagious' in group therapy and specialized inpatient care? Eur Eat Disord Rev. 2011;19(4):289–95.
44. Fairburn CG, Cooper Z, Shafran R, Wilson GT. Eating disorders: A transdiagnostic protocol In: Barlow DH, editor. Clinical handbook of psychological disorders: a step-by-step treatment manual. New York: Guilford Press; 2008. p. 578–614.
45. Lock J, Le Grange D. Treatment manual for anorexia nervosa: a family-based approach. New York: Guilford Publications; 2015.
46. Schmidt U, Magill N, Renwick B, Keyes A, Kenyon M, Dejong H, Lose A, Broadbent H, Loomes R, Yasin H, Watson C. The Maudsley outpatient study of treatments for anorexia nervosa and related conditions (MOSAIC): comparison of the Maudsley model of anorexia nervosa treatment for adults (MANTRA) with specialist supportive clinical management (SSCM) in outpatients with broadly defined anorexia nervosa: a randomized controlled trial. J Consult Clin Psychol. 2015;83(4):796.
47. Brechwald WA, Prinstein MJ. Beyond homophily: a decade of advances in understanding peer influence processes. J Res Adol. 2011;21(1):166–79.
48. Schriber RA, Guyer AE. Adolescent neurobiological susceptibility to social context. Dev Cog Neuro. 2016;19:1–8.
49. Davidson AR, Braham S, Dasey L, Reidlinger DP. Physicians' perspectives on the treatment of patients with eating disorders in the acute setting. J Eat Disord. 2019;7(1):1.

50. Bravender T, Elkus H, Lange H. Inpatient medical stabilization for adolescents with eating disorders: patient and parent perspectives. Eating Weight Disorders-Studies Anorexia, Bulimia Obes. 2017;22(3):483–9.
51. Skårderud F. Shame and pride in anorexia nervosa: A qualitative descriptive study. Eur Eat Disord Rev. 2007;15(2):81–97.
52. Hibbs R, Magill N, Goddard E, Rhind C, Raenker S, Macdonald P, Todd G, Arcelus J, Morgan J, Beecham J, Schmidt U. Clinical effectiveness of a skills training intervention for caregivers in improving patient and caregiver health following in-patient treatment for severe anorexia nervosa: pragmatic randomised controlled trial. BJPsych Open. 2015;1(1):56–66.

4

Attributes of children and adolescents with avoidant/restrictive food intake disorder

Helene Keery[1], Sarah LeMay-Russell[1], Timothy L. Barnes[1,2], Sarah Eckhardt[1], Carol B. Peterson[3,4], Julie Lesser[1], Sasha Gorrell[5] and Daniel Le Grange[5,6*]

Abstract

Background: Avoidant/Restrictive Food Intake Disorder (ARFID) is a comparatively new DSM-5 diagnosis. In an effort to better understand this heterogeneous patient group, this study aimed to describe the physical and psychological attributes of children and adolescents with ARFID, and to compare them to patients with full-threshold or atypical anorexia nervosa (AN).

Methods: Children and adolescents aged 7-to-19 years ($N = 193$) were examined upon presenting at a pediatric eating disorder center between July 2015 and December 2017. Data included diagnosis assessed via the semi-structured Eating Disorder Examination interview along with measures of anthropometrics, depression, anxiety, self-esteem, perfectionism and clinical impairment.

Results: Compared to AN and atypical AN ($n = 87$), patients with ARFID ($n = 106$) were significantly younger (12.4 vs. 15.1 years, $p < .0001$), male (41% vs. 15%, $p < .0002$), and were more likely to be diagnosed with at least one co-morbid DSM-5 diagnosis (75% vs. 61%, $p = .04$). Patients with ARFID were less likely to be bradycardic (4.7% vs. 24.1%, $p < .0001$), amenorrheic (11.1 and 34.7%, $p = .001$), admitted to the hospital (14.2% vs. 27.6%, $p = .02$), and have a diagnosis of depression (18.9% vs. 48.3%, $p < .0001$). Patients with ARFID were significantly less likely to experience acute weight loss vs. chronic weight loss as compared with those with AN or atypical AN ($p = .0001$). On self-report measures, patients with ARFID reported significantly fewer symptoms of depression, anxiety, perfectionism, clinical impairment, concerns about weight and shape, and higher self-esteem than patients with AN or atypical AN (all $ps < .0001$). No differences were observed by race, anxiety disorder, orthostatic instability, suicidal ideation, and history of eating disorder treatment.

Conclusions: Study results highlight the clinical significance of ARFID as a distinct DSM-5 diagnosis and the physical and psychological differences between ARFID and AN/atypical AN. The novel finding that ARFID patients are more likely than those diagnosed with AN to experience chronic, rather than acute, weight loss suggests important related treatment considerations.

Keywords: Avoidant/restrictive food intake disorder, Anorexia nervosa, Atypical anorexia nervosa, Pediatric eating disorder

* Correspondence: Daniel.LeGrange@ucsf.edu
[5]Department of Psychiatry, University of California, San Francisco, CA, USA
[6]Department of Psychiatry and Behavioral Neuroscience, The University of Chicago, Chicago, IL, USA
Full list of author information is available at the end of the article

Plain English summary

This study describes physical and psychological attributes of children and adolescents with DSM-5 Avoidant/Restrictive Food Intake Disorder (ARFID) and compares them to patients with full-threshold or atypical anorexia nervosa (AN). Estimates of the percentage of patients with ARFID range from 5 to 41%. Comparisons to patients with AN have yielded inconsistent findings, but generally indicate that patients with ARFID are more likely to be younger, male, and have longer duration of illness. This is the largest study ($n = 106$) describing patients diagnosed with ARFID using formal DSM-5 criteria. By comparing patients with ARFID to those with AN/atypical AN, this study supports the separation of the diagnosis from other eating and feeding disorders. Findings also underscore the critical necessity of better understanding this unique patient population, which will ultimately improve early detection, and treatment efforts.

Introduction

Avoidant/Restrictive Food Intake Disorder (ARFID) is a comparatively new eating disorder diagnosis in the Diagnostic and Statistical Manual of Mental Disorder, Fifth Edition (DSM-5) [1]. Historically, while patients with Food Avoidance Emotional Disorders were distinguishable from patients with anorexia nervosa (AN) thirty years ago [2], still relatively little is known about this heterogeneous group of patients and the extent to which ARFID may be similar or different from other types of restricting eating disorders [3]. ARFID was included in the DSM-5 to better capture the range of developmental feeding and eating problems as well as to more accurately diagnose patients who previously were diagnosed with an Eating Disorder Not Otherwise Specified or Feeding Disorder of Infancy or Early Childhood in earlier versions of the DSM [4, 5]. While patients with ARFID often present as underweight due to either long-term malnutrition or restriction of intake that causes a significant amount of weight loss, they do not experience the body image disturbance that is characteristic of patients with AN or atypical AN. Accumulating clinical data also suggest that ARFID may have distinct "subtypes." However, these subtypes have not been formalized, and different studies have proposed varying categorizations, including selective eating, generalized anxiety, medical, food allergies, Autism Spectrum/Developmental Disorder, and food avoidant emotional disorder [1, 6–8], and more recently, the three categories of limited intake, limited variety, and aversive [9].

Recent research has provided information about the prevalence of ARFID as well as how children and adolescents with this diagnosis are similar to or different from those with AN. One study estimated the prevalence of ARFID in school children aged 8–13 years at 3.2% [10]. In outpatient adolescent medicine eating disorder clinics, estimates of patients diagnosed with ARFID range from 5 to 41% [3, 11–13]. Another study found that the prevalence of ARFID was 39% in an adolescent eating disorder day treatment program [14], and even higher (43%) in a sample of patients aged 6–12 years presenting with significant weight loss to an eating disorder clinic [15]. Comparisons to patients with AN generally indicate that ARFID patients are more likely to be younger, male, and have a longer duration of illness [3, 13, 15]. ARFID patients also have been found to be equally or more likely to have an anxiety disorder diagnosis and less likely to have a diagnosis of depression than those with AN [3, 14]. Finally, patients who fit criteria for ARFID tend to be underweight, although not to the same degree as patients with AN [3, 11, 14, 15].

Most of the previous studies comparing ARFID and AN/atypical AN have been retrospective chart reviews and used the proposed DSM-5 criteria for ARFID [3, 11–14]. A retrospective chart review published in 2018 used the formal DSM-5 criteria to identify 31 patients (8.4%) with an ARFID diagnosis but did not compare these patients with another group (i.e., AN) [16]. A recent overview of patients with ARFID in tertiary care was restricted by the younger age of its sample (i.e., under age 13) [17]. A description of patient characteristics based prospectively on the current criteria is warranted as this diagnosis gains more attention. Efforts to enhance our understanding of a still largely unknown diagnostic syndrome are of critical importance in improving early detection of ARFID, as well as in informing the development of tailored treatment interventions for this unique disorder. The aim of the present study was to compare ARFID with other restrictive eating disorders (AN and atypical AN) among patients presenting at a specialist community-based eating disorder service. This objective placed ARFID in context with broader eating disorder diagnoses, used both physical and psychological measures, and assessed patients at the time of presentation using DSM-5 criteria.

Methods

This study examines baseline data from a longitudinal study designed to evaluate the effectiveness of evidence-based outpatient treatments for eating disorders. This study was approved by the Children's Minnesota Institutional Review Board.

Setting and participants

The Center for the Treatment of Eating Disorders (CTED) is a service within Children's Minnesota that offers a multi-disciplinary approach to provide specialized care for eating disorders. The outpatient clinic treats patients aged 7 years and older, while the inpatient service treats those aged 7–21 years. Over 250 patients present for evaluation at CTED annually. Owing to a known special interest in treating ARFID, CTED receives increased referrals for this specific patient population from local medical providers (e.g., gastrointestinal specialists).

To be eligible for participation in the study, a patient had to: 1) be 7–19 years old; 2) present for an intake evaluation of eating disorder symptoms; 3) be diagnosed with a DSM-5 feeding or eating disorder; and 4) agree to participate in outpatient treatment. Study data were collected between July 2015 and December 2017. All eligible patients presenting for treatment were approached for participation in the study, and after obtaining informed consent (assent for patients < 18 years), research staff collected data from patients via interviews, pen-and-paper assessments, and electronic health records.

Assessment and measures

Enrolled patients were evaluated by a psychiatrist, psychologist or clinical social worker, and trained assessors who administered measures at the time of the family's first encounter with our service (inpatient or outpatient). Patients were admitted to the inpatient unit if they were determined to be medically unstable by the attending psychiatrist according to recommended guidelines of the American Academy of Pediatrics and the Society of Adolescent Medicine [18].

Patients completed age-appropriate self-report measures, and parents were given standardized assessments to complete about their child. The *intake questionnaire* included questions about eating disorder treatment history, current psychotropic medications, and medical history together with other medical conditions, including gastrointestinal and endocrine disorders. To determine eating disorder diagnosis, patients ages 12 years and older completed the EDE [19], which was also used to assess eating disorder symptom frequency severity as well as concerns about eating, weight, and shape. Patients younger than 12 years old were given a diagnosis agreed upon by the clinicians involved in the assessment after their diagnostic evaluations. Psychiatric assessment included *MINI-Kid* [20] to evaluate self-harm and suicidal ideation, the *Child Depression Inventory 2nd Edition* (CDI-2 [21]) to assess depressive symptoms, and the *Rosenberg Self-Esteem Scale* (RSE [22]) to assess self-esteem. The *Beck Anxiety Inventory* (BAI) [23] was used to assess anxiety, the *Clinical Impairment Assessment* [24] (CIA) to assess the psychosocial impact of the eating disorder, and the *Clinical Perfectionism Questionnaire* (CPQ [25]) to assess perfectionism outside of eating, weight or appearance. Parent reports of their child's anxiety and depression were assessed using the internalizing scale of the *Child Behavior Check List* (CBCL) [26].

DSM-5 eating disorder and comorbid diagnoses were agreed upon by providers based on results from the EDE, semi-structured diagnostic assessment, MINI-Kid, and patient/parent report of symptoms. When patient and parent report differed, objective medical data regarding growth, weight loss, and medical stability were used to inform the diagnostic decision.

Medical assessment, including orthostatic vitals (supine and standing pulse rate and blood pressure), and weight were measured by a medical assistant or nurse. Bradycardia was defined as supine pulse rate of < 50 beats per minute, hypotension as < 90 mmHG, and orthostatic instability as difference in supine and standing heart rate of > 20 beats per minute or difference of > 10 mm HG in supine and standing blood pressure [17]. Amenorrhea was defined as the absence of menarche in girls age 15 years or older (primary) or the lack of menses for the past 3 months (secondary) [27].

AN cases were identified using a weight threshold of < 89% of expected body weight (%mBMI = BMI/50th percentile BMI for age and gender × 100) [28]. Patients who met all DSM-5 diagnostic criteria for AN and had a weight of $\geq$ 90%mBMI were identified as atypical AN [29]. There was no upper level cut-off in BMI for an atypical AN diagnosis.

Statistical analyses

All demographic, medical, and psychological measures were calculated as means and standard deviations for continuous variables and proportions for categorical variables. Initial analyses for demographic and weight presentation consisted of comparing measures across all three diagnoses. Analysis of variance (ANOVA) was applied for continuous variables (e.g., age, weight, and BMI) and $\chi 2$ or Fisher's exact test was used, when appropriate, for categorical variables. Post hoc pairwise comparisons between individual eating disorder groups were also utilized to denote significance. As demonstrated by previous analyses by Sawyer and colleagues [30], data suggested that patients with AN and atypical AN differ by weight at presentation but do not differ significantly on other variables of interest. Further, although patients with AN and atypical AN differed significantly on weight presentation in our cohort, their scores on other medical and psychological measures did not differ significantly. As a result, and due to concerns about small sample sizes in stratified analyses, all further analyses compared the ARFID group to the AN and atypical AN patients combined (AN/atypical AN group; $n = 87$). Patients with ARFID were compared with those with AN and atypical AN by using independent t-tests for continuous variables (mean difference) and $\chi 2$ or

Fisher's exact tests for categorical variables (odds ratios). Between-group differences were assessed with a significance threshold of $p < .05$. All statistical analyses were performed in SAS 9.4 (Cary, NC).

Results

Of the 404 patients who presented for evaluation at CTED during the study period, 338 (84%) met initial eligibility. After evaluation, 266 (66%) were verified as eligible, of which 243 patients were diagnosed with a DSM-5 eating disorder and enrolled in the present study. Of the 243 enrolled patients, 54 patients were diagnosed with AN, 36 with atypical AN, and 111 patients with ARFID (Table 1). Of those enrolled, certain exclusion criteria precluded their inclusion in analyses. Specifically, after accounting for individuals with binge/purge eating disorders who were not underweight (n = 17), individuals diagnosed with unspecified feeding and eating disorders (n = 24), and patients with missing data (n = 8), the final data set for analyses consisted of 193 patients. Within the 193 cases included in analyses, 52 (26.9%) met criteria for AN, 35 (18.1%) met criteria for atypical AN, and 106 (54.9%) met criteria for ARFID. Demographic characteristics are presented in Table 2. The mean age for patients with ARFID was 12.4 years compared to 15.1 years for AN and 15.2 years for atypical AN groups, respectively ($p < .0001$). Over 40% of patients with ARFID were male, compared to 15 and 11% of patients with AN/atypical AN (p = .0002). Most patients (≥ 80%) were White/Caucasian, with no significant differences across racial groups except for Hispanic ethnicity. When examining weight, patients with ARFID presented with a lower weight (37.6 kg, SD = 12.0 kg) on average compared to the AN/atypical AN group (44.4 kg, SD = 8.5 kg, and 56.7 kg, SD = 7.5 kg, respectively). In addition, the ARFID group presented with a significantly lower BMI, BMI z-score, and %mBMI compared to the AN/atypical AN group. While lower weight might be expected given the lower average age of those diagnosed with ARFID, these patients were the least likely to experience acute weight loss (vs. chronic weight loss) (14.9%), as compared with AN (40.0%) and atypical AN (50.0%) (p = .0001).

When comparing patients with ARFID to the AN/atypical AN group, significant differences between vital signs and medical instability were observed (Table 3). Pulse rate (78.8 vs. 63.4, $p < .0001$) and systolic blood pressure (113.1 vs. 109.7, p = .02) were all significantly higher for the ARFID than for the AN/atypical AN group. The ARFID group was significantly less likely to be bradycardic (OR = 0.16, $p < .0001$), amenorrheic (OR = 0.24, p = .001), and admitted to the hospital (OR = 0.43, $p < .02$) compared to the AN/atypical AN group. ARFID and AN/atypical AN groups did not differ on measures of hypotension, orthostatic instability, or history of prior eating disorder treatment (all $ps > .05$).

Using χ2 analyses, patients with ARFID were less likely than the AN/atypical AN group to be diagnosed with depression (OR = 0.25, $p < .0001$), but more likely to have an existing psychiatric comorbidity (OR = 1.88, p = .04) (Table 4). Furthermore, nearly 24% of patients with ARFID had a diagnosis of attention-deficit/hyperactivity disorder (ADHD) compared to only 1.15% in the AN/atypical AN group ($p < .0001$). Compared to the AN/atypical AN group, patients with ARFID scored significantly lower on the Global EDE (0.34 vs. 2.56, $p < .0001$) and corresponding subscales. In addition, patients with ARFID scored significantly lower on the self -report CDI-2 (53.2 vs. 62.0, $p < .0001$), the CPQ (19.4 vs. 25.8, $p < .0001$), the CIA (10.2 vs. 22.4, $p < .0001$), and BAI Total Score (10.2 vs. 16.1, p = .002). Patients with ARFID also scored significantly higher on the Rosenberg Self-Esteem (21.9 vs. 15.2, $p < .0001$) compared to the AN/atypical AN group. There were no statistical significant differences on the parental report of CBCL Internalizing T-Score (61.8 vs. 63.6, p = .34) or self-report on self-harm/suicidal ideation (9.4 vs. 13.6, p = .47).

Table 1 Distribution of total eating disorder diagnoses at CTED, July 2015 – December 2017 (n = 243)

Diagnosis	n	%
Anorexia Nervosa (AN)	54	22.2
Bulimia Nervosa (BN)	9	3.7
Binge Eating Disorder (BED)	2	0.8
Avoidant/Restrictive Food Intake (ARFID)	111	45.7
Other specified feeding or eating disorder		
Atypical AN	36	14.8
AN: limited body image/ behaviors	–	–
BN: low frequency duration	1	0.4
BED: low frequency duration	1	0.4
Purging Disorder	4	1.6
Unspecified Feeding or Eating Disorder	24	9.9

Discussion

The aim of this study was to provide a comprehensive comparison of the unique physical and psychological presentation of patients diagnosed with ARFID according to DSM-5 guidelines when compared to patients with AN and atypical AN. First, this study found that while smaller stature may be expected given the younger age of this subgroup, ARFID patients were significantly lower in weight than both AN/atypical AN patients. Additionally, patients with ARFID were equally orthostatic as the AN/atypical AN group, but were less likely to be amenorrheic, admitted to the hospital, or on psychiatric medication. While patients with AN were more

Table 2 Demographic and weight presentation of study participants with AN, Atypical AN, and ARFID ($n = 193$)

	AN $n = 52$ M (SD) or n (%)	Atypical AN $n = 35$ M (SD) or n (%)	ARFID $n = 106$ M (SD) or n (%)	p [a]
Age	15.06 (1.96)*	15.23 (1.88)*	12.39 (2.65)**	<.0001
Gender				
Male	8 (15.38)*	4 (11.43)*	43 (40.57)**	.0002
Female	44 (84.62)	31 (88.57)	63 (59.43)	
Race/Ethnicity				
White/Caucasian	45 (86.54)	28 (80.00)	87 (82.08)	.69
Black/African-American	0 (0)	1 (2.86)	2 (1.89)	.75[b]
Hispanic/Latino	0 (0)**	6 (17.14)*	9 (8.49)*	.005[b]
Asian	4 (7.69)	0 (0)	4 (3.77)	.25[b]
Weight Presentation				
Kilograms	44.41 (8.50)*	56.67 (7.50)**	37.61 (11.97)***	<.0001
BMI	16.63 (1.74)*	20.66 (2.11)**	16.09 (2.67)***	<.0001
BMI z-score	−1.59 (1.00)*	0.21 (0.62)**	−1.49 (1.45)*	<.0001
%mBMI	83.11 (7.75)*	103.33 (11.54)**	86.40 (14.87)*	<.0001
Acute Weight Loss (vs. Chronic)[c]	16 (40.0%)*	12 (50.0%)*	15 (14.9%)**	.0001

[a]Analyzed using Pearson's Chi-square test for categorical variables or ANOVA for continuous variables, unless noted differently. [b] Due to small cell count, analyzed using Fischer's Exact test. [c] Data missing for 28 patients (for AN: $n = 12$, for Atypical AN: $n = 11$, and for ARFID: $n = 5$). Race/Ethnicity excludes patients who declined to respond or selected "other" ($n = 7$). */**/*** Denotes significance between eating disorder groups using pairwise comparisons ($p < .05$)

likely to be older and female, which likely affected comparative rates of amenorrhea among those with ARFID, overall, the physical differences identified in the current study highlight the importance of thorough medical assessments to determine the impact of low presenting weight. In one recent study, latent class analysis was used to silo eating disorder symptoms into groups that reflected the DSM-5 diagnostic categories of AN and ARFID [31]. For the most part, the findings of Pinhas and colleagues [31] align with our results, regarding between-group differences in age, prior hospitalization, eating disorder symptomology, and rates of psychiatric comorbidity. However, in Pinhas et al. [31], AN patients were more likely to have unstable vital signs whereas in

Table 3 Medical presentation of study participants with AN/Atypical AN, and ARFID ($n = 193$)

	AN or Atypical AN ($n = 87$) M (SD) or n (%)	ARFID ($n = 106$) M (SD) or n (%)	OR or Mean Difference	p [a]
Vital Signs				
Pulse rate	63.44 (16.62)	78.80 (15.91)	−15.35	< .0001
Systolic blood pressure	109.7 (12.09)	113.1 (9.42)	−3.35	.04
Diastolic blood pressure	61.57 (6.71)	63.43 (7.70)	−1.86	.07
Medical Instability				
Bradycardia, < 50 beats per minute	21 (24.14)	5 (4.72)	0.16	< .0001[b]
Hypotension, systolic pressure < 90 mmHg	4 (4.60)	2 (1.89)	0.40	.41[b]
Orthostatic Instability, > 20 beats per minute, > 10 mmHg	48 (55.17)	57 (53.77)	0.95	.85
Admitted/In hospital at presentation	24 (27.59)	15 (14.15)	0.43	.02
Amenorrhea[c]	26 (34.67)	7 (11.11)	0.24	.001
Prior Eating Disorder Treatment	33 (37.93)	40 (37.74)	0.99	.98
Psychotropic medication	34 (39.08)	38 (35.85)	0.87	.64
Other medical condition present potentially impacting weight[d]	7 (8.05)	13 (12.26)	1.60	.34

[a]Analyzed using Pearson's Chi-square test for categorical variables or independent t-tests for continuous variables, unless noted differently. [b] Due to small cell count, analyzed using Fischer's Exact test. [c] Excludes males (for AN/atypical AN, 12 excluded; for ARFID, 43 excluded). [d] Conditions considered included gastrointestinal or endocrine disorders including, but not limited to delayed gastric emptying, gastritis, esophagitis, GERD, Grave's disease, Type 1 Diabetes, chronic constipation, food allergies, acid reflux, celiac disease, irritable bowel syndrome, hypothyroidism, Hashimoto's disease, and gastroparesis

Table 4 Psychiatric measures of participants with AN/Atypical AN, and ARFID ($n = 193$)

	AN or Atypical AN ($n = 87$) M (SD) or n (%)	ARFID ($n = 106$) M (SD) or n (%)	OR or Mean Difference	p [a]
Diagnoses				
Psychiatric comorbidity (any DSM-V diagnosis)	53 (60.92)	79 (74.53)	1.88	.04
ADHD	1 (1.15)	25 (23.58)	26.54	< .0001[b]
Autism	1 (1.15)	6 (5.66)	5.16	.13[b]
Depressive Disorder[c]	42 (48.28)	20 (18.87)	0.25	< .0001
Anxiety Disorder[d]	41 (47.13)	61 (57.55)	1.52	.15
Eating Disorder Examination[e]				
Global score	2.56 (1.58)	0.30 (0.34)	2.25	< .0001
Restraint	2.83 (1.77)	0.29 (0.59)	2.55	< .0001
Eating concerns	1.66 (1.52)	0.32 (0.55)	1.33	< .0001
Shape concerns	2.61 (1.83)	0.33 (0.53)	2.28	< .0001
Weight concerns	3.11 (1.95)	0.27 (0.43)	2.85	< .0001
Parent Report				
CBCL Internalizing T-Score[f]	63.56 (10.22)	61.84 (11.53)	1.73	.34
Self-Report Measures				
vSelf-harm/ Suicidal ideation (MiniKid)[f]	10 (15.63)	8 (10.00)	0.60	.31
Children's Depression Inventory (Total T Score)[f]	61.97 (14.59)	53.18 (10.56)	7.87	< .0001
Rosenberg Self-Esteem[f]	15.19 (7.85)	21.85 (6.06)	−6.66	< .0001
Beck Anxiety Inventory Total Score[e]	16.07 (11.50)	10.17 (9.24)	5.90	.001
Clinical Impairment Assessment[e]	22.39 (13.03)	10.15 (8.98)	11.24	< .0001
Clinical Perfectionism Questionnaire[e]	25.75 (6.85)	19.38 (4.84)	6.37	< .0001

[a]Analyzed using Pearson's Chi-square test or for categorical variables or independent t-tests for continuous variables. [b] Due to small cell count, analyzed using Fischer's Exact test. [c] Patient is considered to have diagnosis of depression if they were diagnosed with Dysthymia, Major Depressive Disorder, Other Specified Depressive Disorder, and/or Unspecified Depression. [d] Patient is considered to have an anxiety diagnosis consists if they were diagnosed with OCD, PTSD, Social Anxiety Disorder, Agoraphobia, Generalized Anxiety Disorder, Panic Disorder, Separation Anxiety Disorder, Specific Phobia, Other Specified Anxiety Disorder, and/or Unspecified Anxiety. [e] Restricted to patients age ≥ 12 (for AN: $n = 81$, for ARFID: $n = 63$) and existing values for EDE subscales, BAI, CIA, and BAI (for AN: $n = 75$, for ARFID: $n = 53$). [f] Removed missing values for internalizing *t*-score, self-harm, total *t*-score, and RSE (for AN: 23 excluded, for ARFID: 26 excluded)

our sample, vital signs were comparable with the exception of bradycardia. Patients with ARFID in the current sample were also less likely to experience acute weight loss, suggesting that future study may benefit from examining rates of weight loss and related consequences for vital sign stability among children and adolescents with ARFID.

Given that the ARFID classification was more recently established in the DSM-5 [1], relatively little research has been published on this population to date. Previous studies describing this population have used retrospective chart reviews and/or assigned patients an ARFID diagnosis based on the proposed DSM-5 criteria [3, 11–15], while our data was prospectively collected and was based on a DSM-5 ARFID diagnosis via a clinician interaction with each patient. Other recent study using the latest diagnostic criteria has been limited by either a restricted age range (i.e., only those aged 13 and younger) [17] or had a substantially smaller sample ($n = 31$) and did not include a comparison group [16]. With an adequately powered sample across a broad age range (i.e., 7–19), our study shows consistency in weight status with previous literature that has characterized patients diagnosed either retrospectively or prospectively with ARFID. Of note, in the current study, patients with ARFID had a lower %mBMI than those diagnosed with AN, which lies in contrast to evidence from prior work indicating patients who fit criteria for ARFID tend to be less underweight than patients with AN [3, 11, 14, 15]. Our findings may be partially explained by the fact that those diagnosed with ARFID in the current sample were also on average, younger in age, and therefore expected to present smaller in stature. However, %mBMI is calculated based upon metrics correspondent to age and height, suggesting that our findings would benefit from replication in future investigation. Patients with ARFID in our sample were also more likely than the AN/atypical AN group to be younger and male [3, 12]. Diagnosis with a comorbid DSM-5 disorder was a common feature between our findings and those of other studies as well

[3, 16]. With regard to our inclusion of atypical AN, we saw similarity to a previous study; patients in our study with AN and atypical AN were observed to have similar levels of psychopathology despite the significant differences in their %mBMI [30]. Notably, those with ARFID were significantly more likely to be diagnosed with ADHD than either AN or atypical AN. While this difference is perhaps reflective of elevated population rates of ADHD among males, future research might investigate this specific comorbidty as a clinical feature of ARFID, with particular attention paid to the impact of stimulant medication use on appetite and clinical presentation. Further, given the significantly higher rates of ADHD evidenced among those diagnosed with ARFID in the current study, and the known comorbidity between ADHD and Autism Spectrum/Developmental Disorder, future work should more specifically investigate this potential shared diagnostic risk.

There are several limitations to this study. First, the sample is primarily white, which limits generalizability. Also, we combined AN and atypical AN because of power concerns; however, as demonstrated by Sawyer et al. [30] and our own analyses, no significant group differences were observed on medical and psychological variables. Further, due to the small sample size of children 12 and younger, we were not able to compare the children aged 12 and under on a measure of anxiety. Finally, lack of information on duration of illness did not allow for between-group comparisons. While the current study indicates that those with ARIFD were more likely to experience chronic vs. acute weight loss, it is noteworthy that assessment of duration of illness in ARFID patients can be difficult given that on average, patients meeting criteria for this disorder have extended duration of illness compared to patients diagnosed with AN, atypical AN and bulimia nervosa [3, 13, 15]. Further, assessment measures specifc to ARFID have been slow to emerge; while this study used a rigorous method with which to determine ARFID diagnosis, future study should rely upon empirically validated measures, specifically oriented toward a determination of this diagnosis.

The current study uniquely identified differences across disorders in acute vs. chronic weight loss. Specifically, those with ARFID were less likely to experience acute vs. chronic weight loss as compared with AN and atypical AN counterparts. Restrictive eating disorders and weight loss have a significant negative impact on both the physical and psychological functioning of children and adolescents [27]. Research suggests that in patients with AN, weight loss and malnutrition are associated with a number of significant life-threatening medical complications including hypotension, bradycardia, and hypothermia [32]. Weight loss in patients with AN has also been associated with atrophy of the brain and decreased cognitive functioning [32]. Similarly, Sawyer et al. demonstrated that adolescents diagnosed with atypical AN have similar medical and psychological impairments as patients with full-threshold AN [30]. However, there are not yet any published studies investigating the physical and psychological effects of weight loss and malnutrition in patients with ARFID; this would be an important area for future study following the descriptive work in the evidence base to date. Learning that patients with ARFID were significantly *less* likely to experience acute weight loss vs. chronic weight loss as compared with those with AN or atypical AN, may be critical in informing future screening efforts. For example, it is possible that a sizeable portion of ARFID patients might be missed if we focus only on those who present at low weight, or those who appear to have lost weight precipitously. Evidence that patients who meet criteria for ARFID are significantly younger than youth with AN and atypical AN, along with potential health consequences associated with sustained low weight, underscores a critical line of future inquiry in this unique patient population.

This study provides additional data to support the validity of separating ARFID from other eating and feeding disorders including AN and atypical AN. Given the relative newness of the diagnosis, ARFID patients may not be detected as early or often as those with more traditionally described AN/atypical AN, leading to reduced access to care. Early detection of ARFID may lead to faster mobilization of treatment efforts and potentially better illness prognoses. As such, our findings based on formal DSM-5 criteria in a sizable sample of individuals with ARFID provide an important foundation for future efforts to better define this clinical syndrome and to ultimately tailor precision interventions for this population.

Conclusions

The current study was uniquely able to examine clinical features of a large treatment-seeking sample of children and adolescents diagnosed with ARFID. Findings from this study highlight the clinical significance of ARFID as a distinct DSM-5 diagnosis and describe the physiological and psychological presentation of this disorder. The novel finding that ARFID patients are more likely than those diagnosed with AN to experience chronic, rather than acute, weight loss should be further investigated, along with associated health consequences. Given the medical and psychiatric heterogeneity of this population, further research is also needed to examine potential differences between ARFID subgroups, as well as to development reliable and valid assessment measures for ARFID that can further improve understanding of this clinical syndrome. The current study provides an important foundation in understanding medical and psychological features of children and adolescents presenting for treatment with ARFID.

Abbreviations

ADHD: Attention-deficit/hyperactivity disorder; AN: Anorexia nervosa; ANOVA: Analysis of variance; ARFID: Avoidant restrictive food intake disorder; BAI: Beck Anxiety Inventory; BMI: Body mass index; CBCL: Child Behavior Check List; CDI-2: Child Depression Inventory 2nd Edition; CIA: Clinical Impairment Assessment; CPQ: Clinical Perfectionism Questionnaire; CTED: Center for the Treatment of Eating Disorders; DSM-5: Diagnostic and Statistical Manual of Mental Disorder, Fifth Edition; EDE: Eating Disorder Examination; FAED: Food avoidant emotional disorder; MINI-Kid: Mini International Neuropsychiatric Interview for Children and Adolescents; RSE: Rosenberg Self-Esteem Scale

Acknowledgments

We acknowledge the generous financial support from the Goven Family Foundation.

Authors' contributions

HK conceptualized and designed the study, drafted the initial manuscript and approved the final manuscript as submitted. SLR carried out the data collection and management, contributed to the initial manuscript draft, reviewed and revised the manuscript, and approved the final manuscript as submitted. TLB carried out the data analyses, drafted the initial manuscript, reviewed and revised the manuscript, and approved the final manuscript for submission. SE assisted with interpretation of data and reviewed and revised the manuscript. CBP provided assessment training and oversight, revised the manuscript, and approved the final manuscript for submission. JL assisted in the conceptualization and design of the study and reviewed and revised the manuscript. SG reviewed and revised the manuscript. DLG assisted in the conceptualization and design of the study and assisted with the interpretation of data, and reviewed and revised the manuscript. All authors approved the final manuscript as submitted and agree to be accountable for all aspects of the work.

Competing interests

Dr. Le Grange receives royalties from Guilford Press and Routledge, and is Co-Director of the Training Institute for Child and Adolescent Eating Disorders, LLC. All other authors have no competing interests or financial relationships to disclose.

Author details

[1]Center for the Treatment of Eating Disorders, Children's Minnesota, Minneapolis, MN, USA. [2]Children's Minnesota Research Institute, Children's Minnesota, Minneapolis, MN, USA. [3]Department of Psychiatry, University of Minnesota, Minneapolis, MN, USA. [4]The Emily Program, St. Paul, MN, USA. [5]Department of Psychiatry, University of California, San Francisco, CA, USA. [6]Department of Psychiatry and Behavioral Neuroscience, The University of Chicago, Chicago, IL, USA.

References

1. Association AP. Diagnostic and statistical manual of mental disorders fifth edition DSM-5. Arlington: American Psychiatric Association; 2013.
2. Higgs JF, Goodyer IM, Birch J. Anorexia nervosa and food avoidance emotional disorder. Arch Dis Child. 1989;64(3):346–51.
3. Fisher MM, Rosen DS, Ornstein RM, Mammel KA, Katzman DK, Rome ES, et al. Characteristics of avoidant/restrictive food intake disorder in children and adolescents: a "new disorder" in DSM-5. J Adolesc Health. 2014;55:49–52.
4. Norris ML, Spettigue WJ, Katzman DK. Update on eating disorders: current perspectives on avoidant/restrictive food intake disorder in children and youth. Neuropsychiatr Dis Treat. 2016;12:213–8.
5. Zimmerman J, Fisher M. Avoidant/restrictive food intake disorder (ARFID). Curr Probl Pediatr Adolesc Health Care. 2017;47(4):95–103.
6. Bryant-Waugh R, Markham L, Kreipe RE, Walsh TB. Feeding and eating disorders in childhood. Int J Eat Disord. 2010;43(2):98–111.
7. Mairs R, Nicholls D. Assessment and treatment of eating disorders in children and adolescents. Arch Dis Child. 2016;101(12):1168–75.
8. Bryant-Waugh R, Kreipe RE. Avoidant/restrictive food intake disorder in the DSM-5. Psychiatr Ann. 2012;42(11):402–5.
9. Norris ML, Spettigue W, Hammond NG, Katzman DK, Zucker N, Yelle K, et al. Building evidence for the use of descriptive subtypes in youth with avoidant restrictive food intake disorder. Int J Eat Disord. 2018;51(2):170–3.
10. Kurz S, van Dyck Z, Dremmel D, Munsch S, Hilberg A. Early-onsent restrictive eating disturbances in primary school boys and girls. European Child Adolesccent Psychiatry. 2015;24:779–85.
11. Ornstein RM, Rosen DS, Mammel KA, Callahan T, Forman S, Jay MS, et al. Distribution of eating disorders in children and adolescents using the proposed DSM-5 criteria for feeding and eating disorders. J Adolesc Health. 2013;53:303–5.
12. Norris ML, Robinson A, Obeid N, Harrison M, Spettigue W, Henderson K. Exploring avoidant/restrictive food intake disorder in eating disordered patients: a descriptive study. Int J Eat Disord. 2014;47:495–9.
13. Forman S, McKenzie N, Hehn R, Monge MC, Kapphahn CJ, Mammel KA, et al. Predictors of outcome at 1 year in adolescents with DSM-5 restrictive eating disorders: report of the national eating disorders quality improvement collaborative. J Adolesc Health. 2014;55:750–6.
14. Nicely TA, Lane-Loney S, Masciulli E, Hollenbeak CS, Ornstein RM. Prevalence and characteristics of avoidant/restrictive food intake disorder in a cohort of young patients in day treatment for eating disorders. J Eat Disord. 2014;2(1):21.
15. Wallin U, Rastam M. Childhood anorexia nervosa compared with low weight food intake disorder without weight and shape-related psychopathology: a retrospective study of 102 patients. Eur Eat Disord Rev. 2016;24:329–33.
16. Cooney M, Lieberman M, Guimond T, Katzman DK. Clinical and psychological features of children and adolescents diagnosed with avoidant/restrictive food intake disorder in a pediatric tertiary care eating disorder program: a descriptive study. J Eat Disord. 2018;6:7.
17. Lieberman M, Houser ME, Voyer AP, Grady S, Katzman DK. Children with avoidant/restrictive food intake disorder and anorexia nervosa in a tertiary care pediatric eating disorder program: a comparative study. Int J Eat Disord. 2019;52(3):239–45.
18. Pediatrics AAo. Policy statement: identifying and treating eating disorders. Pediatrics. 2003;111:204–11.
19. Fairburn CG, Cooper Z, O'Conner M. Eating disorder examination. In: Fairburn CG, editor. Cognitive behavior therapy and eating disorders. New York: Guliford Press; 2014.
20. Sheehan D, Shytle D, Milo K. M.I.N.I. kid: Mini international neuropsychiatric interview for children and adolescents; 2006.
21. Kovacs M. Children's depression inventory 2nd edition technical manual. Ontario: Multi-Health Systems; 2011.
22. Rosenberg M. Society and the adolescent self-image. Rahway: Quinn & Boden Company; 1965.
23. Osman A, Kopper BA, Barrios FX, Osman JR, Wade T. The Beck anxiety inventory: reexamination of factor structure and psychometric properties. J Clin Psychol. 1997;53(1):7–14.
24. Bohn K, Doll HA, Cooper Z, O'Conner M, Palmer RL, Fairburn CG. The measurement of impairment due to eating disorder psychopathology. Behav Res Ther. 2008;46:1105–10.
25. Shafran R, Cooper Z, Fairburn CG. Clinical perfectionism: a cognitive-behavioural analysis. Behav Res Ther. 2002;40(7):773–91.
26. Achenbach TM. Achenbach system of empirically-based assessment (ASEBA). Burlington: University of Vermont, Research Center for Children, Youth & Families; 2000.
27. Practice Committee of the American Society for Reproductive Medicine. Current evaluation of amenorrhea. Fertil Steril. 2006;86(5):S148–55.
28. Le Grange D, Doyle PM, Swanson SA, Ludwig K, Glunz C, Kreipe RE. Calculation of expected body weight in adolescents with eating disorders. Pediatrics. 2012;129(2):e438–46.
29. Hughes EK, Le Grange D, Court A, Sawyer SM. A case series of family-based treatment for adolescents with atypical anorexia nervosa. Int J Eat Disord. 2017;50(4):424–32.
30. Sawyer SM, Whitelaw M, Le Grange D, Yeo M, Hughes EK. Physical and psychological morbidity in adolescents with atypical anorexia nervosa. Pediatrics. 2016;137(4):e20154080.
31. Pinhas L, Nicholls D, Crosby RD, Morris A, Lynn RM, Madden S. Classification of childhood onset eating disorders: a latent class analysis. Int J Eat Disord. 2017;50(6):657–64.
32. Mehler PS, Brown C. Anorexia nervosa - medical complications. J Eat Disord. 2015;3:11.

5

A conceptual comparison of family-based treatment and enhanced cognitive behavior therapy in the treatment of adolescents with eating disorders

Riccardo Dalle Grave[1*], Sarah Eckhardt[2], Simona Calugi[1] and Daniel Le Grange[3,4]

Abstract

Background: The aim of this paper is to give a conceptual comparison of family-based treatment (FBT), a specific form of family therapy, and enhanced cognitive behavior therapy (CBT-E) in the management of adolescents with eating disorders.

Main text: FBT and CBT-E differ in the conceptualization of eating disorders, the nature of involvement of parents and the child/adolescent, the number of treatment team members involved, and evidence of efficacy. FBT is the leading recommended empirically- supported intervention for adolescents with eating disorders. Data from randomized controlled trials indicate that FBT works well with less than half of the parents and adolescents who accept the treatment, but cannot be used with those who do not have available parents, or for those with parents who are not accepting of a FBT model, or are unable to participate in a course of this treatment. CBT-E has shown promising results in cohort studies of patients between ages 11 and 19 years, and has recently been recommended for youth with eating disorders when FBT is unacceptable, contraindicated, or ineffective.

Conclusion: There is a need to compare these two treatments in a randomized controlled trial to assess their acceptability, effectiveness, relative cost and cost-effectiveness, and to explore moderators of treatment response.

Keywords: Eating disorders, Anorexia nervosa, Treatment, Family-based treatment, Enhanced cognitive behavior therapy

Plain English summary

Family-based treatment (FBT) is the current leading empirically-supported intervention for adolescents with eating disorders. As this treatment has certain limitations, alternative approaches are needed. The National Institute for Health and Care Excellence (NICE) has recently recommended cognitive behavior therapy (CBT) for eating disorders in children and young people when family therapy is unacceptable, contraindicated, or ineffective. This recommendation was supported by promising results demonstrated by the enhanced version of CBT (CBT-E), adapted for adolescents with eating disorders.

Given the importance of the NICE recommendation, this paper gives a brief overview of FBT and CBT-E, describes the main conceptual differences between these two treatments, and emphasizes the need to compare these two treatments in a randomized controlled trial to assess their acceptability, effectiveness, relative cost and cost-effectiveness, and to explore moderators of treatment response.

Background

A specific form of family therapy, termed family-based treatment (FBT) [1], or at times referred to as the Maudsley method/Maudsley approach [2], is the current leading empirically-supported intervention for adolescents with eating disorders. As this treatment has certain limitations, alternative approaches are needed. The

* Correspondence: rdalleg@gmail.com
[1]Department of Eating and Weight Disorders, Villa Garda Hospital, Via Montebaldo 89 1-37016 Garda (VR), Verona, Italy
Full list of author information is available at the end of the article

National Institute for Health and Care Excellence (NICE) has recently recommended cognitive behavior therapy (CBT) for eating disorders in children and young people when family therapy is unacceptable, contraindicated, or ineffective [3]. This recommendation was supported by promising results demonstrated by the enhanced version of CBT (CBT-E), adapted for adolescents with eating disorders [4, 5] in cohort studies of patients aged 11 to 19 years.

Given the importance of the NICE recommendation, the aim of this paper is to give a brief overview of FBT and CBT-E and a narrative review of the efficacy and effectiveness of the two treatments, and to describe the main conceptual differences between these two treatments.

An overview of family-based treatment (FBT)

Family therapy for adolescent anorexia nervosa was originally developed in the late 1970s by a team of researchers at the Institute of Psychiatry and the Maudsley Hospital in London [2]. A behaviorally focused version of this original therapy has been described in detail [6], and has been manualized and named family-based treatment (FBT) [1]. In general, FBT does not align with a particular therapeutic approach, but instead integrates techniques from a variety of schools of psychotherapy, including systemic, strategic, narrative, and structural family therapy. The overall philosophy of FBT is that the adolescent with anorexia nervosa is embedded in the family, and that the parents' involvement in the therapy is necessary for treatment success. Indeed, the overall perspective of FBT for adolescent anorexia nervosa is to see the family as a resource in the treatment of their child or adolescent [1].

FBT differs from other treatments of adolescent eating disorders for three main reasons [1]. First, the adolescent is not considered to be in control of his or her behavior, rather the treatment posits that the eating disorder controls the adolescent. The adolescent is seen as functioning as a much younger child in need of significant support from their parents. Second, the goal is to correct this position by improving the parents' control over their adolescent's eating. Frequently this control is abdicated, in part because parents either experience guilt for believing they have caused the adolescent's eating disorder, or because the eating disorder symptoms have frightened them into inactivity or acting indecisively. Third, FBT focuses its effort on the task of weight restoration and to get the adolescent back onto a normal developmental trajectory, particularly in the first phase of the treatment, using an adaptation of the therapeutic family meal developed by the structural family therapy of Minuchin and his colleagues [7]. The primary goal is to keep parents focused on refeeding their adolescent, thus freeing the adolescent from the control of the eating disorder. This therapy is designed to consider adolescent developmental processes and return the adolescent to their developmental trajectory, though only after the patient has re-established a steady upward path.

A key aspect of the treatment is to separate the illness from the patient (i.e., to externalize the illness, or not identify the patient with the illness itself), in order to enable parents to take firm action against the eating disorder as opposed to acting against their daughter or son. FBT favors parents adopting an uncritical acceptance of the adolescent in their struggle against his or her symptoms. Parents are exonerated from blame for the patient's illness and are congratulated on their earlier parenting skills. With few exceptions, parents are also encouraged to work out for themselves how to refeed their child with anorexia nervosa, and to view the therapist as a consultant who supports them in this effort. An important principle of FBT is therefore an agnostic view of the potential causes of anorexia nervosa, to help parents decrease guilt, and use their best resources to facilitate the patient's recovery. The task of full parental engagement in treatment is achieved by appropriately raising their level of anxiety, by emphasizing the seriousness of the illness, which includes the risk of dying, and/or the difficulty of recovery.

Conjoint FBT involves the entire family (parents and siblings) attending each session, along with the unwell adolescent, although a version of this treatment has been delivered to parents alone while the adolescent meets with a nurse for no more than about 10 min at the start of each session (called parent-focused therapy (PFT)) and has been shown to be just as effective [8]. Whether delivered in conjoint or separated format, FBT typically includes no more than 20 sessions, each 50–60 min in length, with the exception of the second session, the family meal, which may for some families last up to 90 min.

There are three phases in FBT (see Fig. 1). In Phase I, usually lasting about 3–4 months with sessions at weekly intervals, parents are charged with the responsibility of correcting their adolescent's disordered eating behaviors and low weight. The therapist's principal task is to assist the parents in developing and refining their strategies around this process. Once eating disorder behaviors are significantly reduced, control over food consumption is transferred back to the adolescent in an age appropriate fashion (in Phase II), and the sessions are gradually reduced from weekly to every second or even third week. In Phase III, once normal body weight (i.e., 95% median body mass index [BMI]) and eating behavior have been achieved, more general issues of adolescent development are addressed, and sessions are scheduled every third week or even at monthly intervals. A main theme in the

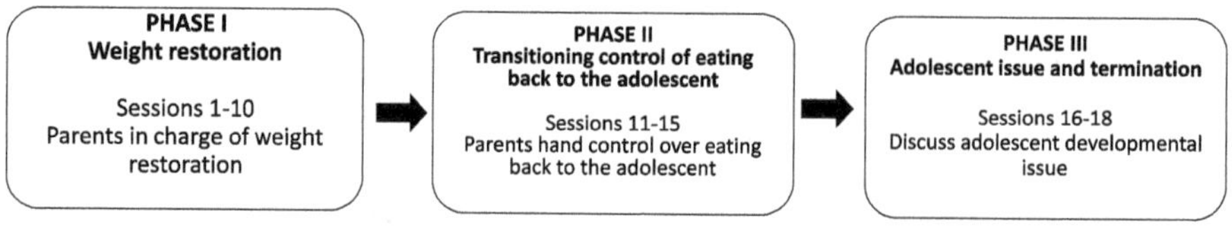

Fig. 1 The three phases of family-based treatment

last phase of this treatment is the creation of a healthy adolescent-parent relationship, which no longer requires the eating disorder as the basis of interaction. This requires increasing the adolescent's autonomy, establishing appropriate intergenerational family boundaries, and helping the parents to recognize the need to reorganize their lives given their child's pending departure from the family home [1].

The treatment team includes a primary clinician (e.g., child and adolescent psychiatrist, psychologist or social worker/family therapist), and a consulting team that could consists of a pediatrician, nurse, and dietitian [1], who meets with parents/patient as needed. Efforts should be made to concentrate the treating team within the same facility whenever possible, as close communication between providers is critical to the treatment's success. For this reason, FBT may best be viewed as a complex and coordinated intervention, and although the most prominent component of the treatment is the focused psychotherapeutic intervention in terms of weight restoration, several sessions with a physician with extensive experience in medical treatment of adolescents with anorexia nervosa should be a key and indispensable component of this treatment. This is especially pertinent should the adolescent show signs of vital sign instability and a period of hospitalization, albeit briefly, should be required [9]. Similarly, a dietitian can be involved to help families with home-based refeeding, and to facilitate greater energy density and food variety [10].

The efficacy of FBT for adolescents

The efficacy of manualized FBT for anorexia nervosa in adolescents has been tested in six randomized controlled trials (RCTs). Findings from these studies demonstrate an average remission rate, when this is defined as percent median BMI > 94% of expected for age, height, and gender, *and* an eating disorder examination score [11] within one standard deviation of population means, as < 40% for all participants at the end of treatment. On the other hand, treatment response, when this is broadly defined as an improvement in weight and eating-related psychopathology, averages near 75% [12]. Of note, no more than 15% of patients participating in FBT are typically hospitalized for acute medical instability for a mean duration of 7–10 days, before returning to the outpatient service for ongoing FBT [13]. Only one of the RCTs utilizing manualized FBT compared this therapy to an active individual comparison treatment, i.e., adolescent focused psychotherapy. On average, FBT is not significantly superior to individual adolescent treatment at post-treatment, but it does achieve greater symptom reduction by 6- and 12-month post-treatment follow-up [12]. For the most, the remaining RCTs utilizing FBT have compare it to different forms of family engagement in treatment. At this time there are no studies which have compared FBT to CBT-E.

FBT for bulimia nervosa has been compared across two RCTs; FBT-BN vs. individual supportive psychotherapy [14], and FBT-BN vs. CBT adapted for adolescents (CBT-A), a treatment derived from the CBT for bulimia nervosa [15, 16]. In the 2007 study, participants in FBT-BN, remitted at significantly higher rates at end of treatment (39% versus 18%), and at 6-month follow-up (29% versus 10%). For the 2015 study, participants in FBT-BN achieved significantly higher abstinence rates than in CBT-A at end of treatment (39% versus 20%), and at 6-month follow-up (44% versus 25%), but abstinence rates between these two groups were no longer statistically significant at 12-month follow-up (49% versus 32%).

An overview of enhanced cognitive behavior therapy

CBT-E is an evidence-based treatment that has been developed for addressing the psychopathology of all eating disorders, as opposed to the specific diagnoses outlined in the Diagnostic and Statistical Manual of Mental Disorders (DSM-5) [17]. Although originally designed for adults, it has now been adapted for adolescents with eating disorders [4, 5].

Whereas FBT is based on the concept that the problem or symptoms belong to the entire family [1], CBT-E views the problem as belonging to the individual. CBT-E is therefore designed to treat the eating disorder as part of the patient, and encourages the patient, not their parents, to take control. CBT-E treatment procedures involve patients actively in all phases of treatment, with the aim of promoting a feeling of self-control; it is the patient that has the final say, not only in the decision to start treatment, but also which problems to address, and which procedures will be used to address them.

CBT-E is a collaborative approach to overcoming problems with eating (collaborative empiricism), whatever they may be. Patients are encouraged to actively participate in the process of change, and to consider the treatment a priority. The CBT-E therapist always keeps their patients fully apprised of what is happening, informing them that it will not be easy, but it will be worthwhile to take steps to overcome their eating problem. In order to avoid increasing any resistance to change, there are no "coercive" or "prescriptive" procedures involved in CBT-E; patients are never asked to do things that they do not agree to. Indeed, one of the four major goals of CBT-E for adolescents is to engage them in the treatment, involving them actively in the process of change.

The second major goal of CBT-E is to deal with the eating disorder psychopathology. This will involve addressing patients' concerns about shape, weight and eating, as well as any dietary restraint and restriction (and low weight if applicable), and extreme weight control behaviors. As part of this process, patients are encouraged to understand and disrupt the mechanisms maintaining their eating disorder psychopathology—the third major treatment goal—which are illustrated to them through the collaborative creation of a personal formulation. This is a key strategy, as it highlights the targets of the treatment to come, and thereby helps guide a made-to-measure approach for addressing the evolving psychopathology of each individual patient. As part of this approach, patients are educated about the processes that characterize their personal formulation, which can be modified mid-course to address any emerging processes, and actively involved in the decision to tackle them. This promotes self-empowerment, and helps them to conclude that they have a problem that needs addressing.

Once the patient has reached this conclusion, which is an essential prerequisite of such a collaborative form of treatment, they are gradually introduced to a flexible set of sequential cognitive and behavioral strategies and procedures, as well as further education, designed to progressively address their personal eating disorder psychopathology and its maintenance mechanisms. These strategies will need to be practiced at home, and it is what the patient does between sessions that will determine the treatment outcome. To achieve cognitive change, patients are encouraged to observe how the processes in their personal formulation operate in real life. This is achieved through real-time self-monitoring. Strategically planned homework tasks, making gradual behavioral changes and analyzing their effects and implications on their way of thinking, are also central to the treatment, but need to be integrated with care, as they may provoke anxiety. To keep the patient on track, the therapist therefore needs to be both empathetic and firm about what needs to be achieved.

The fourth major goal of CBT-E is for the patient to achieve lasting change. Hence, in the later stages of CBT-E, the treatment shifts to a future-oriented approach. When the main maintenance processes outlined in the patient's personal formulation have been disrupted, and they experience periods of no concerns about their shape, weight, and eating, they can be educated about their eating disorder mindset, and helped to become aware of the signs that this is reactivating. They can then be provided with strategies designed to help them decenter from it quickly, and thereby ward off relapse [18].

CBT-E for adolescents starts with two sessions designed to assess the patient's needs and prepare them for treatment. The treatment is then delivered by a single therapist in three main Steps (see Fig. 2), each with a different emphasis. The first is geared towards patients' reassessing their current state, and how what they do affects them. Patients are then asked to consider the pros and cons of tackling their low weight (if applicable). In the second Step, patients (if willing) are provided with the tools they will need to address their eating-disorder psychopathology by alleviating concerns about shape and weight, and assisted with weight restoration (if necessary). In the final Step of CBT-E, the emphasis is on helping patients to develop personalized strategies for rapid recovery from setbacks, and thereby to maintain the changes that they have achieved in the long term.

In patients with a BMI between the 3rd and 25th centile, treatment is generally delivered over the course of 30–40, 50-min sessions, whereas those with a BMI > the 25th centile attend 20 such sessions. As in CBT-E for adults [18], however, the treatment duration is flexible, as it will depend on the items that need to be addressed. Hence, in a review session held after 4 weeks in non-underweight patients, or in one of the review sessions in Step 2 in underweight patients, the decision is taken to use either the "focused" form, which addresses only the specific features of eating-disorder psychopathology, or the "broad" form, which is designed to address any "external" mechanisms, i.e., clinical perfectionism, core low self-esteem, mood intolerance, and/or interpersonal difficulties, that may be operating. These are tackled using specific, additional CBT-E modules, and will therefore require the treatment to be extended. In most patients, the focused form is appropriate, but the broad form should be considered if in the review sessions it is concluded that one or more of the external mechanisms maintaining the eating disorder psychopathology [4]: (i) are pronounced; (ii) appear to be maintaining the eating disorder; and (iii) seem likely to interfere with the response to treatment.

Naturally, parents are not excluded from participating in their child's treatment, but their involvement is limited to helping create a family environment conducive to recovery. To this end, during the first two weeks of treatment, they are invited to attend a single one-hour

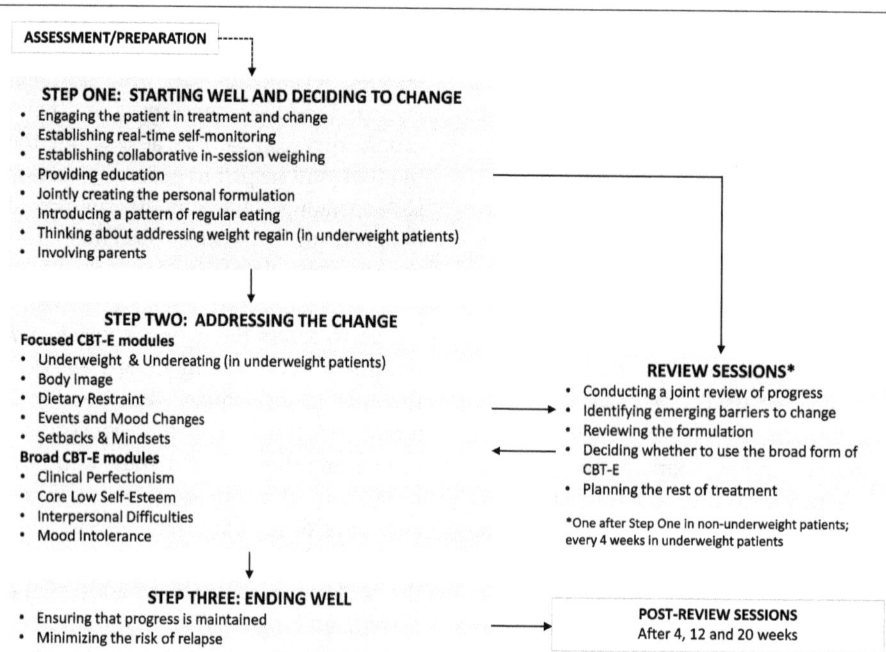

Fig. 2 The enhanced cognitive behavior therapy (CBT-E) map for adolescents with eating disorders

assessment session, held immediately after an individual session with the patient, with the aim of identifying family-related factors capable of undermining their child's efforts to change. This session is held with the parents alone, but is followed by subsequent sessions (four to six times in not-underweight patients, eight to twelve in those who present as underweight) each lasting 15–20 min, with the patient and parents together at the end of a patient's individual session. In general, a date is set for the first joint parent-patient session after the introduction of the regular eating procedure, both in underweight and not underweight patients; this session should be dedicated to explaining how parents may help the patient to implement it. Other joint sessions may be set up when the underweight patient has made the decision to address weight restoration, in order to discuss the parents' role before, during, and after meals. Finally, it may be helpful to involve parents in order to help the patient implement some procedures of the CBT-E broad modules, both in underweight and not underweight patients. During these sessions, parents are kept abreast of how treatment and their child are progressing, and anything they can do to help. In order to promote a sense of self-determination, anything that will be discussed in these sessions is negotiated with and agreed to by the patient beforehand.

The effectiveness of CBT-E for adolescents

To date, four different cohort studies, on patients aged between 11 and 19 years, have been conducted to assess outpatient CBT-E for adolescents. Findings from these studies showed that in patients with anorexia nervosa who complete the treatment (60–65%) about 60% achieved a full response (i.e., BMI centile corresponding to an adult BMI of ≥18.5 kg/m^2 and an eating disorder examination interview score [11] within one standard deviation of population means).

Three of the four studies investigated the effects on patients with anorexia nervosa, and one on non-underweight adolescents with other eating disorders. In the first study, 49 adolescents with anorexia nervosa were given 40 outpatient CBT-E sessions, and a significant increase in BMI-for-age percentile, from 3.36 (SD = 3.73) to 30.3 (SD = 16.7), along with a marked improvement in eating-disorder psychopathology and general psychiatric features, was seen in two-thirds of completers [19]. At 60-week follow-up, these positive outcomes remained almost unchanged despite minimal subsequent treatment. These encouraging findings were mirrored by a subsequent study of outpatient CBT-E involving 68 non-underweight adolescents with an eating disorder [20], three-quarters of whom completed the full 20-session program. Intent-to-treat analysis revealed that, at the end of treatment, 68% of patients displayed only minimal residual eating-disorder psychopathology, and half of those with prior episodes of binge-eating or purging reported no longer having them.

Interestingly, a comparative study of CBT-E efficacy in 46 adolescents and 49 adults with anorexia nervosa [21] revealed that weight normalization occurred in considerably more adolescents than adults (65.3% vs. 36.5%).

Furthermore, weight restoration was achieved roughly 15 weeks earlier on average by adolescents vs. adults. These findings provide compelling evidence not only that CBT-E is even more effective in adolescent patients, but also that positive outcomes may be achieved in a shorter time frame than that required by adults.

Finally, a more recent study set out to assess the outcomes and determine the predictors of change in a cohort of 49 adolescent patients with marked anorexia nervosa, treated with outpatient CBT-E in a real-world setting [22]. More than 95% of patients accepted the treatment and 71.4% completed it, displaying a large increase in weight, together with a marked decrease in eating-disorder and general psychopathology, and clinical impairment scores. These changes were maintained at six-month follow-up, suggesting that CBT-E is a promising treatment for adolescents with anorexia nervosa when it is also delivered in a real-world setting, even though no baseline predictors of drop-out and treatment outcome were found. The percentage of drop-out was higher than those reported in most recent FBT studies (15–20%) [13], but this difference could be in part explained by the criteria used to define drop-out - e.g., 15% of the patients hospitalized during the course of the treatment were included as completers in the FBT study [13], whereas all the hospitalized patients (8.2%) were considered drop-outs in the present study. It also underlines that BMI percentile for age and gender at end of treatment and 20-week follow-up was broadly similar to that reported in the recent FBT studies.

Major differences between FBT and CBT-E

FBT and CBT-E differ in the conceptualization of eating disorders, the nature of involvement of parents and child/adolescent, the number of treatment team members involved, and evidence of efficacy (see Table 1).

Conceptualization of eating disorders

In FBT, the problem or symptoms belong to the entire family, and therapy works to separate the illness from the patient (externalization), enabling parents to temporarily take control of their child or adolescent's eating. Several schools of thoughts contributed to the type and style of this treatment. The family meal, for example, is derived from Structural Family Therapy [7], which postulates that the child is physiologically vulnerable, and has a critical role in the family's avoidance of conflicts that acts as a powerful reinforcement of symptoms. Through family meals parents reinforce the effectiveness of their own parental dyad and the adolescent's emotional involvement with her/his parents is reduced. The strategy of maintaining an agnostic view regarding the causes of anorexia nervosa is derived from Strategic Family Therapy [23, 24], and has the aim of limiting the impact of the symptoms on the patient and family, and to focus the therapy on the problematic patterns that are maintaining the eating disorder. Additionally, the strategy of encouraging the parents to find solutions that work for them, rather than relying on the outside authority of the therapist, while the therapist holds the family and their efforts in a positive and noncritical way, are derived from the Milan Systems Therapy [25]. This school of thought postulates that the family is a rigid organized homeostatic mechanism, resistant to change from the outside. Separating the illness from the adolescent, or externalization, comes from Narrative Therapy [26], and finally, feminist theory, emphasizing the need for partnership and shared control of the therapeutic process [23], has been used to form a sincere partnership between the therapist and the parents with the healthy part of the adolescent's growth process, even if it defiles parental will.

The initial focus of FBT is the task of weight restoration through the parents' efforts at home. Once this is achieved the focus gradually shifts toward adolescent issues with the family, and the therapist encourages the family to examine the relationship between adolescent issues, working towards increased personal autonomy for the adolescent, and establishing more appropriate intergenerational boundaries. Toward the end of treatment, the therapist will check with the parents, if appropriate for the age and developmental stage of the children, regarding their need to reorganize their life together after the child's prospective departure from the

Table 1 Principal differences between family-based treatment (FBT) and enhanced cognitive behavior therapy (CBT-E)

	FBT	CBT-E
Conceptualization of eating disorders	The problem belongs to the entire family The illness is separated from the patient	The problem belongs to the individual It does not separate the illness from the patient
Adolescent's involvement	Not actively involved	Actively involved
Parents' involvement	Vitally important	Useful but not essential
Treatment team	Multidisciplinary	Single therapist
Sessions (n)	18 family sessions Sessions with the consulting team (paediatrician or nurse) in case of need for hospitalization (~ 15%)	20 individual sessions (non-underweight patients) 30–40 individual sessions (underweight patients)

family home [1]. FBT does not directly address the underlying theoretical constructs of CBT-E, such as overvaluation of shape and weight, event and moods influencing eating, and external clinical features (e.g., clinical perfectionism, core low self-esteem, mood intolerance, interpersonal problems), although it strongly encourages peer social interaction.

CBT-E, on the other hand, views the illness as belonging to the individual. Cognitive behavioral theory postulates that these patients have a shared but distinctive self-evaluation scheme based on their overvaluation of shape and weight which plays a central role in maintaining all eating disorders [17]. This "core psychopathology" gives rise, directly or indirectly, to the other clinical features of the disorder, whatever its DSM-5 classification. These clinical features are therefore explored with the patient and laid down in an evolving personal formulation. These clinical "expressions" of the patient's eating disorder and the mechanisms that act to reinforce them are then targeted by a progressive series of well-specified CBT strategies and procedures designed to help patients to change their behavior and reflect on the consequences of these changes. The ultimate aim is to train patients how to decentre from and overcome their difficulties, and, thus, for them to learn to control their eating-disorder mindset, rather than the mindset controlling them [18].

Involvement of parents and adolescent

Parents' involvement in FBT is vitally important for the ultimate success of the treatment. Moreover, in FBT, parents must defer working on other family conflicts or disagreement until the eating-disorder behaviors are resolved. Parents' involvement in CBT-E is useful but not essential. The role of parents, as described above, is only simply to support the implementation of the one-to-one treatment. Both treatments pay attention to adolescent development, however, in FBT the adolescent is not viewed as being in control of his/her behavior (the eating disorder controls the adolescent), and this is corrected by improving the parental control over eating in the first phase of the treatment. On the contrary, in CBT-E the adolescent is helped to learn how to control his/her behavior, and parents may be involved in helping the adolescent in pursuing this task. In FBT the adolescent is initially not actively involved, and plays a more passive role, although his/her role becomes more active in the last phase of the treatment, while in CBT-E the adolescent is encouraged form the beginning to become actively involved in the treatment.

Treatment team

FBT is made up of a variety of key components, each of which may contribute to its effects. Most prominent is the psychotherapeutic element, focusing on weight restoration, and is delivered by a primary clinician (e.g., child and adolescent psychiatric, psychologist or social worker/family therapist). In the most recent FBT trials, this involved no more than 20 one-hour family sessions over about nine months [1]. Another component are the sessions with a physician with expertise in the medical management of adolescents with anorexia nervosa. These meetings usually start out weekly, before tapering off to monthly or six-weekly, as is clinically indicated. Hospitalization for medical instability should be pursued when indicated.

CBT-E is provided by a one therapist (e.g., psychologist or a health professional trained in the treatment) who is substituted when they have to be absent. It is delivered in 20 treatment sessions over 20 weeks (in not underweight patients) and 30–40 sessions over 30–40 weeks (in underweight patients). The treatment also involves a 90-min assessment session with only the parents and some 15–20 min sessions with the patient and parents together (see above). No additional therapeutic input, either from physicians, dieticians, or other health professionals, other than an initial assessment by a physician to check that the patient is suitable for outpatient treatment and reassessment if there were physical concerns (e.g., due to weight loss or frequent purging), is required. Patients who are hospitalized are not included in the outcome as they are considered non-responders to the treatment.

Similarities between FBT and CBT-E

Despite several differences, the general strategy of FBT and CBT-E is to address the maintaining mechanism of the eating disorder psychopathology, as opposed to an exploration of any potential causes of the eating disorder psychopathology. Indeed, both treatments take an agnostic view of the cause of the illness (i.e., no assumptions are made about the potential origins of eating disorders).

A major focus of both treatments is to help the adolescent patient to normalize body weight and to support the adolescent's return to a normal developmental trajectory of weight. Both FBT and CBT-E, although using different procedures, include regular weighing of the patients within each session. The focus of both FBT and CBT-E in addressing dietary restriction and low weight has led to suggest that perhaps one common mechanism of action of the two treatments might be exposure (and habituation) to feared food and its consumption [27].

Another possible mechanism of action shared by FBT and CBT-E is how they might indirectly reduce the over-evaluation of shape and weight once the patient has normalized weight: CBT-E helps the patient to enhance the importance of other domains of life (e.g., school, social life, hobbies, etc.), while FBT works toward increased personal autonomy for the adolescent.

Finally, both FBT and CBT-E set out to manage comorbid psychiatric diagnoses by involving a psychiatrist as part of the care team. Hospitalization, for psychiatric or medical acuity, is recommended only when the patients present with clinical severity that cannot or should not be managed in an outpatient setting.

Conclusions

FBT is the current evidence-based treatment for eating disorders in adolescents, as its efficacy has been assessed by several RCTs. However, the treatment presents a number of challenges. First, there are no direct comparisons of FBT with CBT-E or with other psychological treatments combined with nutritional rehabilitation aimed at weight restoration. Second, the current research evidence suggests that FBT works well with about two third of the parents and adolescents who accept the treatment, although less than 40% achieve a full remission. However, it cannot be used with those adolescents who do not have available parents, or for those with parents who are not accepting of a family-based treatment model. Third, even among those who do accept the treatment, there are sometimes difficulties implementing FBT given the expectation that all members of the family be actively involved, which may necessitate parents taking time away from work, disrupting sibling's schedules and creating complicated travel arrangements.

CBT-E is recommended for adolescents when FBT is unacceptable, contraindicated, or ineffective [3]. This recommendation is based on the promising findings derived by some cohort studies, and it is reinforced by a recent study in a real-world setting, showing outcome data similar to those reported by FBT [22].

The availability of two effective treatments for adolescents with eating disorders now opens the chance to compare them in a randomized controlled trial. Key variables of interest would include the acceptability of the two treatments, their short- and long-term efficacy, their cost cost-effectiveness, and the treatment response moderators that might allow the matching of adolescent patients to CBT-E or FBT. This is not improbable as they differ markedly in their strategies, procedures and postulated mechanisms of action. The atheoretical nature of the FBT [28] might suggest that it is well suited to the needs of younger adolescent patients. In contrast, CBT-E might have its greatest effect in older adolescent patients in whom the mechanisms that maintain eating disorder psychopathology are fully operating [17]. Older adolescents might also better accept an "adult" form of treatment rather than a family style one. However, these hypotheses require testing through a future RCT.

Authors' contributions
All the authors made substantial contributions to the paper, and all approved the final version.

Competing interests
The authors declare that they have no competing interests.

Author details
[1]Department of Eating and Weight Disorders, Villa Garda Hospital, Via Montebaldo 89 1-37016 Garda (VR), Verona, Italy. [2]Center for the Treatment of Eating Disorders, Children's Minnesota, Minneapolis, MN, USA. [3]Department of Psychiatry, University of California, San Francisco, CA, USA. [4]Department of Psychiatry and Behavioral Neuroscience, The University of Chicago, Chicago, IL, USA.

References

1. Lock J, Le Grange D. Treatment manual for anorexia nervosa: A family-based approach. 2nd ed. New York: Guilford Press; 2013 2013.
2. Russell GF, Szmukler GI, Dare C, Eisler I. An evaluation of family therapy in anorexia nervosa and bulimia nervosa. Arch Gen Psychiatry. 1987;44(12): 1047–56.
3. National Guideline Alliance (UK). Eating Disorders: Recognition and Treatment. London: National Institute for Health and Care Excellence (UK); 2017. (NICE Guideline, No. 69).
4. Dalle GR. Cognitive-behavioral therapy in adolescent eating disorders. In: Hebebrand J, Herpertz-Dahlmann B, editors. Eating disorders and obesity in children and adolescents. Philadelphia: Elsevier; 2019. p. 111–6.
5. El Ghoch M, Benini L, Sgarbi D, Dalle GR. Solitary rectal ulcer syndrome in a patient with anorexia nervosa: a case report. Int J Eat Disord. 2016;49(7): 731–5.
6. Le Grange D. Family therapy for adolescent anorexia nervosa. J Clin Psychol. 1999;55(6):727–39.
7. Minuchin S. Families and family therapy. London: Tavistock Publications; 1974.
8. Le Grange D, Hughes EK, Court A, Yeo M, Crosby RD, Sawyer SM. Randomized clinical trial of parent-focused treatment and family-based treatment for adolescent anorexia nervosa. J Am Acad Child Adolesc Psychiatry. 2016;55(8):683–92.
9. Katzman DK, Peebles R, Sawyer SM, Lock J, Le Grange D. The role of the pediatrician in family-based treatment for adolescent eating disorders: opportunities and challenges. J Adolesc Health. 2013;53(4):433–40.
10. Lian B, Forsberg SE, Fitzpatrick KK. Adolescent anorexia: guiding principles and skills for the dietetic support of family-based treatment. J Acad Nutr Diet. 2019;119(1):17–25.
11. Fairburn CG, Cooper Z, O'Connor M. In: Fairburn CG, editor. Eating Disorder Examination. New York: Cognitive behavior therapy and eating disorders Guilford Press; 2008. p. 265–308.
12. Lock J, Le Grange D. Family-based treatment: where are we and where should we be going to improve recovery in child and adolescent eating disorders. Int J Eat Disord. 2018.
13. Lock J, Le Grange D, Agras WS, Moye A, Bryson SW, Jo B. Randomized clinical trial comparing family-based treatment with adolescent-focused individual therapy for adolescents with anorexia nervosa. Arch Gen Psychiatry. 2010;67(10):1025–32.
14. Le Grange D, Crosby RD, Rathouz PJ, Leventhal BL. A randomized controlled comparison of family-based treatment and supportive psychotherapy for adolescent bulimia nervosa. Arch Gen Psychiatry. 2007;64(9):1049–56.
15. Fairburn C. A cognitive behavioural approach to the treatment of bulimia. Psychol Med. 1981;11(4):707–11.
16. Le Grange D, Lock J, Agras WS, Bryson SW, Jo B. Randomized Clinical Trial of Family-Based Treatment and Cognitive-Behavioral Therapy for Adolescent Bulimia Nervosa. J Am Acad Child Adolesc Psychiatry. 2015;54(11):886–94.e2.
17. Fairburn CG, Cooper Z, Shafran R. Cognitive behaviour therapy for eating disorders: a "transdiagnostic" theory and treatment. Behav Res Ther. 2003; 41(5):509–28.

18. Fairburn CG. Cognitive behavior therapy and eating disorders. New York: Guilford Press; 2008.
19. Dalle Grave R, Calugi S, Doll HA, Fairburn CG. Enhanced cognitive behaviour therapy for adolescents with anorexia nervosa: an alternative to family therapy? Behav Res Ther. 2013;51(1):R9–R12.
20. Dalle Grave R, Calugi S, Sartirana M, Fairburn CG. Transdiagnostic cognitive behaviour therapy for adolescents with an eating disorder who are not underweight. Behav Res Ther. 2015;73:79–82.
21. Calugi S, Dalle Grave R, Sartirana M, Fairburn CG. Time to restore body weight in adults and adolescents receiving cognitive behaviour therapy for anorexia nervosa. J Eat Disord. 2015;3:21.
22. Dalle Grave R, Sartirana M, Calugi S. Enhanced cognitive behavioral therapy for adolescents with anorexia nervosa: Outcomes and predictors of change in a real-world setting. Int J Eat Disord. 2019;0(0).
23. Madanes C Strategic family therapy. San Francisco, CA: Jossey-Bass; 1981.
24. Haley J. Uncommon therapy: the psychiatric techniques of Milton H. Erickson. New York: Norton; 1973.
25. Selvini-Palazzoli M. Self-starvation: from the Intrapsychic to the transpersonal approach to anorexia nervosa. London: Chaucer; 1974.
26. White M. Negative explanation, restraint, and double description: a template for family therapy. Fam Process. 1986;25(2):169–84.
27. Hildebrandt T, Bacow T, Markella M, Loeb KL. Anxiety in anorexia nervosa and its management using family-based treatment. Eur Eat Disord Rev. 2012;20(1):e1–16.
28. Loeb KL, Lock J, Le Grange D, Greif R. Transdiagnostic theory and application of family-based treatment for youth with eating disorders. Cogn Behav Pract. 2012;19(1):17–30.

6

Engaging primary care providers in managing pediatric eating disorders: a mixed methods study

Jocelyn Lebow[1,2*], Cassandra Narr[3], Angela Mattke[3], Janna R. Gewirtz O'Brien[4], Marcie Billings[3], Julie Hathaway[1], Kristin Vickers[1], Robert Jacobson[2,3] and Leslie Sim[1]

Abstract

Background: The primary care setting offers an attractive opportunity for, not only the identification of pediatric eating disorders, but also the delivery of evidence-based treatment. However, constraints of this setting pose barriers for implementing treatment. For interventions to be successful, they need to take into consideration the perspectives of stakeholders. As such, the purpose of this study was to examine in-depth primary care providers' perspective of challenges to identifying and managing eating disorders in the primary care setting.

Methods: This mixed methods study surveyed 60 Pediatric and Family Medicine providers across 6 primary care practices. Sixteen of these providers were further interviewed using a qualitative, semi-structured interview.

Results: Providers (n = 60, response rate of 45%) acknowledged the potential of primary care as a point of contact for early identification and treatment of pediatric eating disorders. They also expressed that this was an area of need in their practices. They identified numerous barriers to successful implementation of evidence-based treatment in this setting including scarcity of time, knowledge, and resources.

Conclusions: Investigations seeking to build capacities in primary care settings to address eating disorders must address these barriers.

Keywords: Anorexia nervosa, Bulimia nervosa, Eating disorder, Primary care, Adolescent

Plain English summary

The primary care setting offers an attractive opportunity for, not only the identification of eating disorders in children and adolescents, but also the delivery of interventions that can shorten the course of these life-threatening illnesses. However, due to the unique nature of primary care, effective interventions must be designed specifically to fit within this setting. As such, the purpose of this study was to examine primary care providers' perspective of challenges to identifying and managing eating disorders in the primary care setting. We surveyed 60 Pediatric and Family Medicine providers across 6 primary care practices. Sixteen of these providers were further questioned using more in-depth interview. Providers acknowledged the potential of primary care as a point of contact for early identification and treatment of pediatric eating disorders. They also expressed that this was an area of need in their practices. They identified numerous barriers to successful treatment in this setting including limited time, knowledge, and resources. Researchers seeking to build eating disorder interventions in primary care settings must address these numerous barriers.

* Correspondence: lebow.jocelyn@mayo.edu
[1]Department of Psychiatry and Psychology, Mayo Clinic, Mayo Clinic School of Medicine, 200 First Street SW, Rochester, MN 55905, USA
[2]Mayo Clinic Robert D. and Patricia E. Kern Center for the Science of Health Care Delivery, Rochester, MN, USA
Full list of author information is available at the end of the article

Introduction

Two of the highest priorities in the field of pediatric eating disorders are early identification and expanding access to evidence-based treatment [1]. Because delayed detection and treatment are associated with poor prognosis, prompt access to care is vital [2–4]. The substantial physical morbidity and mortality associated with eating disorders makes this agenda especially urgent [5]. Given the impact of the global COVID-19 pandemic on increasing rates and severity of eating disorders, the need for expanded options to identify eating disorders and access care is particularly salient [6].

Primary care offers several advantages for improving efficient and effective treatment of child and adolescent eating disorders. The majority of young patients with eating disorders present first to their primary care provider, often with complaints such as abdominal pain, fatigue, or menstrual abnormalities [7]. Although previous research suggests that primary care providers converge in identifying eating disorders as an area of concern, they express varying degrees of comfort with identification and management of these patients [8], and diverge on whether they feel this identification and management is within their scope of practice [9]. This discrepancy may lead to missed opportunities for early identification and intervention.

When pediatric and family medicine providers are given the expertise and direction to include eating disorders on their differential, they are well-positioned to identify these potentially life-threatening disorders early in the illness trajectory. In addition, primary care providers are well-suited to address patient and parent ambivalence in accepting an eating disorder diagnosis, a common barrier to treatment. Given the expertise of primary care providers in coaching families to engage in difficult but essential health behaviors (e.g. vaccinations, inhaler use, medication adherence), they are well-equipped to help patients and families transition from pre-contemplation to action in implementing behavior change.

Primary care providers may also bolster adherence through their often-longstanding relationships with families that can be leveraged to efficiently move families towards accepting the eating disorder diagnosis and preparing them to engage in intervention. In particular, research suggests that primary care providers' conversations with patients about health behaviors are linked to patient confidence in their ability to follow through on treatment recommendations [10]. As such, primary care providers may have a distinct ability to mobilize families to begin the lengthy and difficult process of addressing their child's eating disorder.

In spite of such advantages, implementation of eating disorder screening and intervention in primary care is complicated by numerous barriers, including scarcity of resources and time, as well as physician confidence and/or interest in treating these disorders [11]. Previous surveys of primary care physicians across the United States and Canada have found while up to 91% of pediatricians and family physicians feel that it is their role to assess for and identify eating disorders, they often fail to identify these conditions [9, 12]. For example, one study found that 68% of primary care providers only screened for eating disorders when it was associated with the patient's specific presenting problem [11].

When asked about eating disorder intervention, primary care providers were even less confident, with less than half reporting they felt they had the necessary skills to intervene with these disorders in their practice [11, 13]. In one study surveying a group of 70 pediatricians, only 21.5% reported feeling comfortable providing treatment for eating disorders [13]. In fact, the number of pediatricians who felt comfortable treating eating disorders was lower than for any other behavioral health problem including anxiety, depression, somatic symptom disorders, and attention deficit/hyperactivity disorder [13]. With regards to primary care training, less than half of family medicine and pediatric residents report receiving what they feel is adequate training in eating disorders during residency, and over 70% in each group expressed a desire to have more training in this area [14].

In order to successfully leverage the resources of the primary care setting, we must engage primary care provider stakeholders to help identify and address critical system-wide barriers. Though there have been several surveys of primary care providers' needs, comfort, and preferences in diagnosing and/or treating eating disorders, all these studies have been restricted to broad quantitative surveys, which limits a deeper understanding of opportunities for system-wide changes to enhance the identification and treatment of this population within primary care.

This mixed method study is the first attempt to clarify the perspectives of primary care providers on the identification and treatment of eating disorders in their practices using the combination of a broad survey with in-depth follow-up interviews to assess the attitudes and opinions of primary care providers representing both Family Medicine and Pediatrics, including physicians, nurse-practitioners and physician's assistants. Questions focused on their assessment of the need and feasibility for eating disorder care in a primary care setting, their level of confidence for managing children and adolescents with eating disorders in their practice, their view on what resources were needed to assist these patients in primary care, and their opinions on barriers that currently exist to providing effective management.

Methods

All primary care providers in six Midwestern practices who treated children (N = 132) were contacted to participate in a survey regarding managing pediatric eating disorders in their daily work. The primary care practices were all associated with an academic medical center and consisted of 5 separate clinics located in a midsize city and one clinic located in a rural community approximately 10 miles outside of the city. Along with a consent document, the paper survey was sent to 132 providers in the Division of Community Pediatrics and Adolescent Medicine (CPAM) and the Department of Family Medicine. Of these providers, 60 (45%) completed the survey. Primary care providers responded to a survey item regarding their willingness to participate in an in-person semi-structured interview to assess perceived needs and barriers for treating eating disorders within primary care. Twenty-five (42%) stated they would be willing to participate and, of these individuals, 16 providers participated in the semi-structured interviews before theoretical saturation [15] was reached.

The number of patients with an eating disorder that each provider estimated they saw each year varied widely from 2 to 15. Given the variability in experience and skills to identify eating disorders, this is not likely to represent the true prevalence of eating disorders but instead reflects how many they suspect present to their practice. The study was approved by the Mayo Clinic Institutional Review Board.

Measures

Recognizing the numerous competing demands on primary care providers' time, the 8-item quantitative survey was designed to be brief. Questions included Likert-scale ratings of confidence in identifying, medically managing, and advising families around decision-making for the treatment of pediatric eating disorders, as well as a question about the makeup of their patient panel. Primary care providers were also asked to evaluate a case study of a young patient with an eating disorder and discuss their clinical response in an additional item. Finally, providers were asked about their interest in new tools and strategies for addressing disordered eating in their practices. Since no reliable and valid tools exist to assess knowledge or confidence in treating eating disorders among primary care providers, based on a review of the literature, experts in the fields of eating disorders and qualitative research (J.L, L.S., K.V.) developed survey items and interview questions [8, 9, 11–14].

Provider interviews were conducted in-person by an experienced qualitative interviewer (JH) who was not involved with the primary care providers' clinical practice, and took an average of 15–20 min. The interviewer followed a semi-structured interview script that was designed with consideration of guidelines for minimizing bias and increasing the reliability and validity of interview data [16, 17]. Questions for primary care providers included close-ended prompts designed to gauge the provider's familiarity and comfort-level with eating disorder management and assessment, as well as open-ended questions regarding their needs, preferences, and potential barriers to be considered in the development of a primary-care based eating disorder intervention. Interviews were audio-recorded and transcribed verbatim. This interviewer also kept concurrent field notes to help with transcript interpretation. See Supplementary Material for both the quantitative survey and qualitative interview guide.

Analysis

Quantitative analysis of survey items was completed, including descriptive statistics appropriate for this level of data, using IBM Statistical Package for the Social Sciences, version 25. Qualitative data were coded using thematic analysis to identify core categories. Dominant themes, as determined based on multiple participants repeating similar experiences, attitudes, or needs, were identified and a coding strategy was developed. Two investigators (KV, JL) coded all qualitative interviews using content analysis, a systematic process of deductively sorting information based on previously identified themes [18, 19]. After investigators independently coded all qualitative data, predominant categories were agreed upon and representative quotes were identified. When discrepancies in coding occurred, the two analysts met and reviewed the full interview transcript to better understand meaning through examination of the original context.

Results

Quantitative data: brief provider perspective survey

Sixty out of the 132 primary care providers contacted (45% response rate) completed the 8-item survey examining self-reported confidence and interest in delivering eating disorder treatment in the primary care setting (Table 1). Participants included 14 providers from CPAM (23.3%), 37 from Family Medicine (61.7%) and 9 providers who declined to report their Department. In terms of education and role, 36 were physicians (MD or DO; 60%), 20 were nurse practitioners (33.3%), and 4 were physician assistants (6.7%,).

On a 10-point scale, where scores less than 5 were considered low, scores between 5 and 8 were considered moderate, and scores above 8 considered high, primary care providers endorsed moderate confidence in their

Table 1 Primary Care Provider Confidence and Interest in Delivering Eating Disorder Treatment ($N = 60$)

At this time ...	Mean (SD)
How confident are you in your ability to evaluate a patient for the presence of disordered eating in your daily practice? (0 = Not very confident; 10 = Very confident)	5.53 (2.09)
How confident are you in your ability to manage disordered eating in your daily practice? (0 = Not very confident; 10 = Very confident)	3.68 (2.20)
How confident are you in your ability to provide diagnostic feedback to families about the presence of an eating disorder/disordered eating in your daily practice? (0 = Not very confident; 10 = Very confident)	4.34 (2.26)
How confident are you in your ability to advise and support a patient and their family in making decisions about his/her eating disorder treatment? (0 = Not very confident; 10 = Very confident)	4.15 (2.11)
How interested would you be in learning new tools or strategies for addressing disordered eating in your practice? (0 = Not very interested; 10 = Very interested)	8.52 (1.83)
How interested would you be in the development of a new ICS [Integrated Community Specialty: specialists embedded in the practice] for addressing eating and weight disorders? (0 = Not very interested; 10 = Very interested)	8.81 (1.82)

** 2 additional items included a case example and a question about patient panel makeup

ability to evaluate a patient for an eating disorder (mean 5.53, SD 2.09), but low confidence in their ability to manage disordered eating in pediatric patients in their practices (means < 5 for all responses, SDs 2.11–2.26). Respondents rated themselves highly (means > 8, SDs 1.82–1.83) with respect to interest in learning new tools or strategies for eating disorder treatment in their clinical area and also in working with an eating disorder specialist integrated into their practice.

Qualitative data predominant themes: resource needs and feasibility concerns

Sixteen primary care providers (13 females, 81%) participated in interviews including 10 from Family Medicine and 6 from CPAM. Of these providers, 11 were physicians, and 5 were either nurse practitioners or physician assistants.

Interviews from these 16 providers revealed themes consistent with the survey data, in that providers value eating disorder treatment, have low confidence in their own ability to manage eating disorders in their clinical setting, and would be interested in receiving support from eating disorder experts in managing their patients with these complex problems. However, providers identified significant challenges providing care for patients with disordered eating within the constraints of the existing system. Here we organize the predominant themes in two sections. The first set of themes demonstrate provider recognition that current identification and care of pediatric patients with eating disorders is suboptimal in their primary care setting related to current practice barriers. The second set of themes reveal the complexities of successfully implementing and maintaining a new model of care for treatment of pediatric eating disorders in primary care. The resounding primary themes across all interviews and woven within all identified sub-themes are the debilitating impact of insufficient time and the competing demands for that limited time, as experienced by all primary care providers interviewed.

Current barriers to optimal eating disorder management in primary care

Providers described personal, professional, and system-level issues that contribute to a status quo of sub-optimal identification and treatment of pediatric eating disorders, as well as the complexities associated with these disorders themselves. Most providers do not feel there is sufficient time or a simple process to identify young patients with eating disorders: "In primary care, we have X amount of time with patients and our nurses have multiple things to screen for. There's educational factors, there's exercise, there's tobacco exposures, there's health exposures, there's screen time. There are so many things to screen for that we end up diluting what we do effectively. So, time is the enemy in multiple screening. How do you decide to spend your time screening for eating disorders versus convincing them to get HPV vaccination?" (participant 014). Some feel they lack sufficient knowledge to intensify their treatment of these patients, and given limited time and the perception of eating disorders being a less frequent problem, they focus on other important mental health and physical health issues. None diminish the importance of eating disorder treatment: "Honestly probably not interested in training on this. Just that I'm stretched too thin right now and I'm working on saying no to things. I care about this issue and I would like to see better services for our patients." (participant 001).

In contrast to an existing process at 3 of these 6 practices for screening adolescents with depression and connecting them to onsite treatment, there is no systematic approach to eating disorder identification or treatment in their setting. Primary care providers view eating disorder management as complex, and cite aspects such as challenging family dynamics, patients resisting treatment, and provider concerns about the potential to harm the patient/provider relationship if a diagnosis or treatment is pushed: "It's very difficult to have success with people with eating disorders" (participant 013); "It's something that we are not specifically trained in;" and "It's super emotional and can get ugly and there's that impact on the trust and relationship" (participant 001).

Further, if patients do require specialty care, there is a troubling lack of local treatment options. In fact, primary care providers explained that local eating disorder treatment options have decreased, with the few specialists unable to meet the current demand. There is an implicit theme of emotional exhaustion among providers at the thought of trying to do more for these complex patients as a non-specialist when access to more intensive, medically-necessary treatment is unavailable.

Future challenges in implementing system change for pediatric eating disorder management in primary care setting

Though providers appreciated the importance of eating disorder identification and treatment, they expressed mixed views about the feasibility of a program meant to support eating disorder treatment in primary care. Some primary care providers expressed an interest in an integrated model of care, in which providers would receive training in eating disorders and then provide direct care in collaboration with a specialist: "Anything. I'd be interested in anything. Lectures, conferences, webinars." (participant 015).

Though many primary care providers recognized a need to better serve patients with eating disorders, most providers described ambivalence, and some were pessimistic about model implementation without addressing key barriers, such as inadequate time and limited resources." I guess we could do it but we can't do it without scheduled time. We already have so much that we do that is not scheduled that it's ridiculous already." (participant 012). Some expressed concerns about compatibility with the workflow and the relative advantage of implementing a new program, rather than continuing with the status quo of referring elsewhere, "It's not completely reasonable honestly and it concerns me. If the choice is nothing or that, then it's probably a good thing to do... or let the [established eating disorder program 90 miles away provide eating disorder care]." (participant 001). Others suggest that there are a few providers that want to do more of this work: "I think probably like three of us that are working on it or interested. There might be a couple more." (participant 015).

Although not a major theme, some providers made comparisons to existing programs in primary care that include the integrated care program for adolescent depression, and there was appreciation for standardized, brief screening tools and onsite support. Others say that these same resources are spread too thin currently, and access remains a problem, which may contribute to lack of enthusiasm for a new care model for eating disorder treatment. Sustainability of a new program and affordability to patients were also mentioned as concerns.

Discussion

This mixed methods study is the first to take an in-depth look at the attitudes, perceived needs, and barriers primary care providers face in implementing screening and/or eating disorder management in primary care. These results suggest that, in line with previous broad-based survey studies [11, 12], though providers are aware that they need additional support in addressing eating disorders, they are frustrated by the lack of resources and real barriers to care, such as competing demands for limited time and lack of processes to best serve young patients with eating disorders. They emphasize that implementation of any primary care-based eating disorder interventions must be thoughtful and strategic, or risk repeating failures of past programs.

Similar to previous studies, primary care providers reported that they lack the time, training, and skills to provide or access appropriate eating disorder care for their patients. Providers are willing to follow guidelines, but have limited awareness regarding clinical best practices. Also resonant with other surveys [9, 11, 13], they endorse low levels of confidence in their ability to identify and manage eating disorders, which they view as complex and challenging illnesses. Although they endorse a strong desire to improve their skills to help these patients, they identify numerous barriers to doing so, including limited time for provider training and implementation. Finally, providers expressed concern about the lack of validated, effective, and efficient screening tools for pediatric patients, as well as concerns about the realities of implementing any type of universal screening in their already overburdened and brief visits. Though eating disorder screeners exist, most (e.g. the SCOFF) [20] are not validated for pediatric patients. The few screeners that are validated for younger populations (e.g. the Eating Attitudes Test (EAT-26) [21]) are relatively lengthy for integration into a busy primary care practice, especially at the level of universal screening.

The lack of eating disorder resources was a source of significant dissatisfaction for providers. They expressed negative emotion around the lack of resources including shame and frustration that, even at a well-known, highly-resourced institution, there were few treatment options to offer pediatric patients with eating disorders. They also discussed the tremendous burden this places on patients and their families of having to seek treatment at an outside program, frequently outside the region or state.

There was consensus that the current status of eating disorder resources is insufficient to care for young patients in their community. Primary care providers expressed a clear desire to help these patients and a need for support to do so. Because they frequently encountered these patients in their practice, they believed that the primary care setting has considerable potential for the early intervention of these conditions. Yet, they stated for this to happen, the intervention must fit within the constraints of the practice. In the context of the current system, a primary care-based program for pediatric eating disorders might be at risk for failure were it not to consider these barriers during planning and implementation. In other words, primary care providers voiced a rational ambivalence about offering screening, intervention, and management of eating disorders in primary care. Although they feel this is an important and an underserved area, they are concerned about stretching their already overtaxed resources to address these complex and challenging patients, without practice-level changes and supports.

This is particularly important at present. On one hand, the global COVID-19 pandemic has led to increased numbers of patients with eating disorders struggling to access care [6], and thus, there is great need for additional avenues to identify and treat patients with eating disorders, such as could be implemented through primary care. On the other hand, however, the pandemic has exponentially multiplied the demands on health care providers' time, energy, and other resources. For programs to be successful, it is important for the specialist hoping to enter the primary care setting to understand the landscape. Specialists need to address the actual barriers to eating disorder management, including the scarcity of time, provider discomfort with the illness, and the perceived complexity of the disorder. It is tempting for eating disorder specialists to assume the main barrier to primary care-based eating disorder care is a knowledge gap, and that effective intervention will begin (and potentially end) with psychoeducation about eating disorder detection and management. This lack of cultural humility gravely misunderstands the actual barriers in primary care, and, at best, will result in the provision of redundant information to a group that is already aware of the dangers of eating disorders. At worst, knowledge-based interventions run the risk of increasing already-present feelings of guilt and shame in primary care providers without providing any sort of workable solution.

Primary care is not a setting where it is feasible for a specialist to enter, implement an intervention program (even one with a strong evidence base), and leave. Workable solutions begin with relationship-building among stakeholders, and should be informed by implementation science. It is not sufficient to attempt to implement a model that has worked in a specialty setting; specialists must spend time developing an innovative intervention that is effective and sustainable within the primary care system.

In general, possessing onsite resources greatly increases the chance of a referral, even if that resource was not tailored for eating disorders. As part of the quantitative survey providers stated they would be very likely to refer identified eating disorder patients to existing social workers embedded in the practice, even though this resource is not set up to deliver eating disorder treatment. This speaks to the major demands on providers' time that necessitate a convenient resource. Consequently, attempts to engage primary care providers in eating disorder management would be wise to rely on existing processes including convenient and onsite resources if at all possible.

Primary care providers particularly favored a design wherein a few colleagues in the practice are given extra training and identified as experts or "superusers" [22]. Specifically, this core team would provide assurance that the identifying provider will receive assistance throughout the treatment and the patient will not be the sole responsibility of the identifying provider. Having this core team could potentially improve screening and detection even without additional training for the practice. It is possible that, once a motivated few are in place as experts, confidence and knowledge of the entire practice could grow and fear might decrease. Importantly, this also serves to improve assessment and detection, because providers know they have a resource to which to refer if needed.

Findings must be interpreted within the context of several limitations. In particular, while the quantitative survey was sent to all primary care providers who worked with children at the 6 practices, concerns about maintaining confidentiality of respondents meant that differences between responders and nonresponders were not able to be evaluated. Though the quantitative and qualitative surveys were developed by content and methodological experts, we were unable to assess the validity of these measures. Further, providers self-selected for the qualitative interview, which may have influenced the generalizability of our results. Additionally, providers were all practicing in clinics serving largely rural or suburban populations, it is unclear how these results would generalize to providers in other settings, including those that serve within urban centers. Finally, results may be influenced by the particular treatment resources available to this sample of primary care provider participants. As noted, this medical center has numerous mental health resources, including embedded pediatric mental health services and social work and, as such, providers are perhaps more sensitized to the potential for integrating mental health intervention within the primary care setting.

Conclusions

Despite these limitations, this study fills an important gap both in confirming primary care providers' perceptions of the potential of primary care as a point of assessment and triage for young patients with eating disorders, and exploring barriers that need to be addressed in order to successfully integrate these services into the setting. Specialists in the field of eating disorders should attend to the findings that primary care providers see improving eating disorder detection and education as an area of need, and one that is important to their practice. Equally salient is the idea that all interventions are not created equal, and that attempts to leverage this setting to improve early detection and intervention for eating disorders must take into account the noted barriers and needs of the primary care setting. Further research is needed to develop programs of eating disorder education and intervention that meet the needs and fill the gaps identified by primary care providers and to examine the feasibility and efficacy of these programs for treating pediatric patients with eating disorders.

Abbreviations

CPAM: Community Pediatrics and Adolescent Medicine; EAT-26: Eating Attitudes Test

Acknowledgements

The authors would like to thank the primary care providers in the Community Pediatric and Adolescent Medicine and Family Medicine divisions at Mayo Clinic for contributing their invaluable perspectives to this study.

Authors' contributions

JL conceptualized the study, designed the survey/interview questions, helped analyze/code the data and was a major contributor in writing the manuscript. CN, AM, JGO, MB and RJ helped conceptualize the study, reviewed the study materials, and helped recruit participants. JH conducted and transcribed all qualitative interviews and contributed to the manuscript. JH conducted all qualitative interviews and analyzed the quantitative data. KV coded all qualitative data and spearheaded the qualitative data analysis as well as contributing to the manuscript. LS conceptualized the study and was a major contributor in writing the manuscript. All authors read and approved the final manuscript.

Competing interests

The authors declare they have no competing interests.

Author details

[1]Department of Psychiatry and Psychology, Mayo Clinic, Mayo Clinic School of Medicine, 200 First Street SW, Rochester, MN 55905, USA. [2]Mayo Clinic Robert D. and Patricia E. Kern Center for the Science of Health Care Delivery, Rochester, MN, USA. [3]Department of Pediatric and Adolescent Medicine, Mayo Clinic School of Medicine, Rochester, MN, USA. [4]Department of Pediatrics, University of Minnesota, Minneapolis, MN, USA.

References

1. Project HEAL, top mental health experts outline priorities for eating disorder field moving forward [news release]. Mountain View, CA: Project HEAL; September 7, 2016. http://theprojectheal.org/5643-2/. Accessed September 27, 2016.
2. Le Grange D, Lock J, Agras W, Moye A, Bryson S, Jo B, et al. Moderators and mediators of remission in family-based treatment and adolescent focused therapy for anorexia nervosa. Behav Res Ther. 2012;50:85–92.
3. van Son G, van Hoeken D, van Furth E, Donker G, Hoek H. Course and outcome of eating disorders in a primary care-based cohort. Int J Eat Disord. 2010;43(2):130–8.
4. Steinhausen H. Outcome of eating disorders. Child Adolesc Psychiatr Clin N Am. 2009;18(1):225–42.
5. Arcelus J, Mitchell AJ, Wales J, Nielsen S. Mortality rates in patients with anorexia nervosa and other eating disorders: a meta-analysis of 36 studies. Arch Gen Psychiat. 2011;68(7):724–31.
6. Termorshuizen J, Watson H, Thornton L, Borg S, Flatt R, MacDermond B, et al. Early impact of COVID-19 on individuals with self-reported eating disorders: a survey of ~1,000 individuals in the United States and the Netherlands. Int J Eat Disord. 2020;53(11):1780–90.
7. Hoek HW. Incidence, prevalence and mortality of anorexia nervosa and other eating disorders. Curr Opin Psychiatr. 2006;19(4):389–94.
8. Clarke I, Polimeni-Walker I. Treating individuals with eating disorders in family practice: a needs assessment. Eat Disord. 2004;12:293–301.
9. Stein R, McCue Horowitz S, Storfer-Isser A, Heneghan A, Olson L, Eaton Hoagwood K. Do pediatricians think they are responsible for identification and management of child mental health problems? Results of the AAP periodic survey. Amb Peds. 2008;8(1):11–7.
10. Vickers K, Kircher K, Smith M, Petersen L, Rasmussen N. Health behavior counseling in primary care: provider-reported rate and confidence. Fam Med. 2007:730–5.
11. Linville D, Brown T, O'Neil M. Medical providers' self-perceived knowledge and skills for working with eating disorders: a national survey. Eat Disord. 2002;20(1):1–13.
12. Robinson AL, Boachie A, Lafrance GA. Assessment and treatment of pediatric eating disorders: a survey of physicians and psychologists. J Canad Acad Child Adolesc Psychiatr. 2012;21(1):45–52.
13. Winders Davis D, Honaker SM, Jones VF, Williams PG, Stocker F, Martin E. Identification and management of behavioral/mental health problems in primary care pediatrics: perceived strengths, challenges, and new delivery models. Clin Peds. 2012;10:978–82.
14. Leigh H, Stewart D, Mallios R. Mental health and psychiatry training in primary care residency programs: part II. What skills and diagnoses are taught, how adequate, and what affects training directors' satisfaction? Gen Hosp Psychiatr. 2006;28(3):195–204.
15. Sandelowski M. Theoretical saturation. In: Given LM, editor. The SAGE encyclopedia of qualitative research methods. Thousand Oaks: Sage; 2008. p. 875–6.
16. Denzin N, Lincoln Y. Handbook of qualitative research. 2nd ed. SAGE: Thousand Oaks; 2000.

17. Kirk J, Miller M. Reliability and validity of qualitative research. SAGE: London; 1986.
18. Neuendorf K. The content analysis guidebook. 1st ed. SAGE: Thousand Oaks; 2001.
19. Patton M. Qualitative evaluation and research methods. SAGE: Newbury Park; 1990.
20. Morgan J, Reid F, Lacey JH. The SCOFF questionnaire: a new screening tool for eating disorders. West J Med. 2000;172(3):164–5.
21. Garner D, Olmsted M, Bohr Y, Garfinkel P. The eating attitudes test: psychometric features and clinical correlates. Psych Med. 1982;12:871–8.
22. Yuan C, Bradley E, Nembhard I. A mixed methods study of how clinician 'super users' influence others during the implementation of electronic health records. BMC Med Inform Decis. 2015;15(1):26.

7

Diabetes and disordered eating behaviours in a community-based sample of Australian adolescents

Kirrilly M. Pursey[1], Phillipa Hay[2,3], Kay Bussey[4], Nora Trompeter[4], Alexandra Lonergan[4], Kathleen M. Pike[5], Jonathon Mond[6,7] and Deborah Mitchison[2,8*]

Abstract

Background: People with diabetes have been shown to be at risk for disordered eating compared to their non-diabetic peers. However, the majority of studies have been conducted in relatively small samples drawn from clinical diabetes settings or registries. Community-based samples are required to better understand disordered eating behaviours in this population. In a large community-based population sample of Australian adolescents, this study aimed to (1) investigate disordered eating behaviours in adolescents reporting a diagnosis of diabetes compared to their non-diabetic peers and (2) test associations between disordered eating behaviours and insulin restriction.

Methods: Secondary school students ($n = 4854$; mean (SD) age 14.4 (1.6) years; 47% boys) completed an online survey, including self-reported presence of diabetes, demographics, weight status, substance use, insulin restriction and disordered eating behaviours. Clinically meaningful cut-offs for disordered eating behaviours were generated for analysis.

Results: Disordered eating behaviours, specifically self-induced vomiting (diabetes 19.2%, no diabetes 3.3%; $p < 0.001$), laxative use (diabetes 15.4%, no diabetes 2.1%; $p < 0.001$), use of cigarettes (diabetes 26.9%, no diabetes 4.3%; $p < 0.001$) and other drugs (diabetes 28.9%, no diabetes 4.0%; $p < 0.001$), cleanse/detox (diabetes 30.8%, no diabetes 10.5%; $p < 0.001$) and extreme weight loss diets (diabetes 13.5%, no diabetes 4.7%; $p < 0.003$) were higher in those reporting a diagnosis of diabetes. In addition, 17% of those with diabetes reported frequent insulin restriction (≥ once per week), and insulin restriction was associated with more frequent disordered eating behaviours.

Conclusion: There was a high rate of disordered eating behaviours in adolescents with diabetes compared to their peers without diabetes. The findings of this study may have the potential to inform future health promotion, prevention, and early intervention approaches for those with comorbid diabetes and disordered eating behaviours. Future longitudinal studies are required to evaluate disordered eating behaviours in those with diabetes over time in community-based samples.

Keywords: Disordered eating behaviours, Diabetes, Eating disorders, Adolescence

* Correspondence: deborah.mitchison@westernsydney.edu.au
[2]Translational Health Research Institute, School of Medicine, Western Sydney University, Sydney, NSW, Australia
[8]Department of Psychology, Macquarie University, Sydney, NSW, Australia
Full list of author information is available at the end of the article

Plain English summary

People with diabetes are at increased risk of developing disordered eating behaviours compared to people without diabetes. However, studies in the general community are needed to better understand disordered eating in adolescents with diabetes. We conducted an online survey in a large group of adolescents. This study found that several disordered eating behaviours were more common in adolescents with diabetes, including self-induced vomiting, laxative use, use of cigarettes and other illicit drugs, detox and extreme weight loss diets. This study may help to inform future treatments and prevention of disordered eating behaviours in adolescents with diabetes.

Introduction

Eating disorders are complex mental health disorders and have one of the highest mortality and suicide rates of any mental illness [1, 2]. Meta-analytical data has shown that the prevalence of disordered eating behaviours are increasing in the general population [3–5] and a recent study found the point prevalence of any clinical or subclinical eating disorder to be 22% in Australian adolescents [6]. Another common health problem in adolescence is diabetes, predominantly Type 1 Diabetes (T1D) [7]. T1D is an auto-immune condition where the pancreas does not produce insulin. It is one of the most common chronic conditions in childhood and management requires careful monitoring of dietary intake and insulin use. In Type 2 Diabetes (T2D), the body becomes resistant to insulin or the pancreas does not produce adequate insulin. T2D is linked to modifiable lifestyle factors such as diet and exercise and is more common in adulthood; however, it is increasingly occurring in children and adolescents. Although there is no nationally representative data as to the proportion of adolescents affected by T1D in Australia, it is estimated that approximately 6400 Australian children and adolescents aged up to 14 years had T1D in 2016 [8]. While T2D is increasing in adolescence, it represents a far smaller proportion of adolescent diabetes, with an estimated prevalence of 0.01% in those aged 10–14 years and 0.04% in Australians aged 15–19 years [9].

People with diabetes have been shown to be an at-risk group for the development of disordered eating behaviours and consequently eating disorders compared to their non-diabetic peers [10]. Managing diabetes during adolescence can be challenging due to developmental and hormonal changes associated with this life stage [10]. This age also coincides with the peak incidence of eating disorders [11]. In a meta-analysis of 13 studies, 7% of adolescents with T1D were classified as having a diagnosable eating disorder, compared to 2.8% of adolescents without diabetes. Disordered eating behaviours such as self-induced vomiting, excessive exercise and laxative use have also been shown to be significantly more frequent among adolescents with T1D compared to those without diabetes [12]. While the cause of disordered eating in people with T1D is unclear, it may be due to several factors including the greater emphasis placed on monitoring dietary intake and maintaining a healthy weight, as well as insulin-related weight gain and resultant body dissatisfaction [12]. In T1D in particular, intentional insulin restriction is a unique disordered eating behaviour and method for rapid weight loss and caloric purging without the need for severe food restriction. While disordered eating patterns, particularly binge eating, have been identified in people with T2D [13], the majority of scientific literature has focused predominantly on binge eating behaviour in adults. Disordered eating behaviour including insulin restriction in people with diabetes is particularly concerning as it is associated with short-term physical complications including deteriorating glycaemic control and diabetic ketoacidosis, as well as long-term complications such as retinopathy, neuropathy, and premature death [14]. In addition, disordered eating behaviours are associated with impaired psycho-social functioning [15]. Given the ubiquity of disordered eating in diabetes and severity of associated complications, there is a need for a better understanding of this phenomenon to inform future intervention strategies, particularly during adolescence which is a developmental period of significant biological and social changes.

To date, the majority of studies investigating associations between diabetes and eating disorders have been conducted in relatively small samples drawn from clinical diabetes settings or registries [16], which may affect representativeness of the samples and generalisability to the broader population. Findings have also been mixed with regards to the impact of disordered eating on metabolic status [17] and very few studies have investigated community-based and population samples [18, 19]. Moreover, the majority of research has not assessed a broad spectrum of disordered eating behaviours [20], rather focusing on single aspects such as narrowly defined eating disorder diagnoses. Evaluating a range of disordered eating behaviours is needed to better characterise problematic eating patterns in this population, given the transdiagnostic nature of most eating disorder behaviours. Further, these behaviours may occur prior to eating disorder onset, and thus evaluating disordered eating in adolescents with T1D is important if we are to improve current treatment approaches, as well as screening and early intervention models to reduce the likelihood of progression to a diagnosable eating disorder. Studies in the general population, as opposed to clinical settings, are particularly timely and important to inform future community-based prevention and health promotion approaches that include vulnerable subgroups, such as those individuals with diabetes. Finally, community-based samples are required to fully understand the scope of the disordered eating among adolescents with diabetes in comparison to the non-diabetic population. Barriers to such an endeavour to date include the feasibility of recruiting large enough samples to allow detection of a sufficient group of participants with diabetes to facilitate meaningful analysis. The large, community-based sample in the present study provides a unique opportunity to undertake such an investigation.

The aim of this study was to evaluate a range of disordered eating behaviours in adolescents reporting a diagnosis of diabetes compared to their non-diabetic peers in a large community-based population sample of Australian adolescents, as well as to evaluate disordered eating behaviours according to insulin restriction in adolescents reporting diabetes. It was hypothesised that eating disorder behaviours would be higher in adolescents reporting diabetes compared to those without, and that insulin restriction would be associated with greater disordered eating behaviours.

Methods

This is a secondary data analysis as part of the first wave of the EveryBODY study, a longitudinal investigation of eating disorders and body image concerns among Australian adolescents. Full details of the study are published elsewhere [6, 21]. Briefly, school principals and welfare staff of 50 secondary schools in the Hunter region, NSW, Australia, were contacted for participation. In an effort to improve ethnic diversity and representativeness, seven Sydney schools were subsequently invited to participate in the study. A final sample of thirteen schools participated in the study ($n = 12$ Hunter region, $n = 1$ Sydney). Government schools accounted for 67% of participating schools, followed by 33% Independent schools. Total enrolments across participating schools ranged from 514 to 1305 students, with approximately 70% of enrolled students at each school participating in the study. The school Index of Socio-Educational Advantage (ISCEA) of participating schools was close to the general population mean, however, there was less variation in socioeconomic status than the general population [21].

All students from participating school year groups were invited to participate in the online survey, which was completed at school under the supervision of teachers. Information regarding the study was provided to both parents and students in advance of testing. A passive parental consent procedure was used, whereby consent was assumed if parents did not actively opt their child out of the study. Students were required to provide online assent for participation on the day of the survey. At the end of the survey, students were provided with handouts, which contained information regarding resources and referral pathways for disordered eating and general mental health. All students who agreed were entered into a prize draw to win one of ten $100 gift cards. Ethics approval was received from the Macquarie University ethics committee and the New South Wales Department of Education.

Measures

The online survey was comprised of self-reported items including demographics, self-reported height and weight, eating disorder behaviours, appearance-related scales, quality of life, mental health outcomes, social media activity, bullying and sexual and gender identities. The survey was pilot tested prior to its release to ensure the survey language was appropriate and could be completed within a 50-min class. As part of the current analysis, only variables relating to reported presence of diabetes, demographics, weight status, and disordered eating behaviours were included.

Demographics

Demographic variables were assessed including sex, age, country of birth, and postal code. Postal code was used to estimate participants area-level socioeconomic status (SES) using the Socioeconomic Index for Areas (SEIFA) Index of Relative Socioeconomic Advantage and Disadvantage (IRSAD), which classifies postcodes into deciles from 1 (most disadvantaged/least advantaged) to 10 (least disadvantaged/most advantaged) [22].

Self-reported diabetes diagnosis

Due to the community-based nature of the survey, as well as the age and comprehension levels of the adolescent sample recruited, a single dichotomous question was used to assess the presence of diabetes: "Have you ever been told by a doctor that you have diabetes?". The question did not differentiate between T1D and T2D. Presence of diabetes (response options: yes/no) was used to categorise participants for analysis.

Anthropometrics

Participants were asked to self-report height (in centimetres) and weight (in kilograms), which was used to calculate body mass index (BMI) centile, adjusted for child age and gender. Online self-reported height and weight has previously been found to be valid for both adolescents and young adults [23, 24].

Eating disorders examination questionnaire

The Eating Disorders Examination Questionnaire (EDE-Q) was used to assess weight/shape concerns and disordered eating behaviours. The EDE-Q is a 28-item tool that assesses eating disorder pathology over the previous 28-days. The questions are scored using a 7-point Likert scale, with higher scores indicating greater eating disorder pathology. For the current study, only the weight and shape concern subscales (combined) and behavioural items were included.

The weight and shape concern subscales include 12 items in total, which are averaged such that scores range from 0 to 6, with higher scores indicating more severe weight/shape concerns. This combined weight/shape concern scale has previously been validated in Australian adolescents [25]. Disordered eating behaviours for the purposes of weight or shape control that were assessed as part of the EDE-Q included objective binge eating, subjective binge eating, self-induced vomiting, use of laxatives, and driven exercise. Respondents are asked to indicate the frequency of these behaviours over the past 28 days using a free response format.

Other and atypical weight control Behaviour's including insulin omission

Several additional behavioural frequency items were developed by the research team to assess other behaviours used for weight control purposes including: fasting for eight hours or more, cigarette smoking, other drug use, detoxes or cleanses, and strict weight loss diet. In addition, insulin restriction was assessed for those with diabetes using the following question: *"Over the past 4 weeks (28 days) how many times have you used less insulin (if you are diabetic) than you should have as a means of controlling your shape or weight?"*. Disordered eating behaviours were reported as frequency over the past 28 days. Frequency of at least once per week (i.e. 4 occasions per 28 days) was interpreted as frequent insulin restriction for the current study in line with the frequencies used for other behavioural symptoms in bulimia nervosa and binge eating disorder [26].

Data analysis

A dedicated data set was derived of complete data for the main study variables in this study. Thus, from a total of 5191 participants who completed the survey, 337 respondents were excluded due to missing data on the variables of interest, resulting in a final sample of 4854 students for the current analyses. Participant characteristics were analysed descriptively, with data presented as frequencies for categorical data, mean (SD) for parametric data, and medians (IQR) for non-parametric data. To generate clinically meaningful cut-offs, disordered eating behaviours were transformed into a dichotomous variable. Consistent with previous research [6, 15, 25], the following cut-offs were used to categorise variables: *Any occurrence (≥1 time in past 28 days):* cigarette smoking, other drugs, detox/cleanse; *Weekly occurrence (≥4 times in past 28 days):* fasting, objective binge eating, subjective binge eating, self-induced vomiting, laxative use, insulin omission; *Greater than 3 days per week (≥13 times in past 28 days):* strict weight loss diet; *Five days per week or greater (≥20 times in past 28 days):* driven exercise.

For demographic comparisons between adolescents with and without diabetes, *t*-tests were used for continuous variables, while chi-squared tests were used for categorical variables. Univariate logistic regression models adjusted for age, sex and BMI centile were used to calculate odds ratios for disordered eating behaviours according to presence of diabetes. Data were grouped into younger (11–14 years) and older (15–19 years) adolescents to assess if there were any associations between disordered eating behaviours and age. Due to the low numbers of participants with diabetes who reported restricting insulin, Mann Whitney-U tests for continuous data and Fishers Exact tests for categorical data were used to compare these participants to those with diabetes who did not report restricting insulin.

Results

Participant characteristics are presented in Table 1. The mean age of participants was 14.4 (±1.6) years (range 11–19 years) and 47% were boys. Little's MCAR test demonstrated data were not missing at random ($p < 0.001$). Compared to the current study sample, survey non-completers had a higher proportion of males (completers 47%, non-completers 59%; $p < 0.001$), were older (completers 14.4 years, non-completers 15.2 years; $p < 0.001$) and had a higher BMI centile (completers 54.1, non-completers 58.8; $p = 0.03$). The majority of participants were in Grade 7 ($n = 1069$), followed by Grade 10 ($n = 1047$), Grade 8 ($n = 1011$), Grade 9 ($n = 915$), Grade 11 ($n = 543$) and Grade 12 ($n = 269$). The mean BMI centile was 54.1 (± 30.9) with 65% classified as normal weight. Participants were from a range of socioeconomic backgrounds with a mean SEIFA decile of 5 (range 1–10). A total of 52 (1.1%) adolescents self-reported receiving a diagnosis of diabetes from a doctor. The diabetes group had a higher proportion of participants within the obese BMI category ($p < 0.001$).

Disordered eating behaviours

Disordered eating behaviours according to diabetes status are presented in Table 2. Those with diabetes reported higher frequency of disordered eating behaviours including self-induced vomiting, laxative use, use of cigarettes and other drugs for weight or shape control, and cleanse/detox and extreme weight loss diets, compared to those with no diabetes. Adolescents with diabetes had between 2.7 and 6.3 greater odds of reporting several disordered eating behaviours, especially those associated with weight control. The behaviours that were most strongly associated with diabetes, controlling for demographic differences, were the use of cigarettes, laxatives and other drugs for weight control purposes. Weight and shape concerns, fasting, driven exercise and binge eating were also higher in participants reporting diabetes, however this did not reach statistical significance.

Table 1 Participant characteristics according to presence of diabetes

	Total sample ($n = 4854$)	Diabetes ($n = 52$)	No diabetes ($n = 4802$)	p
	Mean (SD)			
Age *mean (SD)*	14.4 (1.6)	14.5 (1.9)	14.4 (1.6)	0.55
BMI percentile *mean (SD)*	54.1 (30.9)	61.7 (27.7)	54.0 (30.9)	0.14
SEIFA *mean (SD)*	985.0 (42.0)	977.9 (41.3)	985.1 (42.0)	0.24
SEIFA decile *mean (SD)*	5.3 (1.9)	5.6 (1.6)	5.3 (1.9)	0.30
	% (n)			
Sex [boys]	47.0 (2282)	59.6 (31)	46.9 (2251)	0.07
Weight category				
Underweight	7.5 (366)	3.9 (2)	7.6 (364)	
Normal Weight	64.8 (3144)	51.9 (27)	64.9 (3117)	
Overweight	12.6 (612)	7.7 (4)	12.7 (608)	
Obese	15.1 (732)	36.5 (19)	14.9 (713)	**<.001**
Country of birth				
Australian	89.6 (4347)	84.6 (44)	89.6 (4303)	
European	2.1 (102)	1.9 (1)	2.1 (101)	
Asian	5.5 (267)	5.8 (3)	5.5 (264)	
Other	2.8 (138)	7.7 (4)	2.8 (134)	0.26

Notes: *BMI* body mass index, *SEIFA* Socioeconomic Index for Areas

No significant associations were identified between disordered eating behaviours and age group.

Insulin restriction

Nine participants (17%) reporting diabetes reported regular insulin restriction for the purpose of weight loss (frequency of ≥1 per week). There were no significant differences between groups for age or BMI centile. Disordered eating behaviours were significantly higher in those reporting insulin restriction compared to those not restricting insulin including (all Fishers Exact) fasting (33.3% vs 4.7%, respectively; $p = 0.03$), objective binge eating (77.8% vs 14.0%, respectively; $p < 0.001$), subjective binge eating (77.8% vs 9.3%, respectively; $p < 0.001$), self-induced vomiting (66.7% vs 9.3%, respectively; $p = 0.001$), laxative use (77.8% vs 2.3%, respectively; $p < 0.001$), driven

Table 2 Frequency and odds of eating disorder behaviours, weight and shape concern according to reported presence of diabetes

	Total sample ($N = 4854$)	Diabetes ($n = 52$)	No diabetes ($n = 4802$)	x^2 (p) [a]	Odds ratio (95% CI) [b]
	% (n)				
EDE Q Disordered eating behaviours					
Fasting	10.5 (511)	9.6 (5)	10.5 (506)	0.1 (0.83)	0.2 (0.03, 1.7)
Objective binge eating	17.4 (844)	25.0 (13)	17.3 (831)	2.1 (0.15)	1.1 (0.5, 2.5)
Subjective binge eating	17.2 (834)	21.2 (11)	17.1 (823)	0.1 (0.45)	0.4 (0.1, 1.4)
Self-induced vomiting	3.5 (170)	19.2 (10)	3.3 (160)	**38.5 (< 0.001)**	3.9 (1.3, 11.3)
Laxative use	2.2 (108)	15.4 (8)	2.1 (100)	**41.8 (< 0.001)**	4.7 (1.4, 15.7)
Driven exercise	5.5 (268)	3.9 (2)	5.5 (266)	0.3 (0.60)	1.0
Cigarette use	4.6 (222)	26.9 (14)	4.3 (208)	**60.2 (< 0.001)**	4.8 (1.9, 11.7)
Illicit drug use	4.2 (206)	28.9 (15)	4.0 (191)	**78.3 (< 0.001)**	6.3 (2.7, 14.7)
Detox or cleanse diet	10.7 (519)	30.8 (16)	10.5 (503)	**22.2 (< 0.001)**	2.7 (1.2, 6.2)
Extreme weight loss diet	4.8 (232)	13.5 (7)	4.7 (225)	**8.7 (0.003)**	1.8 (0.5, 6.0)
	Mean (SD)				
EDEQ Shape concern *mean (SD)*	1.6 (1.8)	2.1 (2.1)	1.6 (1.8)	0.08 [c]	
EDEQ Weight concern *mean (SD)*	1.5 (1.8)	1.9 (2.0)	1.5 (1.8)	0.14 [c]	

Notes: [a] Chi 2 test; [b] Univariate odds ratios adjusted for age, sex and BMI centile; [c] t test p value; *EDEQ* Eating Disorders Examination Questionnaire

exercise (22.2% vs 0%, respectively; $p = 0.03$), cigarette use (77.8% vs 16.3%, respectively; $p = 0.001$), illicit drug use (77.8% vs 18.6%, respectively; $p = 0.001$), detox or cleanse diet (100.0% vs 16.3%, respectively; $p < .0.001$), extreme weight loss diet (44.4% vs 7.0%, respectively; $p = 0.01$). Weight concern [median (IQR); 3.6 (1.4–5) vs 0.6 (0–3.2), respectively; $p = 0.03$] and shape concern [median (IQR); 3 (2–5.5) vs 1.5 (0–3.8), respectively; $p = 0.03$] were also higher in those reporting insulin restriction compared to those not restricting.

Discussion

This study aimed to explore disordered eating behaviours according to reported diagnosis of diabetes and insulin restriction in a general community-based population sample of adolescents. To the authors' knowledge, this study has assessed the broadest spectrum of disordered eating behaviours in the context of diabetes to date. Several disordered eating behaviours were greater in those with a self-reported diagnosis of diabetes, including self-induced vomiting, laxative use, cleanse or detox diets, extreme weight loss diets as well as cigarette and drug use for the purposes of weight or shape control. In addition, frequent insulin restriction was found to be common in those who reported diabetes and was associated with even greater rates of disordered eating.

The behaviours that were particularly common among youth with diabetes compared to their peers included purging behaviours (i.e., self-induced vomiting and laxative use) and atypical substance-related weight control behaviours (use of detoxes, cigarettes and other drugs). The rates of self-induced vomiting (19%) and laxative use (15%) among adolescents with diabetes in this sample were higher than previous studies of adolescents with diabetes in clinical settings (4 and 1%, respectively [27, 28];). This may be attributable to the community-based, anonymous nature of the current survey compared to recruitment from diabetes clinics in previous studies. Further, while purging behaviours have frequently been assessed in people with diabetes, the frequency of purging is often unreported, with studies instead relying on global measures of eating disorder psychopathology [16]. Detoxes and extreme weight loss dieting were frequently reported in adolescents with diabetes in this study. This type of behaviour may be triggered among youth diagnosed with diabetes who are taught to closely monitor their dietary intake and weight during a time where dieting is a known casual risk factor for eating disorder onset among non-diabetic youth [29]. The use of extreme weight control strategies is especially concerning among adolescents with diabetes as this may affect their overall blood glucose management.

The use of cigarettes [30] and other illicit drugs [31–33] for the purposes of weight and shape control has been previously documented in the general population and those with clinical and subclinical eating disorders, however, the frequency of these behaviours among people with diabetes has been understudied. In the current study, we found that adolescents with diabetes were almost 5-times more likely to report cigarette use and more than 6-times more likely to report illicit drug use for weight control purposes compared to their non-diabetic peers. Cigarette smoking in people with diabetes poses increased health risks including eye and nerve problems, hyperglycaemia and poor glycaemic control, while use of illicit drugs may be particularly dangerous for youth with diabetes if they consequently reduce their dietary intake or forget to take insulin, which has the potential to lead to poor glycaemic control. Given the unique medical implications of these disordered eating behaviours for people with diabetes, these findings indicate that it is important to assess a range of disordered eating behaviours in clinical diabetes settings and tailor interventions to be specific to those with diabetes. Adolescents who reported diabetes were not more likely to engage in frequent binge eating behaviour, in both unadjusted and adjusted models that included body mass index. This was contrary to expectations, given the strict dietary control required in diabetes, which is also widely regarded as a risk factor for binge eating [34]. Indeed, previous research has found that among adolescents who intentionally overdose on insulin, the primary reason for this was to allow themselves to binge eat [35]. However, this finding may also be because binge eating is more commonly found in adults, including those with T2D [36], and less prevalent in adolescents. More research is required to determine whether adolescent T1D is associated with greater risk of binge eating or not.

Within the diabetes group, 17% reported insulin restriction at least once per week in order to control weight. Insulin restriction for the purpose of weight or shape control has been widely reported in previous literature ranging from 4 to 58% in people with T1D [37]. Insulin restriction in the current study identified a vulnerable subgroup displaying very high rates of eating disorder behaviours, which is similar to previous studies in male and female adults [38]. Disordered eating behaviours have also been shown to be associated with insulin restriction in adolescents [18, 39]. Furthermore, weight and shape concern were higher in those that reported restricting insulin. The use of insulin can result in weight gain, which may contribute to body dissatisfaction, a leading risk factor for the development of disordered eating [40]. However, due to the cross-sectional nature of the study, we are unable to determine causal pathways for the development of weight and shape concern and disordered eating behaviours among youth with diabetes. Consistent with existing guidelines [10], paediatric diabetes clinics should routinely screen for disordered eating behaviours, including insulin omission. Strategies to address insulin omission including psychoeducation should be employed to minimise likelihood of progression to a diagnosable eating disorder.

This is important given that identification and referral to timely and appropriate care provision may reduce subsequent complications and improve treatment outcomes [41].

The findings of this study may have the potential to inform future health promotion, prevention, and early intervention approaches. Given the differences in disordered eating behaviours according to diabetes status, selective programs for those with diabetes may be preferable, given that there are unique disordered eating behaviours in this group. Alternatively, existing health promotion and universal prevention programs may consider adding diabetes-specific information, such as insulin restriction, given the serious medical complications associated with this behaviour. In addition, education for parents and health care professionals may also be useful to assist in identifying signs of disordered eating behaviours and referral to appropriate treatment pathways.

Strengths of this study include the recruitment of a large, general community-based population sample of adolescents across a broad range of demographic characteristics, with many previous studies recruiting convenience samples of people with diabetes from clinical settings. However, this study has some limitations to acknowledge. The self-reported diabetes question was worded to be age appropriate, but it did not differentiate between T1D and T2D. Given the age of the sample recruited, it can be assumed that the majority of participants had T1D as this is the predominant form of diabetes in this age group. However, the group with diabetes also had a higher BMI, which is associated with increased risk for T2D. Due to the different biological mechanisms, morbidity and management strategies in T1D compared to T2D, future studies should ensure that the type of diabetes is specific in the question, to allow for analyses according to diagnosis. In addition, as this was a secondary analysis as part of a larger study, an eating disorders assessment tool specific to diabetes was not used. Previous research has suggested that prevalence estimates of diagnosable eating disorders should be interpreted with caution in people with diabetes [17], as many eating disorder assessment tools for the general population include questions that pathologise behaviours that are important for management of T1D (for example the focus on food intake) and may inflate the prevalence of disordered eating. To address this limitation, this study specifically explored specific eating disorder behaviours rather than eating disorder diagnosis. The cross-sectional nature of the study precludes inferences about cause and effect with respect to the emergence of diabetes and eating disorders. Future longitudinal community-based studies are required and studies that investigate the impact of disordered eating on metabolic and other indices of physical as well as mental health status in young people with diabetes. The small number of participants in the diabetes group, and particularly the insulin restriction subgroup, is a limitation of the study. However, differences between the two subgroups were nevertheless observed suggesting there was sufficient power in the analyses. Finally, assessment of insulin over-dosing in addition to insulin restriction is recommended in future studies of this kind, given the reported association with binge eating behaviour.

Conclusions

This study found that disordered eating behaviours including self-induced vomiting, laxative use, cleanse or detox diets, extreme weight loss diets as well as cigarette and drug use were higher in adolescents reporting a diagnosis of diabetes in a community-based population sample of Australian adolescents, a particularly vulnerable subgroup due to the rapid biological and social changes during this stage of development. In addition, frequent insulin restriction was found to be common in those who reported a diagnosis of diabetes and was associated with very high rates of disordered eating behaviours and weight and shape concern. Future longitudinal studies are required to evaluate disordered eating behaviours in those with diabetes over time in community-based samples.

Abbreviations

BMI: Body mass index; EDE-Q: Eating Disorders Examination Questionnaire; IRSAD: Index of Relative Socioeconomic Advantage and Disadvantage; SD: Standard deviation; SEIFA: Socioeconomic index for areas; SES: Socioeconomic status; T1D: Type 1 diabetes; T2D: Type 2 diabetes

Acknowledgements

Not applicable.

Authors' contributions

KP conceived of the idea, analysed the data and wrote the manuscript. DM conceived of and leads the EveryBODY Study. DM, NT, AL, KB collected the data. PH, JM, KP consulted on design and interpretation of analyses. All authors contributed to revisions of the draft manuscript. All authors read and approved the final manuscript.

Competing interests

Dr. Mitchison is supported by the National Medical and Health Research Council (GNT 1158276). Professor Hay receives/has received sessional fees and lecture fees from the Australian Medical Council, Therapeutic Guidelines publication, and New South Wales Institute of Psychiatry and royalties/honoraria from Hogrefe and Huber, McGraw Hill Education, and Blackwell Scientific Publications, Biomed Central and PlosMedicine and she has received research grants from the NHMRC and ARC. She is Chair of the National Eating Disorders Collaboration Steering Committee in Australia (2019-) and Member of the ICD-11 Working Group for Eating Disorders (2012-) and was Chair Clinical Practice Guidelines Project Working Group (Eating Disorders) of RANZCP (2012–2015). She has conducted education for psychiatrists and prepared a report under contract for Shire Pharmaceuticals (July 2017). All views in this paper are her own.

Author details
[1]Faculty of Health and Medicine, University of Newcastle, Callaghan 2308, NSW, Australia. [2]Translational Health Research Institute, School of Medicine, Western Sydney University, Sydney, NSW, Australia. [3]Campbelltown and Camden Hospitals, Campbelltown, NSW, Australia. [4]Department of Psychology and Centre for Emotional Health, Macquarie University, Sydney, NSW, Australia. [5]Departments of Psychiatry and Epidemiology, Columbia University Irving Medical Center, New York, NY, USA. [6]Centre for Rural Health, University of Tasmania, Launceston, Australia. [7]School of Medicine, Western Sydney University, Campbelltown, Australia. [8]Department of Psychology, Macquarie University, Sydney, NSW, Australia.

References

1. Arcelus J, Mitchell AJ, Wales J, Nielsen S. Mortality rates in patients with anorexia nervosa and other eating disorders: a meta-analysis of 36 studies. Arch Gen Psychiatry. 2011;68(7):724–31.
2. Pompili M, Girardi P, Tatarelli G, Ruberto A, Tatarelli R. Suicide and attempted suicide in eating disorders, obesity and weight-image concern. Eat Behav. 2006;7(4):384–94.
3. Galmiche M, Déchelotte P, Lambert G, Tavolacci MP. Prevalence of eating disorders over the 2000–2018 period: a systematic literature review. Am J Clin Nutr. 2019;109(5):1402–13.
4. Hay PJ, Mond J, Buttner P, Darby A. Eating disorder behaviors are increasing: findings from two sequential community surveys in South Australia. PloS one. 2008;3(2):e1541.
5. Mitchison D, Hay P, Slewa-Younan S, Mond J. The changing demographic profile of eating disorder behaviors in the community. BMC Public Health. 2014;14:943.
6. Mitchison D, Mond J, Bussey K, Griffiths S, Trompeter N, Lonergan A, et al. DSM-5 full syndrome, other specified, and unspecified eating disorders in Australian adolescents: prevalence and clinical significance. Psychol Med. 2019:1–10.
7. Mayer-Davis EJ, Lawrence JM, Dabelea D, Divers J, Isom S, Dolan L, et al. Incidence trends of type 1 and type 2 diabetes among youths, 2002-2012. N Engl J Med. 2017;376(15):1419–29.
8. Australian Institute of Health and Welfare. Prevalence of type 1 diabetes among children aged 0–14 in Australia 2013. Canberra: Australian Institute of Health and Welfare (AIHW); 2015. Report No.: Diabetes series no. 24. Cat. no. CVD 70.
9. Australian Institute of Health and Welfare. Type 2 diabetes in Australia's children and young people: a working paper. Canberra: Australian Institute of Health and Welfare (AIHW); 2014. Report No.: Diabetes Series no. 21. Cat. no. CVD 64.
10. American Diabetic Association. Comprehensive Medical Evaluation and Assessment of Comorbidities: Standards of Medical Care in Diabetes—2018. Diabetes Care. 2018;41(Supplement 1):S28-S37.
11. Smink FRE, van Hoeken D, Hoek HW. Epidemiology of eating disorders: incidence, prevalence and mortality rates. Curr Psychiatry Rep. 2012;14(4): 406–14.
12. Young V, Eiser C, Johnson B, Brierley S, Epton T, Elliott J, et al. Eating problems in adolescents with type 1 diabetes: a systematic review with meta-analysis. Diabet Med. 2013;30(2):189–98.
13. Allison KC, Crow SJ, Reeves RR, West DS, Foreyt JP, DiLillo VG, et al. Binge eating disorder and night eating syndrome in adults with type 2 diabetes. Obesity. 2007;15(5):1287–93.
14. Colton PA, Olmsted MP, Daneman D, Farquhar JC, Wong H, Muskat S, et al. Eating disorders in girls and women with type 1 diabetes: a longitudinal study of prevalence, onset, remission, and recurrence. Diabetes Care. 2015;38(7):1212–7.
15. Bentley C, Gratwick-Sarll K, Harrison C, Mond J. Sex differences in psychosocial impairment associated with eating disorder features in adolescents: a school-based study. Int J Eat Disord. 2015;48(6):633–40.
16. Pursey K, Hart M, Jenkins L, McEvoy M, Smart C. Screening and identification of disordered eating in people with Type 1 Diabetes: A systematic review. Submitted for publication; 2019.
17. Keane S, Clarke M, Murphy M, McGrath D, Smith D, Farrelly N, et al. Disordered eating behaviour in young adults with type 1 diabetes mellitus. J Eat Disord. 2018;6:9.
18. Araia E, Hendrieckx C, Skinner T, Pouwer F, Speight J, King RM. Gender differences in disordered eating behaviors and body dissatisfaction among adolescents with type 1 diabetes: results from diabetes MILES youth-Australia. Int J Eat Disord. 2017;50(10):1183–93.
19. Sivertsen B, Petrie KJ, Wilhelmsen-Langeland A, Hysing M. Mental health in adolescents with type 1 diabetes: results from a large population-based study. BMC Endocr Disord. 2014;14:83.
20. d'Emden H, McDermott B, Gibbons K, Harris M, Cotterill A. Choosing a screening tool to assess disordered eating in adolescents with type 1 diabetes mellitus. J Diabetes Complicat. 2014;29(1):2–4. https://doi.org/10.1016/j.jdiacomp.2014.09.008.
21. Trompeter N, Bussey K, Hay P, Mond J, Murray SB, Lonergan A, et al. Fear of negative evaluation and weight/shape concerns among adolescents: the moderating effects of gender and weight status. J Youth Adolesc. 2018;47(7):1398–408.
22. Australian Bureau of Statistics. Socio-Economic Indexes for Areas (SEIFA). Canberra Australian Bureau of Statistics 2011. Contract No.: 2033.0.55.001.
23. Pursey K, Burrows TL, Stanwell P, Collins CE. How accurate is web-based self-reported height, weight, and body mass index in young adults? J Med Internet Res. 2014;16(1):e4.
24. Goodman E, Hinden BR, Khandelwal S. Accuracy of teen and parental reports of obesity and body mass index. Pediatrics. 2000;106(1 Pt 1):52–8.
25. Mond J, Hall A, Bentley C, Harrison C, Gratwick-Sarll K, Lewis V. Eating-disordered behavior in adolescent boys: eating disorder examination questionnaire norms. Int J Eat Disord. 2014;47(4):335–41.
26. American Psychiatric Association. Diagnostic and statistical manual of mental disorders (DSM 5). 5th ed. Arlington: American Psychiatric Publishing; 2013.
27. Grylli V, Hafferl-Gattermayer A, Schober E, Karwautz A. Prevalence and clinical manifestations of eating disorders in Austrian adolescents with type-1 diabetes. Wien Klin Wochenschr. 2004;116(7–8):230–4.
28. Howe CJ, Jawad AF, Kelly SD, Lipman TH. Weight-related concerns and behaviors in children and adolescents with type 1 diabetes [corrected] [published erratum apppears in J AM PSYCHIATR NURSES ASSOC 2008 Feb-mar;14(1):70]. J Am Psychiatr Nurse Assoc. 2007;13(6):376–85.
29. Patton GC, Selzer R, Coffey C, Carlin JB, Wolfe R. Onset of adolescent eating disorders: population based cohort study over 3 years. BMJ. 1999;318(7186):765–8.
30. Fulkerson JA, French SA. Cigarette smoking for weight loss or control among adolescents: gender and racial/ethnic differences. J Adolesc Health. 2003;32(4):306–13.
31. Patton GC, Coffey C, Carlin JB, Sanci L, Sawyer S. Prognosis of adolescent partial syndromes of eating disorder. Br J Psychiatry. 2008;192(4):294–9.
32. Stock SL, Goldberg E, Corbett S, Katzman DK. Substance use in female adolescents with eating disorders. J Adolesc Health. 2002;31(2):176–82.
33. Pisetsky EM, Chao YM, Dierker LC, May AM, Striegel-Moore RH. Disordered eating and substance use in high-school students: results from the youth risk behavior surveillance system. Int J Eat Disord. 2008;41(5):464–70.
34. Fairburn CG. Eating disorders: the transdiagnostic view and the cognitive behavioral theory; 2008.
35. Schober E, Wagner G, Berger G, Gerber D, Mengl M, Sonnenstatter S, et al. Prevalence of intentional under- and overdosing of insulin in children and adolescents with type 1 diabetes. Pediatr Diabetes. 2011; 12(7):627–31.
36. Abbott S, Dindol N, Tahrani AA, Piya MK. Binge eating disorder and night eating syndrome in adults with type 2 diabetes: a systematic review. J Eat Disord. 2018;6:36.
37. De Paoli T, Rogers PJ. Disordered eating and insulin restriction in type 1 diabetes: A systematic review and testable model. Eat Disord. 2018;26(4):343–360.
38. Herpertz S, Albus C, Kielmann R, Hagemann-Patt H, Lichtblau K, Kohle K, et al. Comorbidity of diabetes mellitus and eating disorders - a follow-up study. J Psychosom Res. 2001;51(5):673–8.
39. Markowitz JT, Butler DA, Volkening LK, Antisdel JE, Anderson BJ, Laffel LM. Brief screening tool for disordered eating in diabetes: internal consistency and external validity in a contemporary sample of pediatric patients with type 1 diabetes. Diabetes Care. 2010;33(3):495–500.
40. Stice E, Shaw HE. Role of body dissatisfaction in the onset and maintenance of eating pathology: a synthesis of research findings. J Psychosom Res. 2002;53(5):985–93.
41. Hay P, Chinn D, Forbes D, Madden S, Newton R, Sugenor L, et al. Royal Australian and new Zealand College of Psychiatrists clinical practice guidelines for the treatment of eating disorders. Aust N Z J Psychiatry. 2014;48(11):977–1008.

8

An audit of the changes in thiamine levels during higher caloric nutritional rehabilitation of adolescent patients hospitalised with a restrictive eating disorder

Elizabeth Parker[1,2*], Terri Maister[3], Anita Stefoska-Needham[3], Christine Wearne[4], Gail Anderson[5], Linette Gomes[5], Simon Clarke[5,6,7] and Michael Kohn[5,6,7]

Abstract

Background: Routine supplementation of thiamine in patients with restrictive eating disorders prior to initiation of nutritional rehabilitation, is an example of a clinical guideline based on expert opinion rather than evidence-based recommendations. This study investigates whether adolescents hospitalised with a restrictive eating disorder commenced on a higher caloric refeeding regimen, present with or develop thiamine deficiency during their admission.

Methods: An eighteen month retrospective audit of 119 consecutive admissions for nutritional rehabilitation was conducted on patients admitted with an eating disorder in a large tertiary teaching hospital in Western Sydney. Data from paper-based and electronic medical records were collected. Baseline and weekly blood thiamine levels were documented, as well as patient demographic information including admission weight, age, length of stay, percentage median body mass index, weight change throughout admission and caloric prescription.

Results: Sixty admissions met inclusion criteria, mean age 17.2 years (SD 1.2); 88% female; BMI 16.8 kg/m^2 (SD 1.8) on admission. A linear mixed effects model identified that median thiamine levels increased by 9.2 nmol/L per week ($p < 0.001$). No patient developed thiamine deficiency during their admission, one patient was admitted with thiamine levels below the normal range at 62 nmol (normal range 67 – 200 nmol/L) which resolved by the second week of admission. In 15 out of 60 patients (25%), thiamine levels were observed to rise above the upper limit.

Conclusions: Nutritional management of 60 malnourished adolescents hospitalised with an eating disorder was conducted safely with the provision of only 10 mg thiamine in a multivitamin daily, and no additional thiamine supplementation. The high caloric refeeding protocol, inclusive of a daily multivitamin, provided adequate thiamine to prevent thiamine deficiency. Further research should examine thiamine requirements in an exclusive severely malnourished population to assess the need for thiamine replacement in the most vulnerable group.

Keywords: Thiamine, Vitamin B1, Eating disorder, Anorexia nervosa, Nutrition

* Correspondence: Elizabeth.Parker@health.nsw.gov.au
[1]Department of Dietetics & Nutrition, Westmead Hospital, PO Box 533, Wentworthville, NSW 2145, Australia
[2]Sydney School of Health Sciences, Faculty of Medicine and Health, The University of Sydney, Sydney 2006, NSW, Australia
Full list of author information is available at the end of the article

Plain English Summary

This study looks at the change in thiamine (Vitamin B1) levels in 60 adolescent patients admitted to hospital with a restrictive eating disorder. Patients were provided with an oral meal plan with or without nasogastric tube feeding in hospital. Patients received a daily multivitamin providing 10 mg thiamine, however did not receive an additional thiamine supplement during their hospital admission. The results of this study found that no patients developed thiamine deficiency during their hospital admission, and that the average blood thiamine level increased each week. The results of this study suggest that this group of patients hospitalised with an eating disorder received adequate amounts of thiamine through an oral meal plan with or without nasogastric tube feeding, and a daily multivitamin, and did not require an additional thiamine supplement.

Background

Nutritional management, incorporating refeeding and weight restoration (also termed nutritional rehabilitation), is a key pillar of the clinical care pathway of patients with anorexia nervosa (AN) and other restrictive eating disorders [1]. Refeeding complications can include the development the Refeeding Syndrome (RFS), and other metabolic and micronutrient changes. Shifts in electrolytes and fluid in response to increased caloric intake are implicated in the development of these complications [2].

Abnormal levels of phosphate, changes in macronutrient metabolism, as well as low extracellular levels of sodium, magnesium and potassium, are also used as markers of RFS [2]. Recently, Rio et al. (2013) [3] proposed more specific criteria for diagnosing RFS, encompassing electrolyte levels, presence of oedema and respiratory/cardiac dysfunction. In addition to RFS, thiamine deficiency (TD) is also listed as a concern when providing nutritional replenishment to malnourished patients, as severe deficiency can lead to Wernicke's encephalopathy (WE) or Wernicke Korsakoff's syndrome (WKS) [2].

In 2006, the National Institute for Health and Care Excellence (NICE) developed clinical guidelines to identify patients at risk of refeeding complications, including patients with a low body mass index (BMI) < 18.5 kg/m^2, unintentional weight loss > 10% body weight in the last 3–6 months, and a recent history of little of no nutritional intake [4]. The updated NICE guidelines recommend supplementing with 200–300 mg oral thiamine daily prior to commencing feeding and during the first 10 days of feeding in people identified at risk of developing refeeding problems [4]. However, the paucity of scientific evidence underpinning these and other recommendations has been a key criticism of the NICE Clinical Guidelines, in the management of patients with eating disorders [5, 6]. There is also a growing body of evidence that challenges the 'start low, go slow' approach to renourishing patients with a restrictive eating disorder, as it has been shown to lead to the development of 'underfeeding syndrome', whereby malnourished patients are provided with insufficient energy intakes to meet basal metabolic needs and they continue to lose weight [7–12].

Routine supplementation of thiamine in patients with AN prior to initiation of nutritional rehabilitation is an example of a clinical guideline based on expert opinion rather than evidence-based recommendations [2, 4, 13–15]. This practice is based on foundation knowledge of the role of thiamine as an essential cofactor in carbohydrate metabolism, an essential pathway during refeeding [2], and previous research demonstrating thiamine supplementation prior to nutritional rehabilitation may prevent TD and its associated neuropsychiatric conditions WE and WKS [16, 17]. A study of 37 patients with AN reported a 38% prevalence of TD [18], and a systematic review by Oudman E et al. (2018) identified 12 cases of TD causing WE in patients with AN ranging from BMI 12.2 kg/m^2 to 17.4 kg/m^2, including some patients with a history of alcohol and substance abuse [19].

The aim of this study is to investigate whether adolescents hospitalised with a restrictive eating disorder and commenced on a high caloric refeeding regimen, present with or develop thiamine deficiency.

Methods

Study design

A retrospective audit of 119 consecutive admissions between July 2016–December 2017 was conducted. Inclusion criteria were patients diagnosed with a restrictive eating disorder requiring nutritional rehabilitation and at least one thiamine level measured during the admission. Patients were excluded from the study if they did not have a blood thiamine level assessed during admission. Those with repeat admissions were included in the analysis if the inclusion criteria was met for subsequent admissions.

Retrospective data from paper-based and electronic medical records were collected for each admission. This included patient demographics, diagnosis, weekly weight, body mass index (BMI), weekly caloric intake, oral electrolyte supplementation received, length of hospital stay, history of purging and laxative use and any clinical signs and symptoms of refeeding syndrome and thiamine deficiency, including delirium and peripheral oedema. Baseline and weekly blood thiamine levels as well as supplement prescription were also reviewed. This study received ethical approval from the Western Sydney Local Health District Human Research and Ethics committee.

Ward program

On admission, patients were prescribed a standardised nutritional regimen consisting of either (i) continuous nasogastric feeds with oral intake limited to sips of water, (ii) nocturnal nasogastric feeds with an oral meal plan during the day, or (iii) oral meal plan only (Fig. 1).

Patients who were considered medically unstable (presenting with bradycardia, heart rate ≤ 50 bpm, QTc interval on ECG > 440 ms, or significantly hypotensive) were typically commenced on 1 kcal/mL formula of continuous nasogastric (NG) tube feeding to provide 2400 kcal/day at a rate of 100 mL/hour, or a 1.5 kcal formula at a rate of 35 mL/hr. for 12 h and then increased to 70 ml/hr. (providing 1890 kcal on Day 1). All oral intake other than water was restricted during the first 24 h.

Patients with an eating disorder who were assessed as medically stable were commenced on an oral meal plan providing 1800 to 3800 kcal with or without supplementary nocturnal NG feeds (1 kcal/mL formula at 100 mL/hour for 10 h providing 1000 kcal). If a meal was not consumed to completion, patients were provided with additional nutritional supplements to assure prescribed caloric intake.

A patient's caloric intake was increased throughout hospitalisation by increasing meal plans (1800 kcal, 2300 kcal, 2800 kcal, 3300 kcal and 3800 kcal), providing nutritional supplements (300 kcal or 400 kcal), or altering the volume or concentration of enteral feeds (1.0, 1.5, 2.0 kcal/mL formula). The total caloric intake was reviewed at least 3 times/week by the treating medical team, where decisions were made in regards to modifying the total caloric intake.

Typically, patients received prophylactic phosphate supplementation and a daily multivitamin with the commencement of the nutritional regimen. The daily multivitamin provided 10 mg thiamine. The thiamine content in oral meal plans was 2.30–3.62 mg/day, and the thiamine content of Enteral Formula ranged from 1.6–3.2 mg/L. Serum electrolyte levels were monitored 6 h post nutritional intervention commencement and continued regularly until discharge. Biochemical analyses were based on the hospital reference ranges for thiamine 67–200 nmol/L. To measure thiamine levels, a commercial kit Chromsystems™ with combined Vitamin B1/B6 Analysis UHPLC/52952 was used, with an intra-assay coefficient of variation ≤3.8% and inter-assay coefficient of variation ≤6% [20].

Statistical analysis

Descriptive analysis included patient demographics and clinical data. Number (n), range, mean, standard deviation, and percentages are reported. Variables recorded

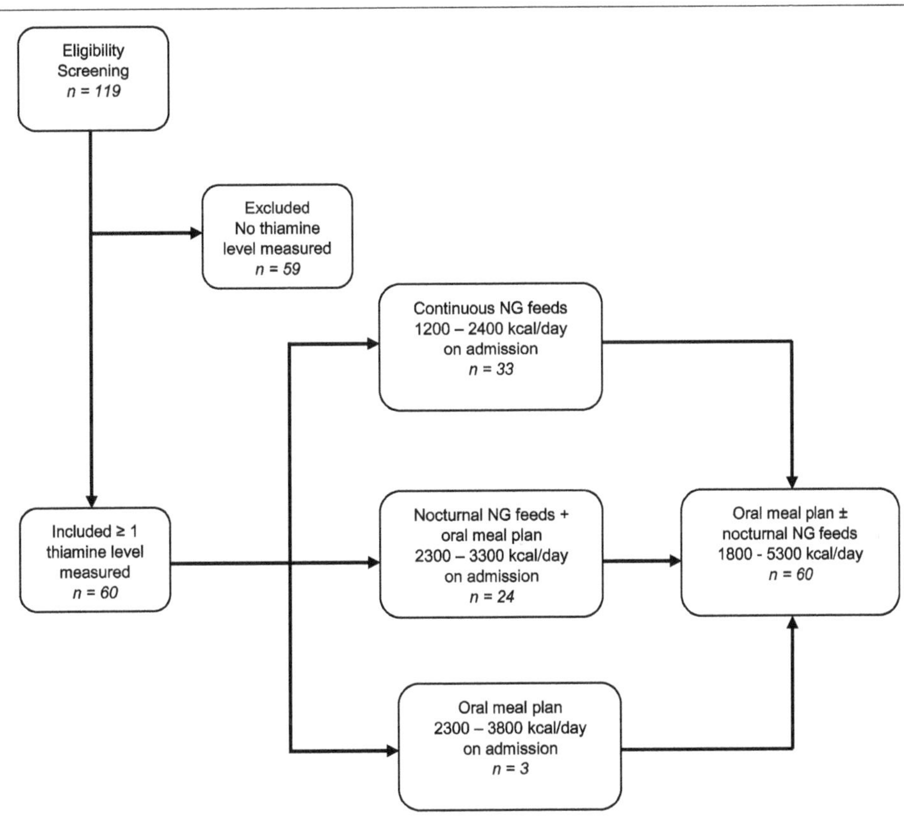

Fig. 1 Nutrition rehabilitation program provided to patients on admission and the progression to oral dietary intake

included caloric prescription on admission, admission weight, weight change, length of hospitalisation. Percentage median BMI (%mBMI), a calculation of the 50th percentile BMI for age and gender, was used as an indicator of malnutrition due to this being a routinely used measure in adolescent and young adult patients [21, 22].

Data were entered into SPSS for Windows Version 21, IBM Corporation and S-Plus for analysis. A linear mixed effects model conducted on thiamine trends during nutrition rehabilitation was used to analyse the data. Blood thiamine levels were assessed through data stacking. The random effect was plotted as week per individual admission. The fixed effect was weekly blood thiamine level and the value and standard error were assessed. Statistical significance was set at p value < 0.05.

Results

During the 18 month study period, 119 consecutive admissions were identified and 60 admissions (50.4%) met the eligibility criteria for analysis (52 patients with 1 admission, 4 patients with 2 admissions). The patient cohort included 37 admissions diagnosed with DSM-5 criteria [23] for anorexia nervosa (restricting type), 14 admissions with anorexia nervosa (binge eating/purging type), and 6 admissions with Avoidant/Restrictive Food Intake Disorder. Three admissions were diagnosed with an Atypical anorexia nervosa. All patients received the daily multivitamin supplement.

Fifty-nine cases were excluded as thiamine level was not tested during their admission. Of the 60 patients included in the study, 88% (n = 53) were female. On admission, mean age was 17.2 years (SD 1.2), percentage mBMI was 80.4% (SD 8.9). Patients were malnourished (11.7% severe, 31.7% moderate, 56.7% mild) [22]. Additional patient characteristics are presented in Table 1.

Initial nasogastric (NG) tube feeding and/or oral intake was introduced and an average of 2482.0 kcal (SD 413.2) was prescribed, and was sequentially increased during the admission (Fig. 2).

The mean thiamine level on admission was 157.5 nmol/L (SD 36.0). During hospitalisation and nutrition intervention, median thiamine levels increased by 9.2 nmol per week (SD 2.4, IQR 4.4–14, p value < 0.001), based on the linear mixed effects model (Fig. 3). There was only one occasion, representing 1.7% of the study sample, when a patient had blood thiamine level recorded below the normal reference range at 62 nmol/L, on admission, prior to nutrition intervention. The remaining thiamine levels on admission were all within the normal reference range of 67 – 200 nmol/L. Over the duration of admission, 15 out of 60 patients (25%) were observed to have a blood thiamine level greater than the upper limit of the normal reference range (200 nmol/L).

Discussion

Adolescents hospitalised with a restrictive eating disorder and commenced on a high caloric prescription did not require additional thiamine supplementation, beyond 10 mg contained within a daily multivitamin, to maintain normal levels of thiamine during nutritional rehabilitation. Blood thiamine levels increased weekly during their admission, most likely due to thiamine intake from a daily oral multivitamin, dietary food intake and enteral feeds.

Neither low thiamine levels nor many of the proposed predisposing factors for low thiamine, are typically present for adolescents with mild to moderate malnutrition presenting with restrictive eating disorders. Nevertheless, guidelines for the nutritional management of

Table 1 Characteristics of adolescent patients hospitalised with a restrictive eating disorder (60 admissions, 56 patients)

Variable	Mean (SD)	Median (LQ-UQ)
Age (years)	17.2 (1.2)	17.2 (16.4–18.1)
Admission Weight (kg)	45.8 (7.3)	45.8 (41.3–51.9)
Discharge weight (kg)	53.4 (6.6)	53.6 (48.9–57.0)
Admission BMI (kg/m2)	16.8 (1.8)	17.1 (15.8–18.3)
Discharge BMI (kg/m2)	19.5 (1.2)	19.7 (18.7–20.2)
Admission %mBMI	80.4 (8.9)	81.3 (75.2–87.2)
Discharge %mBMI	93.2 (6.3)	94.3 (89.4–97.0)
Change in %mBMI	12.8 (6.6)	12.0 (7.4–16.6)
Energy intake on admission (kcal)	2482.0 (413.2)	2400.0 (2400.0–2800.0)
Energy intake on discharge (kcal)	3753.3 (617.7)	3800.0 (3400.0–3800.0)
Total weight gain (kg)	6.9 (4.4)	6.1 (4.2–8.9)
Average weight gain per week (kg)	2.0 (0.8)	2.0 (1.5–2.4)
Average LOS (weeks)	3.6 (2.0)	3.2 (2.2–4.6)

BMI Body mass index, *%mBMI* Percentage median body mass index, *LOS* Length of hospital stay.

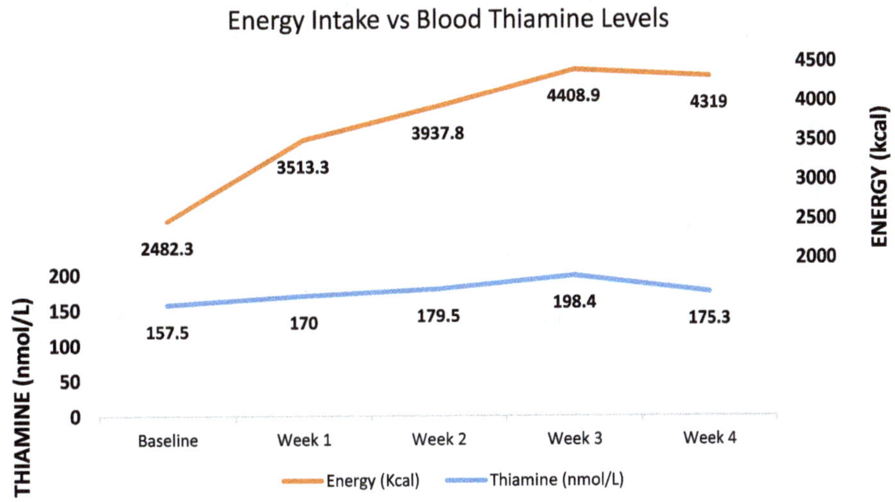

Fig. 2 Changes in energy intake and blood thiamine levels $n = 60$

patients diagnosed with AN include the prophylactic supplementation of 200-300 mg thiamine as a preventative measure for the development of refeeding complications [13]. Restriction of thiamine rich foods, excessive excretion of magnesium, and ethanol toxicity are suggested as causes for low thiamine levels and the development of WE in patients with starvation and restrictive eating disorders [17, 24–28]. There appears to be uncertainty in the literature regarding the prevalence of thiamine deficiency observed in malnourished patients, relating to two different methods of analysis, i.e. erythrocyte transketolase activity versus measurement of blood thiamine.

Low levels of erythrocyte transketolase activity have been reported in as many as 38% of patients diagnosed with AN [18]. In the present study only one patient presented with TD on admission, as measured by blood thiamine level. The higher prevalence of thiamine deficiency in AN reported by Winston AP (2000) [18] may be explained by the use of a different method of

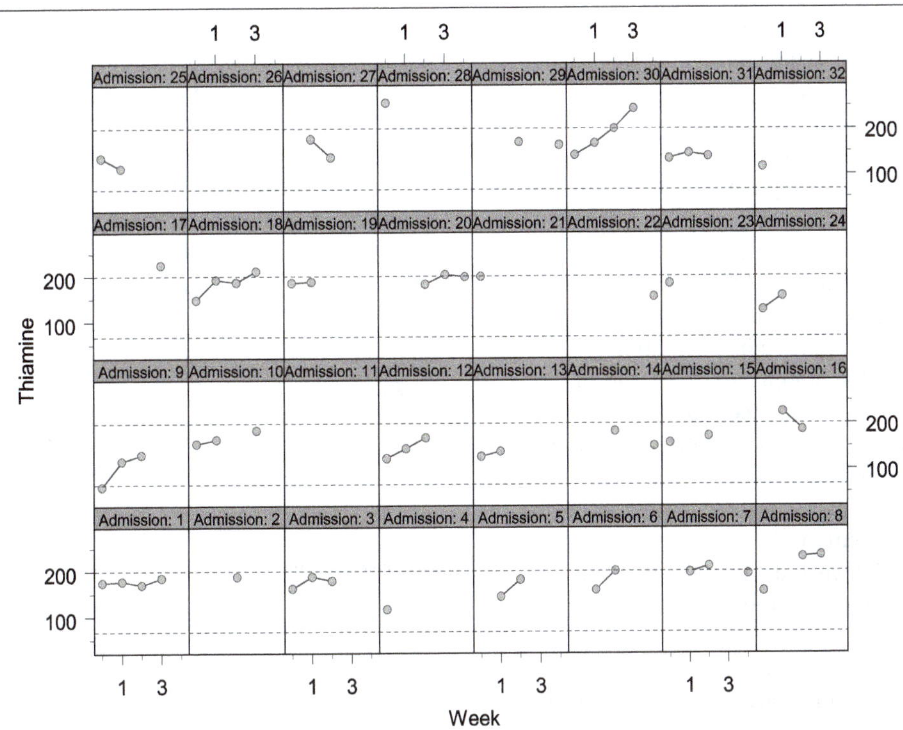

Fig. 3 Linear mixed effects model stacking patient thiamine outcome per week of Patients 1–32

assessment in addition to investigating an older population with possibly a longer duration of illness. In their study of 37 patients, the authors reported no statistical relationship between erythrocyte transketolase activation and age, BMI, duration of restricted oral intake, frequency of vomiting, use of laxatives or alcohol consumption [18]. Reduced erythrocyte transketolase activity is likely a result of malnutrition rather than a refeeding complication, and does not necessarily infer reduced levels of thiamine.

No patients developed TD in this study. Above-RDI levels of thiamine were provided via oral meal plans, daily multivitamin supplementation and enteral feeds, as part of standard-care practices. The RDI for thiamine for patients admitted to the adolescent ward ranges from 1.1 mg/day – 1.2 mg/day, depending on gender and age [29], and the multivitamin alone provided patients with 10 mg of thiamine daily (approximately 10 times the RDI). Comparison of these findings to other studies is difficult because the amount of thiamine consumed from oral intake and enteral feeds is not being routinely reported [18, 19].

Recommendations for the management of TD in malnourished patients continues to be influenced by guidelines for alcohol dependent patients. Thiamine deficiency in alcohol dependent individuals may result from inadequate thiamine intake, however it may also be a complication of ethanol toxicity leading to reduced intestinal absorption and bioavailability of thiamine, as well as increased thiamine requirement needed for the metabolism of alcohol [16, 17]. Furthermore, magnesium depletion has shown effects of aggravating thiamine deficiency, whereby alcohol ingestion leads to increased excretion of magnesium and may expedite the presentation of WE symptoms [24]. Guidelines for preventing refeeding complications [2, 4, 30], including patients with AN [13], recommend 200–300 mg/day thiamine supplementation, which is similar to the lower end of the range recommended in guidelines for preventing and treating TD and WE in alcohol dependent individuals which range from 200 to 600 mg/day thiamine supplementation [17, 31, 32].

A limitation of the present study is the absence of thiamine measurements for 49.6% of the study population, and only one method of analysis was measured. The retrospective collection of data means the study was bound by what information was documented during the admission. The current study did not identify any clinical symptoms of WE such as mental confusion or delirium, however routine assessments for ataxia and ocular motility abnormalities such as nystagmus and opthalmoplegia, are not part of routine care and may have been missed. As part of routine care, if any cases of delirium had been detected during inpatient treatment, the patient would have been referred for further investigation including clinical signs of TD. Another limitation of the study is that patients had predominantly mild to moderate malnutrition. TD and refeeding complications are more likely to develop in those with severe malnutrition, so any recommendations from this study can only apply to mild and moderately malnourished patients.

Future studies would benefit from assessing prospectively the typical symptoms of WE, including ataxia, opthalmoplegia, nystagmus and confusion on admission and throughout nutritional rehabilitation. Furthermore, future studies may consider using multiple methods for assessing thiamine status including measurement of urinary thiamine excretion as well as MRI in suspected cases of WE.

There is scope for this study to be expanded beyond an investigation of thiamine status in adolescent patients with eating disorders to include all patients who present with malnutrition and are at risk of thiamine deficiency and refeeding complications on admission. A greater sample size using a prospective study design will increase the validity of the study. Furthermore, by assessing different ages, genders and contributing comorbidities, the generalisability of the study will be expanded and translation into practice will be more impactful.

Conclusions

In conclusion, the results of the study suggest that providing high doses of thiamine through additional supplementation may be unnecessary in mild and moderately malnourished adolescents hospitalised with a restrictive eating disorder. Considering there were no cases of patients developing TD during the admission, it would suggest that patients received adequate thiamine levels through the nutritional rehabilitation program in the current study, through oral diet, enteral feeds and a daily multivitamin.

Abbreviations

AN: Anorexia nervosa; RFS: Refeeding syndrome; TD: Thiamine deficiency; WE: Wernicke's encephalopathy; WKS: Wernicke-Korsakoff syndrome; BMI: Body mass index; % mBMI: Percentage median body mass index; NG: Nasogastric

Acknowledgements

Not applicable.

Authors' contributions

EP, SC, GA, LG and MK were involved in the development of the study design. TM and EP were involved in data collection and analysis. TM and EP drafted the manuscript, with contributions from ASN, CW and MK. All authors read and approved the final manuscript.

Competing interests
The authors declare that they have no competing interests.

Author details
[1]Department of Dietetics & Nutrition, Westmead Hospital, PO Box 533, Wentworthville, NSW 2145, Australia. [2]Sydney School of Health Sciences, Faculty of Medicine and Health, The University of Sydney, Sydney 2006, NSW, Australia. [3]SMART Foods Centre, School of Medicine, Faculty of Science, Medicine and Health, University of Wollongong, Wollongong, NSW 2522, Australia. [4]Department of Medical Psychology, Westmead Hospital, Westmead, NSW 2145, Australia. [5]Department of Adolescent & Young Adult Medicine, Westmead Hospital, Westmead, NSW 2145, Australia. [6]Sydney School of Medicine, Faculty of Medicine and Health, The University of Sydney, Sydney, NSW 2006, Australia. [7]Centre for Research into AdolescentS' Health (CRASH), Adolescent & Young Adult Medicine, Westmead Hospital, Westmead, NSW 2145, Australia.

References

1. American Psychiatric Association, Practice Guideline for the Treatment of Patients with Eating Disorders. American Psychiatric Association Publishing. 3rd ed; 2006.
2. Mehanna HM, Moledina J, Travis J. Refeeding syndrome: what it is, and how to prevent and treat it. BMJ. 2008;336:1495–8.
3. Rio A, Whelan K, Go L, Reidlinger DP, Smeeton N. Occurrence of refeeding syndrome in adults started on artificial nutrition support: prospective cohort study. BMJ Open. 2013;3(1):1–9.
4. National Institute for Clinical Excellence (NICE). "Nutrition support in adults: oral nutrition support, enteral tube feeding and parenteral nutrition," *NICE Clinical Guideline* 32. London: National Institute for Health and Clinical Excellence; 2006.
5. Kohn MR, Madden S, Clarke SD. Refeeding in anorexia nervosa: increased safety and efficiency through understanding the pathophysiology of protein calorie malnutrition. Curr Opin Pediatr. 2011;23:390–4.
6. Garber AK, Kohn M. Newer approaches to acute nutritional rehabilitation for patients with anorexia nervosa. Adolesc Med. 2018;29:344–58.
7. Garber AK, Sawyer SM, Golden NH, et al. A systematic review of approaches to refeeding in patients with anorexia nervosa. Int J Eat Disord. 2016;49: 293–310.
8. O'Connor G, Nicholls D, Hudson L, Singhal A. Refeeding low weight hospitalized adolescents with anorexia nervosa: a multicenter randomized controlled trial. Nutr Clin Pract. 2016;31:681–9.
9. Smith K, Lesser J, Brandenburg B, et al. Outcomes of an inpatient refeeding protocol in youth with anorexia nervosa and atypical anorexia nervosa at Children's hospitals and clinics of Minnesota. J Eat Disord. 2016;4:35.
10. Parker EK, Faruquie SS, Anderson G, Gomes L, Kennedy A, Wearne CM, Kohn MR, Clarke SD. Higher caloric refeeding is safe in hospitalized adolescent patients with restrictive eating disorders. J Nutr Metab. 2016;2016:5168978. https://doi.org/10.1155/2016/5168978. Epub 2016 May 12.
11. Maginot TR, Kumar MM, Shiels J, et al. Outcomes of an inpatient refeeding protocol in youth with anorexia nervosa: Rady Children's Hospital San Diego/University of California, San Diego. J Eat Disord. 2017;5:1.
12. Peebles R, Lesser A, Park CC, et al. Outcomes of an inpatient medical nutritional rehabilitation protocol in children and adolescents with eating disorders. J Eat Disord. 2017;5:7.
13. The Royal College of Psychiatrists, Physicians and Pathologists, "MARSIPAN: Management of really sick patients with anorexia nervosa," *College Report CR189*, Council of the Royal College of Physicians, 2nd edition, 2014.
14. Hofer M, Pozzi A, Joray M, Ott R, Hahni R, Leuenberger M, Kanel RV, Stanga Z. Safe refeeding management of anorexia nervosa inpatients: an evidence-based protocol. Nutrition. 2014;30:524–30.
15. Sobotka L. Basics in Clinical Nutrition: Refeeding Syndrome. *e-SPEN*. Eur-Journal Clin Nutr Metab. 2010;5:e146–7.
16. Frank LL. Thiamin in clinical practice. JPEN. 2015;39:503–20.
17. Sechi GP, Serra A. Wernicke's encephalopathy: new clinical settings and recent advances in diagnosis and management. Lancet Neurol. 2007;6(5): 442–55.
18. Winston AP, Jamieson CP, Madira W, Gatward NM, Palmer RL. Prevalence of thiamine deficiency in anorexia nervosa. Int J Eat Disord. 2000;28(4):451–4.
19. Oudman E, Wijnia JW, Oey MJ, van Dam MJ, Postma A. Preventing Wernike's encephalopathy in anorexia nervosa: a systematic review. Psychiatry Clin Neurosci. 2018;72:774–9.
20. Chromsystems Instruments & Chemicals GmbH. High Throughput UHPLC, combined Vitamin B1/B6 Analysis – UHPLC. Chomsystems. 2020; [cited 2020 May 27]. Available from https://www.chromsystems.com/high-throughput-uhplc-combined-vitamin-b1-b6-analysis-52952-uhplc.html.
21. Centres for Disease Control and Prevention. Data table of BMI-for-age charts. 2000; Available at: https://www.cdc.gov/growthcharts/data/set1 clinical/cj41l024.pdf. [cited 2020 Mar 5].
22. Golden NH, Katzman DK, Sawyer SM, et al. Position paper of the society for adolescent health and medicine: medical management of restrictive eating disorders in adolescents and young adults. J Adolesc Health. 2015;56:121–5.
23. American Psychiatric Association. Diagnostic and statistical manual of mental disorders. 5th ed. Arlington: American Psychiatric Publishing; 2013.
24. Lonsdale D. Thiamine and magnesium deficiencies: keys to disease. Med Hypotheses. 2015;84:129–34.
25. Renthal W, Marin-Valencia I, Evans PA. Thiamine deficiency secondary to anorexia nervosa: an uncommon cause of peripheral neuropathy and Wernicke encephalopathy in adolescence. Pediatr Neurol. 2014;51:100–3.
26. Pentland B, Mawdsley C. Wernicke's encephalopathy following 'hunger strike'. Postgrad Med J. 1982;58:427–8.
27. Stubbs C. Case study: refeeding syndrome and thiamin deficiency after extended starvation. Aus J Nutr Diet. 1999;56:221–3.
28. Drenick EJ, Joven CB, Swenskid ME. Occurrence of acute Wernicke's encephalopathy during prolonged starvation for the treatment of obesity. N Engl J Med. 1966;274:937–9.
29. National Health and Medical Research Council. Nutrient Reference Values for Australia and New Zealand. Australian Government and Ministry of Health, 2014.
30. Stanga Z, Brunner A, Leuenberger M, Grimble RF, Shenkin A, Allison SP, Lobo DN. Nutrition in clinical practice-the refeeding syndrome: illustrative cases and guidelines for prevention and treatment. Eur J Clin Nutr. 2008;62: 687–94.
31. Galvin R, Brathen G, Ivashynka A, Hillbom M, Tanasescu R, Leone MA. EFNS guidelines for diagnosis, therapy and prevention of Wernicke encephalopathy. Eur J Neurol. 2010;17:1408–18.
32. Haber P, Lintzeris N, Proude E, Lopatko O. Guidelines for the treatment of alcohol problems. Australian Government Department of Health and Ageing; 2009.

9

Outcomes of inpatient psychological treatments for children and adolescents with eating disorders at time of discharge

Leanna Isserlin[1,2*], Wendy Spettigue[1,2], Mark Norris[2,3] and Jennifer Couturier[4]

Abstract

Background: Recommended first line treatment for children and adolescent eating disorders is outpatient therapy. However, a significant number of children and adolescents with eating disorders continue to require inpatient treatment during the course of their illness. The effect of psychological treatments in an inpatient setting on outcomes at the time of discharge remains unclear. This paper presents the results of a review of the literature on outcomes at the time of discharge following inpatient psychological treatment for children and adolescents with eating disorders.

Main body: The majority of studies found were observational and of low quality. The most consistently reported positive outcome of inpatient treatment is weight gain. Results related to symptom change and motivation vary between studies. Within the inpatient setting, there is considerable heterogeneity in the types of treatments offered, goals of treatment, length of stay and outcomes measured.

Conclusion: There remains a paucity of high-quality studies examining the effect of psychological treatments provided to children and adolescents in an inpatient setting. The significant heterogeneity between studies makes it not possible to compare across studies. Future research should aim to resolve these deficiencies in order to better determine the specific factors that contribute to positive outcomes of inpatient treatment for children and adolescents with eating disorders.

Keywords: Child, Adolescent, Humans, Inpatients, Hospitalization, Feeding and eating disorders

Plain English summary

For children and adolescents with eating disorders, outpatient treatment is the type of treatment with the most support in the scientific literature and should be the basis of most treatment plans. However, many children and adolescents will require inpatient treatment at some point in their illness. The effect of inpatient treatment on eating disorder symptoms remains unclear. This paper aims to review the available literature on psychological treatments provided to children and adolescents with eating disorders in an inpatient setting in order to understand what is known to date. Unfortunately, there remain very few studies designed in such a way to be able to answer the question 'what is the best psychological treatment to provide in an inpatient setting to children and adolescents with eating disorders?' and due to considerable variability in the studies available, the

* Correspondence: lisserlin@cheo.on.ca
[1]Department of Psychiatry, Children's Hospital of Eastern Ontario, University of Ottawa, Ottawa, ON K1H 8L1, Canada
[2]Children's Hospital of Eastern Ontario Research Institute, Ottawa, ON K1H 8L1, Canada
Full list of author information is available at the end of the article

only consistent positive result in the studies available is that inpatient treatment is effective in producing weight gain. Further research is needed in order to optimize treatment for children and adolescents with eating disorders in the inpatient setting.

Background

Eating disorders (EDs) are complex disorders that typically appear during childhood and adolescence [1]. Current ED guidelines and expert consensus support outpatient family-based treatment as the first-line recommended treatment for children and adolescents [2–4]. Despite this recommendation, a proportion of patients with potentially life-threatening severe EDs will require higher levels of support, including inpatient stabilization and treatment [5].

Unfortunately, inpatient lengths of stay (LOS) for ED treatment tend to be long in comparison to other medical and psychiatric disorders, with the average LOS in studies from Germany, Japan, Switzerland and Scotland being greater than 7 weeks [6–9]. Modifying factors for LOS in adolescent patients include treatment under the Mental Health Act and nasogastric feeding, both of which appear to be associated with longer LOS [9]. Prolonged LOS is concerning, as it can disrupt adolescent development and engagement in school, family and social life. Further, inpatient treatment is expensive in terms of economic costs and intensive medical resource requirement [10]. In 2013, a review of admissions with a mean length of stay 37.9 days (standard deviation [SD] 19.7 days) to a Canadian tertiary care center for medical stabilization and initial weight rehabilitation for adolescents with AN found that the mean total hospital cost was $51,349 Canadian Dollars (CAD) (SD $26598) with a mean total societal cost of $54,932 CAD (SD $27864) per admission [10]. Similar studies from Portugal and Germany found comparable high costs for eating disorders treatment, in that the average cost per admission in those countries was 5202 to 5883€ and 13,367€ respectively [11, 12].

While three recently published studies examining outcomes across varying treatment settings supports the least intensive management as first line treatment for EDs [13–15], the evidence base that examines best practice for patients who do require inpatient treatment remains scant. The goal of this review is to further explore the scope and benefits of psychological treatments provided to children and adolescents with EDs in inpatient settings at the time of hospital discharge.

Methods

PRISMA systematic review methodology was used to capture all articles on inpatient treatment for EDs in children and adolescents [16]. Our search utilized the following databases: Medline, PsycINFO, EMBASE, Cochrane Database of Systematic Reviews, Cochrane Central Register of Controlled Trials (CENTRAL) and CINAHL, and included the following search terms: Anorexia Nervosa (AN) OR Bulimia Nervosa (BN) OR Binge Eating Disorder (BED) OR Other Specified Feeding and Eating Disorder (OSFED) OR Eating Disorder Not Otherwise Specified (EDNOS) OR Avoidant/Restrictive Food Intake Disorder (ARFID) AND Inpatient Treatment. The search string was developed further and was modified for each database as appropriate (see Additional file 1). Inpatient treatment was defined for the purposes of this review as treatment that involves 24 h/day care in a hospital setting. Reference lists were reviewed for any additional articles. Two reviewers had to agree for inclusion of articles in our review, with a third reviewer resolving any disputes. The initial database search included all years up until March 2017. In November 2018 a forward citation chaining process was completed to search each included article to examine if it had been cited by any additional articles since March 2017 up until November 2018. Newly found articles were then screened to decide whether they matched the inclusion criteria. The forward chaining process involved the use of Google Scholar to locate all articles citing our included articles from the primary search. Inclusion criteria included original peer-reviewed research articles that focused on children and adolescents up to age 18 years, provided a description of an ED-specific treatment as well as weight and/or psychological outcomes at the time of discharge, and were published in English or French. Studies of all different types of methodology were included (randomized controlled trials [RCTs], open trials, case reports). Studies were excluded if they did not distinguish between outcomes for children and adolescents and outcomes for adults, or if they focused only on medical interventions, pharmacotherapy or refeeding protocols aimed at restoring medical stability to facilitate discharge to outpatient treatment.

For each included study, the study type (e.g. prospective or randomised control trial), number of participants included in the analysis, treatment method, primary outcome variable(s), and observed results were summarized.

Given the low quality of the studies, quantitative analysis was not possible. Qualitative review of all included studies was performed, summarizing the outcomes at end of inpatient treatment. We distinguish outcomes across various types of treatment frameworks as well as the evidence supporting the use of adjunctive therapies as part of inpatient treatment.

Two reviewers (LI and JC) independently assessed the risk for bias in the articles using the GRADE (Grading of Recommendations, Assessment, Development and Evaluations) system [17]. The GRADE system incorporates analysis of risk of bias based on various limitations of the studies, including lack of concealment of allocation, blinding, accounting of all participants, and selective reporting of outcomes for RCTs, and lack of an adequate control population, flawed measurement of outcomes, failure to adequately control for confounding factors and incomplete or inadequately short follow-up for observational studies.

Results

The database search initially provided $n = 7136$ citations, as reported in the PRISMA flowchart (Fig. 1). An additional 49 citations were added through review of references and forward citation chaining. After removing duplicates, $n = 6426$ records remained, of which $n = 5881$ were eliminated given that they did not meet the inclusion criteria. Of the 545 full text articles assessed for eligibility, $n = 479$ studies were excluded because they were longitudinal follow-up studies with no information on outcome at the time of discharge, were primarily adult studies, were review or secondary analysis papers, book chapters or guidelines, or did not provide sufficient description of the treatment provided, did not focus on inpatient treatment, or otherwise did not meet the inclusion criteria. Ultimately, $n = 66$ studies were selected for inclusion in this review (See Fig. 1). Quantitative analysis of the results was not possible due to the varying outcome measures used, the low quality of the studies and the high heterogeneity in methods used amongst the studies. Instead a narrative summary of the results is

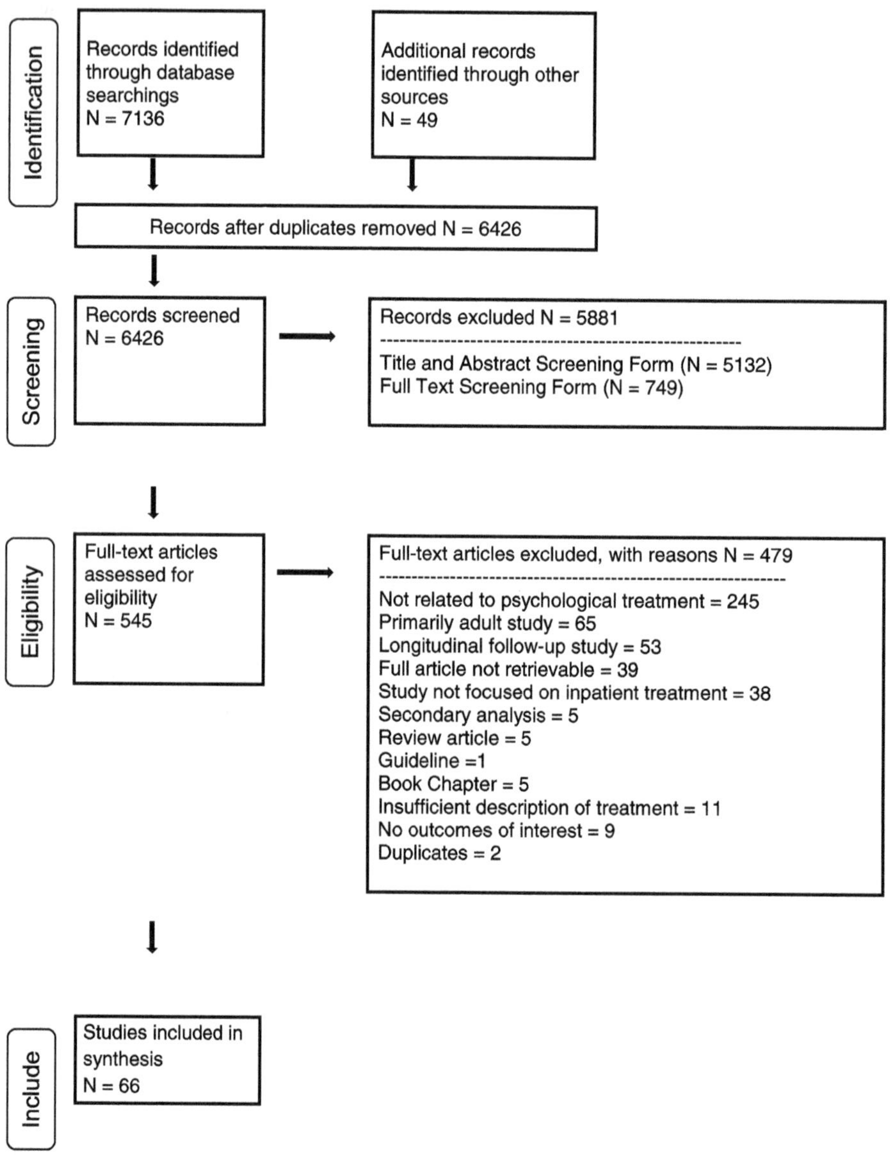

Fig. 1 PRISMA (Preferred Reporting Items for Systematic Reviews and Meta-Analyses) flow diagram of study selection

presented below. The risk of bias as assessed by the GRADE system was deemed as high for all included studies.

Inpatient ED programs for anorexia nervosa

Primary outcome - weight gain

We failed to identify any RCTs exploring outcomes of inpatient treatment specifically for pediatric AN, including atypical anorexia nervosa. We identified twenty studies (total $n = 1091$) describing inpatient treatment based on an integrative approach for AN, including psychiatric, medical, nutritional, and pharmacologic management, as well as individual, group and family therapy along with skilled nursing support [18–37]. None of these studies included control or comparison groups. Various measures of change in weight were used across these studies. Mean change in weight was positive in all studies. Mean LOS ranged widely between studies (Table 1).

Three studies (total $n = 39$) examined inpatient treatment utilizing a family-based approach [38–40], and three papers (total $n = 296$) reported on inpatient treatment utilizing a cognitive behavioural (CBT) approach [41–43]. In all studies patients gained weight in hospital, although measures by which weight changes were reported varied, as did LOS (Table 1).

Fourteen additional studies reported on a behaviour therapy approach (total $n = 218$) [44–57]. Various approaches to reporting change in weight were used, and all studies reported a positive change in weight from admission to discharge (Table 1). Of interest, Collins et al. (1983) reported that LOS was correlated to admission weight and feeding mode (i.e. oral vs nasogastric tube (NGT) feeds), and reported that the highest LOS was in those < 75% Treatment Goal Weight (TGW) at admission and requiring NGT feedings [49]. Another cohort study, by Solanto et al. (1994), reported weight gain under two types of behaviour contracts, varying only with regards to the expected rate of weight gain as measured every 4 days (q4d) (i.e. 0.36 kg/q4d vs 0.55 kg/q4d) [56]. Those treated under the contract with higher weight targets gained weight at a faster rate and gained more weight overall.

Two reports (total $n = 6$) were included in which patients were treated within an inpatient program using a psychodynamic approach [58, 59]. The LOS and weekly weight gain for these patients varied substantially (Table 1).

Finally, two reports examined the effect on weight of admission to a general pediatrics unit with supportive psychotherapy [37, 60, 61]. In both studies patients gained weight (Table 1).

Symptom change

While all of the observational studies of patients with AN using an integrative framework for inpatient treatment reported on change in weight, fewer reported on change in ED symptoms or psychopathology (Table 1). Four studies reported on changes in the Eating Disorder Examination-Questionnaire (EDE-Q) [22, 24, 35, 36]. In only one of these studies, Fennig et al's (2015) [36], a significant pre-post difference ($n = 51$, $p < 0.05$) was found and attributed predominantly to changes in *restraint* and *eating concerns* subscales. Of note, BMI at discharge was higher in the Fennig et al. (2015) study than the other three studies that reported on EDE-Q scores. Three studies (total $n = 126$) reported change in Eating Attitude Test (EAT) scores at admission and discharge [21, 30, 32]. The difference in EAT scores was noted to improve in two of the studies [21, 32]. Fennig et al. (2015), compared scores on the Eating Disorder Inventory-2 (EDI-2) at admission and discharge and found no significant change in total or subscale scores [36].

Schlegl et al. (2016), used a CBT framework for treatment and reported on symptom change using EDI-2 scores [42]. All subscales showed significant improvements (Table 1).

Several studies using a behaviour therapy approach reported on symptom change during admission (Table 1). Cinciripini et al. (1983) described a case report in which purging after meals decreased from 48% of meals/week to 0% of meals per week [47]. Two other studies reported on EAT scores, both of which showed a reduction in scores during admission [44, 57]. Of note, Alessi et al. (1989) reported that EAT scores remained high for the first 7 weeks of treatment (with weight gain of 4.5 kg over the first 7 weeks) and scores then dropped (from total score of 60 to 10) during the last 3 weeks of a 10-week admission. Steinhausen et al. (1985) reported symptom change through EDI scores and noted that the mean "Drive for Thinness" scores decreased significantly over the course of admission ($p = 0.02$) [57].

Measures of change in motivation

Castro-Fornieles et al. (2007) measured motivation for change using the Anorexia Nervosa Stage of Change Questionnaire (ANSOCQ) at admission and discharge in an inpatient program utilizing an integrative framework [21]. Change in mean ANSOCQ score was noted to be statistically significant; however, both admission and discharge scores were characterized as within the "preparation" phase of motivation, and wide confidence intervals were reported (Table 1).

Inpatient programs for mixed ED diagnoses

Weight gain

Three studies using an integrative approach (total $n = 239$) were included and reported on weight gain during inpatient treatment for patients with mixed ED diagnoses [9, 28, 30] (Table 2). The studies included in this

Table 1 Studies of inpatient treatment for children and adolescent patients with anorexia nervosa

First Author, Year	# of Participants <18 yrs. (Diagnosis)	Study Design	Mean Length of Stay	Primary Outcome	Findings
Studies of Inpatient Treatment Based on an Integrative Approach for AN					
Anis, 2016 [18]	59 (47 AN-R[a] and 12 atypical AN[b])	Case series	67.2 days (SD=81.1 days)	Change in weight admission to discharge (BMI[c])	Weight increased from mean BMI 16.3 (SD=1.35) to 17.1 (SD=1.35)
Ayton, 2009 [19]	50 (23 AN-R, 5 AN-B/P[d] and 6 EDNOS[e])	Case control (outcomes compared between those admitted with parental consent vs those formally detained)	240 days or 417 days	Change in weight admission to discharge (BMI)	Weight increased from BMI 14.4 (SD=1.9) to 18.5 (SD=1.6) or 16.6 (SD=2.6) to 19.6 (SD=1.5), difference in weight at admission between groups was significant (p=0.001) and non-significant at discharge.
Bourion-Bedes, 2013 [20]	66 (54 AN-R and 12 AN-B/P)	Case series	Not reported	Change in weight (BMI) and % of participants reaching 90%TGW[f]	Admission BMI 14.8 (SD=1.8) and change in BMI 3.1 (SD=1.4) (p<0.001) 90.9% of patients reached 90%TGW by a mean of 58.2 days (SD=38.3) of admission
Castro-Fornieles, 2007 [21]	49 (37 AN-R and 12 AN-B/P)	Case series	29.8 days (SD=17.6)	Change in weight admission to discharge (mean BMI), change mean EAT-26[g] scores ANSOCQ[h] scores admission to discharge	Weight increased from mean BMI 15.5 (SD=1.4) to 18.4 (SD=0.8) (p<0.001) Mean EAT-26 score decreased from 53.9 (SD=29.9) to 43.5 (SD=29.0) (p=0.002) Mean ANSOCQ score decreased from 53.6 (SD=19.7) to 62.9 (SD=24.5) (p=0.001)
Fennig, 2015 [36]	44 (all AN)	Case series	115.8 days (SD=54.7)	Change in weight admission to discharge (mean BMI), mean EDE-Q[i] scores, mean EDI-2[j] scores	Weight increased from mean BMI 16.2 (SD=1.8) at admission to 19.5 (SD=1.5) at discharge Change in total EDE-Q score was significant (p<0.05) No significant change in EDI-2 scores admission to discharge
Goddard, 2013 [22]	11 (AN or EDNOS)	Case Series	29.0 days (SD=11.9)	Change in weight admission to discharge (mean BMI), mean EDE-Q scores	Weight increased from BMI 15.0 (SD=1.6) at admission to 18.5 (SD=1.3) at discharge (p=0.001) EDE-Q total and subscales improved, but non-significant change admission to discharge
Heinberg, 2003 [23]	40 (27 AN-R, 8 AN-B/P, 2 "low weight" BN, 1 subthreshold AN-R, 1 subthreshold BN[k], 1 atypical ED)	Case control (comparison to adult sample and inpatient to day treatment for adolescent)	20.6 days (SD=13.03)	Weight gain per week	Rate of inpatient weight gain mean 1.86kg/week (SD=0.68) vs adults gained 1.95 kg/week. Day Treatment weight gain 0.99kg/week (SD=0.47)
Hetman, 2017 [24]	51 (44 AN-R, 7 AN-B/P)	Case control (comparison of patients that did not require readmission by one year and those that did require re-admission)	112 days (SD=69.6) and 113.8 days (SD=34.8)	Weight gain admission to discharge (BMI) and Percent from Target Weight (PFTW) at Discharge, change mean EDE-Q scores admission to discharge	No readmission – increase in BMI from 16.4 (SD=1.8) to 19.6 (SD=1.1) vs readmission – increase in BMI from 16.39 (SD=2.0) to 19.89 (SD=1.19) PFTW in group not requiring readmission was 101.2% at discharge vs 98.2% in group requiring readmission (p<0.05) Change in EDE-Q scores did not differ between groups
Kalisvaart, 2007 [25]	39 (28 AN, 11 EDNOS)	Case Series	50.8 (SD=29.6)	Weight gain admission to discharge (%TGW and BMI) and rate of weight gain	%TGW rose from 74.8 (SD=9.4) at admission to 85.1 (SD=5.3) at discharge (p<0.001) BMI rose from a mean of 15.5 (SD=1.9) to 17.6

Table 1 Studies of inpatient treatment for children and adolescent patients with anorexia nervosa *(Continued)*

First Author, Year	# of Participants <18 yrs. (Diagnosis)	Study Design	Mean Length of Stay	Primary Outcome	Findings
					(SD=1.2) at discharge (p<0.001) Mean rate of weight gain was 0.1kg/d (SD=0.06)
Leon, 1985 [26]	31 (19 AN-R, 12 AN-B/P)	Case Control (AN-R vs AN-B/P)	143 (Range 56-276) for AN-R group, 135 (Range 43-242) for AN-B/P group	Weight gain (change in weight in kg admission to discharge)	Weight rose from a mean of 38.4kg (range 28.2-47.3) to 47.2kg (37.3-49.5) for AN-R group and from a mean of 42.0kg (35.0-48.6) to 46.8kg (34.1-54.5)
Lock, 2003 [37]	39 (all AN)	Case series	31.9 (SD=16.5)	Weight gain admission to discharge (%TGW)	Mean %TGW rose from 74.9% (SD=7.0%) at admission to 85.2% (SD=5.8%) at discharge
Lievers, 2009 [27]	268 (217 AN-R, 51 AN-B/P)	Case series	135 (SD=97)	Weight gain admission to discharge (BMI)	Mean BMI rose from 13.5 (SD=1.3) at admission to 17.4 (SD=1.4)
Mekori, 2017 [28]	88 (44 AN-R, 17 AN-B/P, 13 BN, 14 EDNOS-B/P)	Case control (compared patient with AN vs BN or EDNOS-B/P)	204 (SD=91)	Weight gain admission to discharge (BMI)	Mean BMI rose significantly from admission to discharge (15.8, SD=1.9 to 19.8, SD=0.7) for AN group.
Nova, 2008 [29]	14 (all AN)	Case Series	Unclear	Weight gain admission to one month (%TGW, weight in kg)	Mean %TGW rose from 72.2 (SD=7.9) at admission to 78.7 (SD=6.0) after one month (p<0.001) Mean weight at admission was 39.4 (SD=6.1) and rose to 43.0 (SD=4.9) after one month (p<0.001)
Rothschild-Yakar, 2011 [30]	62 (33 AN-R, 10 AN-B/P, 19 BN)	Case control (compared AN-R to AN-B/P and BN combined)	196.2 (SD=68.1) for AN-R group	Change in mean weight from admission to discharge (BMI) Change in EAT -26 scores admission to discharge	Mean BMI rose from 14.94 (SD=1.93) at admission to 19.24 (SD=1.45) at discharge for AN-R group. Mean EAT-26 score for AN-R group decreased from 41.8 (SD=18.6) to 32.2 (SD=22.2), ES (diagnosis x time = 0.23, NS)
Roux, 2016 [31]	83 (all AN)	Case control (compared adolescent to adult patients)	137.6 (SD=101.8)	Change in weight from admission to discharge (BMI)	Mean BMI rose from 14.3 (SD=1.44) at admission to 17.9 (SD=1.7) at discharge
Shugar, 1994 [32]	15 (all AN-B/P)	Case series	91 (range 84-98)	Change in weight admission to discharge (BMI) Change in EAT-26 score from admission to discharge	Mean BMI rose from 38.4 (SD=2.56) at admission to 16.3 (SD=0.98) at discharge Mean EAT-26 score decreased from 48.7 (SD=9.8) at admission to 29.6 (SD=9.7) at discharge
Tasaka, 2017 [33]	41 (all AN-R)	Case series	130.7 (SD=66.2)	Change in weight admission to discharge (BMI and %TGW)	Mean BMI rose from 13.2 (SD=1.6) at admission to 15.3 (SD=1.7) at discharge Mean %TGW rose from 68.3 (SD=7.3) at admission to 78.8 SD=3.6) at discharge
Toms, 1972 [34]	1 (AN)	Case Report	239	Change in weight admission to discharge (kg)	Weight increased from 25.5kg at admission to 42.6kg at discharge
Vall, 2017 [35]	40 (36 AN-R, 4 AN-B/P)	Case Series	20.1 (SD=10.3)	Change in weight admission to discharge (BMI centile) Change in EDE-Q score admission to discharge	Mean BMI centile rose from 9.0 (SD=2.1) at admission to 21.3 (SD=3.1) at discharge Mean total EDE-Q score did not differ significantly from admission to discharge
Stuides Inpatient Treatment Utilizing a Family-Based or Cognitive Behavioural Approach for AN					
Goldfield, 2003 [38]	1 (AN-R)	Case Report	Not Reported	Change in weight from admission to discharge (BMI)	BMI rose from 15.4 at admission to 19.5 at discharge.
Halvorsen,	37 (all AN)	Case Series	144.2 (SD=95.2)	Mean change in weight during	Mean weight rose be 7.5kg (SD=4.4) during

Table 1 Studies of inpatient treatment for children and adolescent patients with anorexia nervosa *(Continued)*

First Author, Year	# of Participants <18 yrs. (Diagnosis)	Study Design	Mean Length of Stay	Primary Outcome	Findings
2018 [39]				admission (kg)	admission.
Matthews, 2016 [40]	1 (AN-R)	Case Report	9	Change in weight admission to discharge (BMI and %TGW)	BMI rose from 16.3 at admission to 17.5 at discharge %TGW rose from 82.0% at admission to 85.8% at discharge
Salbach-Andrae, 2009 [41]	57 (41 AN-R, 16 AN-B/P)	Case series	89.6 (SD=24.5)	Change in weight admission to discharge (BMI centile)	Mean BMI centile rose from 1.46 (SD=2.41) at admission to 9.44 (SD=6.68) at discharge
Schlegl, 2016 [42]	238 (188 AN-unspecified, 42 AN-B/P, 8 atypical AN)	Case series	81.9 (32.0)	Change in weight admission to discharge (BMI) Change in EDI-2 scores admission to discharge	Mean BMI rose from 14.8 at admission to 17.3 at discharge (ES=2.06) EDI-2 Global rose from 296.0 (SD=64.3) at admission to 245.7 (SD=65.1) at discharge (ES= 0.78)
Paul, 2013 [43]	1 (AN-R)	Case report	6	Change in weight admission to discharge (kg)	Weight rose from 36.5kg at admission to 37.6kg at discharge
Studies of Inpatient Treatment Utilizing a Behaviour Therapy Approach for AN					
Alessi, 1989 [44]	1 (AN-R)	Case Report	70	Change in weight admission to discharge (kg) Mean EAT-26 scores admission to discharge	Weight rose from 23.8 kg at admission to 31.8kg at discharge EAT-26 scores remained high until 49 days into admission then decreased (actual absolute values not given)
Blanchet-Collet, 2016 [45]	1 (AN-R)	Case Report	Not Reported	Change in weight admission to discharge (BMI)	BMI rose from 13.5 at admission to 16.5 at discharge
Blinder, 1970 [46]	1 (AN-R)	Case Report	38	Change in weight admission to discharge (kg)	Weight rose from 42.6kg at admission to 51.0kg at discharge
Cinciripini, 1983 [47]	1 (AN-B/P)	Case Report	39	Change in weight admission to discharge (kg) Change in intake admission to discharge (kcal/day)	Weight rose from 44.0kg at admission to 54.0kg at discharge Daily intake rose from 850kcal at admission to 1700kcal at discharge
Clark, 1981 [48]	2 (AN-R)	Case reports	44 days and 56 days	Change in weight admission to discharge (kg)	Case 1: weight rose from 39.4kg at admission to 45kg at discharge Case 2: weight rose from 39kg to 50kg at discharge
Collins, 1983 [49]	37 (AN-R)	Case series	23.9 (range 2-66)	Weight gain admission to discharge (kg)	Mean weight gain was 5.8kg (range 0-12.7kg) from admission to discharge
Garfinkel, 1973 [50]	4 (AN-R)	Case reports	Case 1: 42days Case 2: 42 days Case 3: 56 days Case 4: 21 days	Weight gain while being treated under behavioural therapy framework (kg)	Case 1: 9.0kg Case 2: 8.6kg Case 3: 14.6kg Case 4: 11.9kg
Halmi, 1975 [51]	4 (all AN)	Case reports	Not specifically reported for adolescent patients,	Weight gain admission to discharge (%TGW)	Mean %TGW at admission was 67.5% and at discharge was 84%

Table 1 Studies of inpatient treatment for children and adolescent patients with anorexia nervosa *(Continued)*

First Author, Year	# of Participants <18 yrs. (Diagnosis)	Study Design	Mean Length of Stay	Primary Outcome	Findings
			43.8 days for adults and adolescents combined	Total weight gain during admission (kg)	Mean total weight gain during admission was 8.15kg
Leitenberg, 1968 [52]	2 (both AN)	Case reports	45 days and 39 days	Weight gain while treated under behavioural therapy framework (kg) Increase in intake while treated under behavioural therapy framework (kcal)	Case 1: weight rose 8.2 kg, intake rose from 1700kcal to 4000kcal Case 2: weight rose 11.2kg, intake rose from 1600kcal to 3900kcal
Nygaard, 1990 [53]	84 (all AN)	Case series	23 (range 7-56)	Weight gain admission to discharge (kg)	Mean weight gain from admission to discharge was 1.89 (SD=1.41)
Pertschuk, 1978 [54]	2 (both AN)	Case reports	13	Weight gain while treated under behavioural therapy framework (kg)	Case 1: 4.88 kg Case 2: 3.63 kg
Poole, 1978 [55]	2 (both AN)	Case reports	23	Weight gain while treated under behavioural therapy framework (kg)	Case 1: 12.6 kg Case 2: 15.3 kg
Solanto, 1994 [56]	53 (all AN)	Case control (compared 22 vs 31 patients treated under to different behaviour contracts)	28	Rate of weight gain when treated under each behaviour contract.	Group 1: 0.09kg/d (SD=0.05) Group 2: 0.16kg/d (SD=0.07) Significant effect for contract x day (p<0.009)
Steinhausen, 1985 [57]	24 (17 AN-R, 7 AN-B/P)	Case series	77	Weight gain admission to discharge (%TGW) Change in EAT-26 scores admission to discharge Change in EDI-drive for thinness admission to discharge	Mean weight rose from 65.9%TGW at admission to 87.4%TGW at discharge (p<0.0001) Mean EAT-26 score dropped from 37.1 to 12.7 (p< 0.0001) Mean EDI-drive for thinness dropped from 8.0 to 1.9 (p<0.02)
Studies of Inpatient Treatment Utilizing a Psychodynamic Approach for AN					
Groen, 1966 [58]	5 (all AN)	Case reports	61 (range 30-91)	Weight gain admission to discharge (kg)	Mean weight rose from 36.6 kg (range 29-43kg) at admission to 43kg (range 36-47kg) at discharge
Kronenberg, 1994 [59]	1 (AN-R)	Case report	152	Weight gain admission to discharge (kg)	Weight rose from 35kg at admission to 42kg at discharge
Studies of Inpatient Treatment on Pediatric Unit for AN					
Jenkins, 1987 [60]	21 (16 AN-R, 5 AN-B/P)	Case series	185 (SD=122)	Weight gain admission to discharge (%TGW)	Mean %TGW rose from 68% (5.5) at admission to 99% (SD=7.7) at discharge
Maxmen, 1974 [61]	5 (all AN)	Case reports	40 (range 11-67)	Weight gain admission to discharge (kg)	Mean weight rose from 34.4kg at admission to 43.2 at discharge

[a] *AN-R* anorexia nervosa – restricting subtype
[b] *AN* anorexia nervosa
[c] *BMI* body mass index
[d] *AN-B/P* anorexia nervosa – binge/purge subtype
[e] *EDNOS* eating disorder not otherwise specified
[f] *TGW* treatment goal weight
[g] *EAT-26* eating attitude test
[h] *ANOSOCQ* anorexia nervosa stages of change questionnaire
[i] *EDE-Q* eating disorders examination - questionnaire
[j] *EDI-2* eating disorders inventory
[k] *BN* bulimia nervosa

Table 2 Studies of inpatient treatment for children and adolescents mixed eating disorder diagnoses

Author, Year	# of Participants (Diagnosis)	Study Design	Mean Length of Stay	Primary Outcome	Finding
Mekori, 2017 [28]	88 (44 AN-R, 17 AN-B/P, 13 BN, 14 EDNOS-B/P)	Case control (compared patient with AN vs BN or EDNOS-B/P)	204 (SD = 91)	Weight gain admission to discharge (BMI)	Mean BMI rose significantly from admission to discharge (15.8, SD[a] =1.9 to 19.8, SD = 0.7) and did not increase significantly in the BN/EDNOS group (19.8, SD = 2.1 to 21.1, SD = 1.3); F (group x time) = 88.1, $p < 0.0001$)
Morris, 2015 [9]	89 (70 AN, 2 atypical AN, 1 BN, 16 Unspecified ED)	Case series	141.1 (SD = 125.7)	Weight gain admission to discharge (mean weekly weight gain and BMI)	Mean weekly weight gain was 0.43 kg/week and there was a significant rise in mean BMI admission to discharge ($p <$ 0.001)
Rothschild-Yakar, 2011	62 (33 AN-R, 10 AN-B/P, 19 BN)	Case control (compared AN-R to AN-B/P and BN combined)	196.2 (SD = 68.1) for AN-R group, 178.8 (SD = 69) for AN-B/P and BN	Change in mean weight from admission to discharge (BMI) Change in EAT −26 scores admission to discharge	Mean BMI rose from 14.94 (SD = 1.93) at admission to 19.24 (SD = 1.45) at discharge for AN-R and from 18.80 (SD = 3.99) to 20.15 (SD = 2.29) for AN-B/P and BN. ES (diagnosis x time = 0.59, $p < 0.001$) Mean EAT-26 score decreased for AN-R group from 41.8 (SD = 18.6) to 32.2 (SD = 22.2) and in AN-B/P and BN group from 46.7 (SD = 15.0) to 28.8 (SD = 14.7). ES (diagnosis x time = 0.23, NS)

[a]*SD* Standard deviation

section reported outcomes for various eating disorders (ie AN, BN, OSFED and EDNOS) as a combined group rather than differentiating outcomes by diagnosis. In all 3 studies patients gained weight from admission to discharge. Not surprisingly, in the 2 studies that differentiated anorexia nervosa-restricting subtype (AN-R) from other ED diagnoses, there was a significantly greater increase in Body Mass Index (BMI) for the group containing AN-R patients [28, 30].

Symptom change

Rothschild-Yakar et al. (2013) compared symptom change from admission to discharge in an integrative inpatient treatment program for mixed ED diagnoses, using the EAT-26 in a group of patients with AN-R vs anorexia nervosa binge-purge subtype (AN-BP) or bulimia nervosa (BN) [30]. Overall there was a statistically significant improvement in EAT-26 scores over the course of the admission ($p < 0.001$), and no significant difference in change in EAT-26 scores by diagnosis.

Inpatient programs for bulimia nervosa

We identified only one study that reported outcomes of inpatient treatment specifically for youth with BN [62]. The treatment provided was based on behaviour therapy and outcomes focused primarily on changes from admission to discharge in serotonin levels, as measured by 5-hydroxytriptamine induced calcium release from platelets. As such, this study was limited in that the only reported ED-specific outcome was change in BMI, and weight decreased slightly over admission (Table 3).

Inpatient programs for ARFID

Weight

Three case reports or case series were identified which described inpatient treatment of a total of eight children with ARFID treated using either a family-based or CBT or behavioural therapy approach [63–65]. Weight gain was reported in two studies (Table 4).

Change in Oral intake

Singer et al. (1992) reported on change in caloric intake in kcal/day for three patients with ARFID using a CBT inpatient treatment [64]. Oral intake rose for all three patients over the course of admission (Table 4).

Pitt and Middleman (2018) reported on two cases of adolescents with ARFID [65]. After admission, nasojejunal (NJ) tubes were placed to initiate refeeding when oral feeding was not tolerated. The authors reported that the use of an individualized behaviour plan for each patient providing reinforcements for eating was the critical factor which helped these patients to tolerate oral intake without vomiting and allowed for the removal of the NJ tubes (Table 4).

Table 3 Studies of inpatient treatment for children and adolescent with bulimia nervosa

Author, Year	# of Participants (Diagnosis)	Study Design	Mean Length of Stay	Primary Outcome	Finding
Wockel, 2009 [62]	13 (all BN)	Case series	69 (SD = 24.5)	Weight change admission to discharge (BMI)	Mean BMI decreased by 0.3 kg (SD=1.4) from admission to discharge

Combined inpatient and day treatment programs

Weight gain

Five studies summarized the experience of 264 adolescents with AN treated as inpatients followed immediately by day treatment (DTP), utilizing either an integrative or CBT approach [66–70]. Studies considered as providing combined inpatient and day treatment programs reported on change from the point of admission to an inpatient program through the end of their involvement in day treatment. In these studies, all patients received inpatient treatment directly followed by day treatment services. All five studies included inpatient treatment for medically unstable patients followed by transfer to a DTP once medical stability was attained (Table 5). Total mean LOS (i.e. inpatient and DTP combined) varied substantially between studies. Weight increased in all studies (Table 5).

Symptom change

Symptom change was reported using various scales in two studies of combined inpatient and DTP [66, 68]. Hillen et al. (2015) failed to demonstrate a significant change in EDI-2 scores. Dalle Grave et al. (2014) reported a significant decrease in EDE-Q scores pre to post treatment for global score and for all subscales other than Shape Concern. The percentage of patients with Global EDE-Q scores < 1 SD above the community mean at admission was 2% (+/− 7.7) and at discharge it was 10% (+/− 38.5), suggesting a decrease in ED thoughts and urges with treatment (Table 5).

Motivation

Hillen et al. (2015) reported on change in motivation as measured by the ANSOCQ in 35 patients [68]. Overall mean scores increased by 21.7 points which signified moving from contemplation to preparation phases. Overall, 29.4% (up from 0% at admission) of patients were classified as being in "maintenance phase" and 26.5% (up from 15% at admission) in "action phase" at time of discharge from DTP (Table 5).

Overall outcome

Treat et al. (2008) included 71 patients who combined inpatient and DTP and reported on "overall outcome" [70]. At the end of DTP 35.2% were deemed to have an excellent outcome, 26.8% were deemed to have good outcome,14.1% were deemed below average outcome and 23.9% were described as having a poor outcome, according to definitions assigned by the authors which

Table 4 Studies of inpatient treatment for children and adolescents with avoidant restrictive food intake disorder

Author, Year	# of Participants (Diagnosis)	Study Design	Mean Length of Stay	Primary Outcome	Findings
Spettigue, 2018 [63]	3 (2 ARFID[a]-aversive subtype, 1 ARFID-mixed subtype)	Case reports	53 days	Change in weight gain (%TGW)	Case 1: Weight increased from 83%TGW to 100%TGW. Case 2: Weight increased from 75.8%TGW to 100%TGW. Case 3: Weight increased from 72%TGW to 88%TGW
Singer, 1992 [64]	3 (1 ARFID – aversive subtype, 2 ARFID-mixed subtype)	Case reports	32 days (range 16–60 days)	Change in weight (kg) Increase in caloric intake from admission to discharge (kcal/day)	Case 1: Increase in weight from 21.8 kg to 24.5 kg (over 60 days), intake increased from 1557 kcal/d to 2208 kcal/d) Case 2: Increase in weight from 21.4 kg to 22.6 kg (over 16 days), intake increased from 740 kcal/d to 1500 kcal/d) Case 3: Increase in weight from 17.7 kg to 18.0 kg (over 19 days), intake increased from 1200 kcal/d to 1500 kcal/d
Pitt, 2018 [65]	2 (ARFID – mixed subtype)	Case reports	Not reported	Reduction in vomiting and tolerance of oral intake without emesis	Vomiting frequency reduced and oral tolerance improved although specifics not reported

[a]*ARFID* Avoidant restrictive food intake disorder

Table 5 Studies of inpatient treatment followed by day treatment for children and adolescents with eating disorders

Author, Year	# of Participants (Diagnosis)	Study Design	Mean Length of Stay	Primary Outcome	Finding
Delle Grave, 2014 [66]	27 (all AN[b], subtype not recorded)	Case series	91 days inpatient + 49 days day treatment	Weight gain from admission to inpatient to discharge from day treatment (kg, BMI centile) Change in EDE-Q[a] scores from admission to inpatient until discharge from day treatment	Mean weight rose from 38.5 (SD = 6.1) at admission to 49.7 (SD = 5.6) at discharge Mean BMI centile rose from 2.7 (SD = 4.2) at admission to 34.2 (SD = 15.7) at discharge Mean EDE-Q Global score dropped from 3.7 (SD = 1.3) at admission to 2.1 (SD = 1.2) at discharge ($p < 0.001$)
El Ghoch, 2014 [67]	33 (all AN, subtype not recorded)	Case Control	91 days inpatient + 49 days day treatment	Weight gain admission to inpatient to discharge from day treatment (kg, BMI centile)	Mean weight rose from 38.9 kg (SD = 5.1) to 49.4 kg (SD = 3.9) at discharge (admit to discharge $p < 0.001$, admit vs control $p < 0.001$, discharge vs control $p < 0.06$) Mean BMI centile rose from 1.6 (SD = 4.0) at admission to 31.7 (SD = 10.6) at discharge (admit to discharge $p < 0.001$, admit vs control $p < 0.001$, discharge vs control $p < 0.8$)
Hillen, 2015 [68]	34 (31 AN-R[b], 3 AN-B/P[b])	Case series	105.7 (SD[c]=38.5)	Weight gain admission to inpatient to discharge from day treatment (BMI, %TGW[d]) Change in EDI-2[e] scores admission to inpatient to discharge from day treatment Change in ANSOCQ[f] score admission to inpatient to discharge from day treatment	Mean BMI rose from 15.7 (SD = 1.2) at admission to 18.0 (1.0) at discharge Mean %TGW rose from 77.6% (SD = 5.4%) at admission to 88.5% (SD = 4.4%) at discharge Mean EDI-2 score dropped from 270.9 (SD = 66.6) at admission to 255.5 (SD = 78.1) at discharge ($p < 0.36$) Mean ANSOCQ score rose from 50.2 (SD = 14.8) at admission to 71.6 (SD = 23.0) at discharge ($p < 0.0001$)
Strober, 2006 [69]	99 (all AN, subtype not recorded)	Case series	118 (SD = 27)	Weight gain admission inpatient to discharge from day treatment (BMI)	Mean BMI rose from 12.5 (SD = 1.1) at admission to 18.5 (SD = 0.42) at discharge
Treat, 2008 [70]	71 (all AN, subtype not recorded)	Case series	33.6 days inpatient, 22.3 days day treatment	Weight gain admission to inpatient to discharge from day treatment (%TGW, BMI) Overall outcome as rated by composite of %TGW, weight trajectory and compensatory measures)	Mean %TGW rose from 74.1 (SD = 7.3) to 87.3% (SD = 5.77) at discharge ($p < 0.01$) Mean BMI rose form 15.2 (SD = 1.54) at admission to 17.9 (SD = 1.07) at discharge ($p < 0.01$) Excellent outcome in 25 patients, intermediate in 29 patients and poor in 17 patients at discharge from day treatment

[a]Eating Disorders Examination Questionnaire
[b]Anorexia Nervosa – binge/purge
[c]Standard Deviation
[d]Treatment Goal Weight
[e]Eating Disorders Inventory
[f]Anorexia Nervosa Stages of Change Questionnaire

included a combination of % ideal BMI, maintenance of weight and compensatory behaviours (Table 5).

Adjunctive treatments

Adjunctive cognitive remediation therapy (CRT)

Four studies reported on the addition of CRT to integrative inpatient treatment for patients with AN (total n = 127) [71–74] (Table 6). Herbrich et al. (2017) described no difference in the change in weight between adolescent patients who received 10 sessions of CRT over 10 weeks compared to those who received treatment as usual (TAU) in a quasi-experimental design ($n = 24$ in each group) [74]. The other three studies did not include a control group. Patients (total $n = 79$) gained weight, but it was not possible to determine whether CRT had an impact on weight gain above and beyond what would have been expected by inpatient treatment [71–73].

Three studies of CRT added to inpatient treatment for AN reported on symptom change (Table 6). A report of two cases by Asch et al. (2014) described that total scores on the EAT decreased for one patient and increased in the other patient and Eating Behavior Rating Scale (EBRS) scores decreased slightly for both patients, by the end of 10 weeks [71]. Another study by Harrison et al. (2018), included 70 hospitalized patients who received individual CRT, and noted no change in EDE-Q scores [73].

In a study by Harrison et al. (2018), patients reported on change in motivation as measured by the MSCARED before and after the course of CRT [73]. There was a statistically significant shift in motivation noted ($p < 0.001$), with 42.9% in preparation, action or maintenance stages of change at initiation of CRT, and with 95.7% in one of those stages of change after receiving CRT (Table 6). Due to the design of this study it was not possible to differentiate the effect of inpatient treatment alone from inpatient treatment plus CRT.

Adjunctive multi-family/parent group therapy

A study by Depestele et al. (2017) reported on 112 patients with various ED diagnoses admitted to an inpatient ED unit providing an integrative therapy approach to treatment, who also received either adjunctive multi-family group therapy (MFT, $n = 62$) or adjunctive multi-parent group therapy (MPT, $n = 50$) [75]. Both MPT and MFT interventions "promoted an autonomy-supportive parental attitude and the adolescents' autonomy and self-determination." Results reported a main effect of time on drive for thinness ($p < 0.001$) and body dissatisfaction ($p < 0.001$) as measured by EDI-2. Both scales improved independent of the type of intervention (Table 6).

Adjunctive bright light therapy

A study by Janas-Kozik et al. (2011) examined patients with AN and depressive symptoms (> 17 on Hamilton Depression Rating Scale) who were admitted to a CBT-based inpatient program and treated adjunctively with Bright Light Therapy [76]. In this study patients were randomized to receive either daily 30 min of Bright Light Therapy (BLT) + inpatient treatment ($n = 12$) × 6 weeks, or inpatient treatment only × 6 weeks (n = 12). Patients in both groups had a significant change in their BMI during the 6-week study; however, weight change from baseline was statistically significant by week 3 ($p = 0.038$) in the BLT group but only at week 6 ($p = 0.048$) in the TAU group (Table 6).

Adjunctive meal support

Three studies examined the effect of meal support/supervision as part of inpatient treatment for groups of patients with mixed ED diagnoses [77–79] (Table 6). In the two studies examining weight gain, there were no significant differences between cohorts who received meal support (total $n = 77$) and those who did not (total $n = 78$) on the rate of weight gain per day, although there was a trend towards greater weight gain per day in the group who received meal support [78, 79]. In these two studies, the approach to meals for patients who did not receive meal support was not documented. A separate study by Couturier & Mahmood (2009) reported a significant decrease in the rate of nasogastric tube feeds in the cohort of patients treated on an inpatient unit after the institution of consistent meal support [77].

Selective versus non-selective menus

Leacy & Cane (2012) ($n = 22$) compared the rate of weight gain and EDE-Q scores in patients with AN who received non-selective menus (i.e. meals chosen by a dietician) or selective menus (i.e. meals chosen by the patient, under the direction of a dietician) as part of their inpatient treatment [80]. The non-selective menu group gained weight significantly faster than those in the selective menu group ($p = 0.02$) (Table 6). No significant differences were found on any of the EDE-Q items related to eating concern. Overall change in EDE eating concern scores in this study were low, ranging from −0.6 to 1.1 (Table 6).

Conclusions

The aim of the present review was to identify the scope and benefits of psychological treatment provided to children and adolescents with EDs in inpatient settings. We identified 66 studies that demonstrated considerable heterogeneity in the types of treatment provided and the outcomes reported. While all studies focused on inpatient treatment, in some studies this treatment was

Table 6 Studies of adjunctive treatments in addition to inpatient treatment for children and adolescents with eating disorders

Author, Year	# of Participants (Diagnosis)	Study Design	Mean Length of Intervention	Primary Outcome	Findings
Asch, 2014 [71]	2 (both AN-R)	Case reports	10 weeks	Change in weight (BMI pre/post) Change in EAT-26 score pre/post Change in EBRS[a] score pre/post	Both patients gained weight (Pt 1: BMI 15.3 to BMI 18.1, Pt 2: BMI 13.3 to BMI 17.5) EAT-26 scores for both patients decreased over the intervention EBRS scores for both patients decreased over the intervention
Kuge, 2017 [72]	7 (all AN)	Case reports	4 weeks	Change in weight (BMI and %TGW pre/post)	Mean weight rose over the intervention (mean BMI rose from 14.8 to 16.0, ES[b] 0.80 and mean %TGW rose from 73.6 to 79.4%, ES 0.68)
Harrison, 2017 [73]	70 (66 AN-R, 4 AN-B/P)	Case series	10 weeks	Change in weight (mean %TGW pre/post) Change in EDE-Q score pre/post Change in motivation (MSCARED[c] pre/post)	Weight increased significantly during the intervention (79.3%TGW to 89.0%TGW, $p <$ 0.001) Non-significant decrease in EDE-Q score ($p <$ 0.08) Significant increase in motivational stage of change ($p < 0.001$)
Herbrich, 2017 [74]	48 (36 AN-R, 8 AN-B/P, 4 atypical AN)	Case control	5 weeks	Change in weight (mean BMI centile pre/post)	Significant increase in BMI centile in both groups pre/post ($p < 0.006$), no difference between groups
Depestele, 2017 [75]	112 (45 AN-R, 26 AN-B/P, 24 BN, 16 ED-NOS)	Case control (compared adjunctive multi-family group, n = 62 vs multi-parent group, n = 50)	8.5 weeks	Change in mean EDI-2 scores over time and between interventions Change in frequency of B/P behaviours over time	Significant improvement in mean EDI-2 sub-scales of drive for thinness ($p < 0.001$) and body dissatisfaction ($p < 0.001$). No significant difference between interventions BP behaviours decreased over time for patients with BN ($p < 0.05$) and AN-B/P ($p <$ 0.01)
Janas-Kozik, 2011 [76]	24 (all AN-R)	RCT (inpatient bright light therapy + CBT,[d] n = 12, vs inpatient CBT alone, n = 12)	6 weeks	Mean change in weight during intervention (BMI)	At end of intervention both groups had an increase in BMI of 10%, however significant increase from baseline in bright light group evident at week 3 vs week 6 for no bright light therapy
Couturier, 2009 [77]	21 (19 AN-R, 2 AN-B/P)	Case control (patients treated with meal support, n = 12, versus no meal support, *n* = 9)	61.2 (SD = 37.4) vs 78.0 (SD = 46.5), NS difference ($p < 0.39$)	Mean weekly weight gain Rate of need for NGT[e] feeds	Mean weekly weight gain did not differ between groups (1.2 kg/week +/−1.0 vs 0.6 kg/week +/−0.4, $p < 0.09$) Patients receiving meal support had a significantly lower rate of NGT feeds than those without meal support (11.1% vs 66.7%, $p < 0.02$)
Kells, 2013 [78]	52 (restrictive ED, no specific diagnoses reported)	Case control (patients who received at least one supervised meal/admission, *n* = 13 vs those who received no meal support, n = 39)	8.4 (SD = 7.5) vs 5.9 (SD = 3.5), non-significant difference ($p < 0.66$)	Mean daily weight gain (kg)	No significant difference between groups (0.35 kg+/−0.23 kg/week vs 0.33 kg+/− 0.29 kg/week, $p < 0.65$)

Table 6 Studies of adjunctive treatments in addition to inpatient treatment for children and adolescents with eating disorders *(Continued)*

Author, Year	# of Participants (Diagnosis)	Study Design	Mean Length of Intervention	Primary Outcome	Findings
Kells, 2016 [79]	108 (restrictive ED, no specific diagnoses reported)	Case control (patients with no meal support, $n = 38$ vs delayed meal support, $n = 11$ vs meal support, $n = 54$)	5.9 (SD = 3.5) vs 9.8 (SD = 7.3) vs 6.7 (SD = 3.3), non-significant difference ($p < 0.27$)	Mean daily weight gain (kg)	No significant difference between groups (0.34 +/−0.29 kg/d vs 0.31 +/− 0.26 kg/d vs 0.32 +/− 0.29 kg/d, $p < 0.63$)
Leacy, 2012 [80]	40 (38 AN-R, 2 AN-B/P)	Case control (patients treated with selective menus, n = 22, compared to non-selective menus, $n = 18$)	74.2 (SD = 28.7) vs 60.3 (SD = 22.8), non-significant difference ($p < 0.09$)	Mean weekly weight gain and change in EDE-Q scores	Patients treated with non-selective menus had a significantly higher weekly weight gain (0.95 +/− 0.35 kg/week) than those treated with selective menus (0.72 +/− 0.24 kg/week) ($p < 0.02$) There was no difference in change in EDE-Q scores between groups.

[a] *EBRS* Eating behaviors rating scale
[b] *ES* Effect size
[c] *MSCARED* Motivational stages of change for adolescents recovering from an eating disorder
[d] *CBT* Cognitive behavioral therapy
[e] *NGT* Nasogastric tube

provided on a pediatric unit and in other studies it was provided on a psychiatric unit, either designed specifically for the treatment of patients with EDs or not. The treatment provided also varied with regards to the therapeutic modalities utilized, length of stay in intensive treatment, and the goals or expectations of treatment.

Despite the presence of substantial biases, and lack of control groups, each of the specialized ED inpatient programs and non-specialized general pediatric wards reported success in helping underweight patients with restrictive eating disorders gain weight. Beyond this finding, given the overwhelming heterogeneity of methods described, there is little that can be concluded from the various studies contained within.

Similarly, it is impossible to draw any conclusions as to which adjunctive treatments might be most helpful when treating youth with AN in hospital. While adjunctive treatments were examined, i.e. the use of meal support, selective versus non-selective menus, bright light therapy, CRT, and multi-family versus multi-parent group, the quality of the studies does not allow us to draw any conclusions about the effectiveness of these treatments. There are also some interesting omissions from this literature on adjunctive inpatient treatments, including no papers looking at outcomes of adjunctive yoga, exercise programs, art therapy, journaling, mindfulness, dialectical behaviour skills groups, or individual or group motivational enhancement therapy. Furthermore, there are insufficient studies of inpatient treatment for EDs other than AN, such that no conclusions can be drawn about the effectiveness of inpatient programs for the treatment of BN, ARFID or BED.

Finally, none of these studies serve to identify the specific factors most associated with a successful inpatient program for the treatment of children and adolescents with EDs. Clinical experience often points to a number of factors that appear to have clinical relevance, including a specialized, experienced multidisciplinary treatment team that combines confidence, compassion, consistency and the ability to create a safe environment where it is assumed that patients will take the nutrition they need to recover. These units typically provide skilled meal support and attend to patients' medical, nutritional and psychological needs, with a focus on weight gain, renourishment and symptom interruption. It is widely recognized that families need to be supported and educated, and patients benefit from therapy which helps them to separate from and externalize the illness, thereby improving their motivation for recovery. Unfortunately, few of these factors have been identified, studied or discussed in the literature, there are no RCTs to provide guidance, and it is impossible to compare one inpatient program to another based on studies to date. It is also impossible to discern the optimal LOS, which combination of individual, group or family therapy is essential, or to determine the ideal group therapy content.

Limitations of this review include the inability to complete a meta-analysis or quantitative analysis due to the low quality and high heterogeneity of the studies available, the lack of inclusion of the search term "unspecified feeding and eating disorder" which could have yielded additional studies on this topic, a lack of studies specifically reporting on particular diagnoses including EDNOS, OSFED or atypical anorexia nervosa, and an inability to disaggregate findings based on subgroup such as gender or age (ie children vs adolescents).

Future research should focus on resolving these deficiencies through the use of studies based on high quality research methods, standardized operation of reporting treatment variables and outcomes, and multi-site designs to gather data on larger numbers of participants. Given the paucity of research in this field, the prolonged LOS (and associated costs) often observed, as well as the substantial variability by which treatments are delivered, it is critical that basic indicators of admission and treatment are standardized and reported, in order to continue to move the field forward. Only with improved research methods and reporting will it be possible to identify the key components of successful inpatient treatment and to improve outcomes for children and adolescents with EDs.

Abbreviations

AN: Anorexia nervosa; AN-R: Anorexia nervosa – restricting subtype; AN-B/P: Anorexia nervosa – binge/purge subtype; ANSOCQ: Anorexia nervosa stages of change questionnaire; ARFID: Avoidant restrictive food intake disorder; BED: Binge eating disorder; BLT: Bright light therapy; BMI: Body mass index; BN: Bulimia nervosa; CBT: Cognitive behaviour therapy; CRT: Cognitive remediation therapy; DTP: Day treatment program; EAT-26: Eating attitude test; ED: Eating disorder; EDE-Q: Eating disorder examination – questionnaire; EDI-2: Eating disorder inventory; EDNOS: Eating disorder not otherwise specified; GRADE: Grading of Recommendations, Assessment, Development and Evaluations; MPT: Multi-parent group therapy; MFT: Multi-family group therapy; NGT: Nasogastric tube; NJ: Nasojejunal; OSFED: Other specified feeding and eating disorder; PRISMA: Preferred Reporting Items for Systematic Reviews and Meta-analyses; RCT: Randomized control trial; TAU: Treatment as usual

Acknowledgements

The authors would like to acknowledge the contribution of Neera Bhatnagar (library scientist) who supported the initial abstract search, as well as Cheryl Webb and Dr. Natasha Snelgrove who contributed to this work through screening of abstracts.

Authors' contributions

All authors contributed to the screening of articles for inclusion/exclusion. LI and JC assessed the risk of bias for the articles included. The authors contributed to and approved the final manuscript.

Competing interests
The authors declare that they have no competing interests.

Author details
[1]Department of Psychiatry, Children's Hospital of Eastern Ontario, University of Ottawa, Ottawa, ON K1H 8L1, Canada. [2]Children's Hospital of Eastern Ontario Research Institute, Ottawa, ON K1H 8L1, Canada. [3]Division of Adolescent Health, Department of Pediatrics, Children's Hospital of Eastern Ontario, University of Ottawa, Ottawa, ON K1H 8L1, Canada. [4]Department of Psychiatry & Behavioural Neurosciences, McMaster University, Hamilton, ON L8N3Z5, Canada.

References
1. Le Grange D, Lock J, editors. Childhood and adolescence: looking at eating disorders when they start. New York: Guildford Press; 2011.
2. Hay P, Chinn D, Forbes D, Madden S, Newton R, Sugenor L, et al. Royal Australian and new Zealand College of Psychiatrists clinical practice guidelines for the treatment of eating disorders. Aust N Z J Psychiatry. 2014; 48(11):977–1008.
3. Lock J, La Via MC. American Academy of C, adolescent psychiatry committee on quality I. practice parameter for the assessment and treatment of children and adolescents with eating disorders. J Am Acad Child Adolesc Psychiatry. 2015;54(5):412–25.
4. Wilson GT, Shafran R. Eating disorders guidelines from NICE. Lancet. 2005; 365(9453):79–81.
5. Jauregui-Garrido B, Jauregui-Lobera I. Sudden death in eating disorders. Vasc Health Risk Manag. 2012;8:91–8.
6. Kastner D, Lowe B, Weigel A, Osen B, Voderholzer U, Gumz A. Factors influencing the length of hospital stay of patients with anorexia nervosa - results of a prospective multi-center study. BMC Health Serv Res. 2018;18(1):22.
7. Nozoe SSY, Yoshioka M, Naruo T, Masuda A, Nagai N, Tanaka H. Clinical features of patients with anorexia nervosa: assessment of factors influencing the duration of in-patient treatment. J Psychosom Res. 1995;39(3):271–81.
8. Warnke I, Rossler W. Length of stay by ICD-based diagnostic groups as basis for the remuneration of psychiatric inpatient care in Switzerland? Swiss Med Wkly. 2008;138(35–36):520–7.
9. Morris J, Simpson AV, Voy SJ. Length of stay of inpatients with eating disorders. Clin Psychol Psychother. 2015;22(1):45–53.
10. Toulany A, Wong M, Katzman DK, Akseer N, Steinegger C, Hancock-Howard RL, et al. Cost analysis of inpatient treatment of anorexia nervosa in adolescents: hospital and caregiver perspectives. CMAJ Open. 2015;3(2):E192–7.
11. AM C, M G-P, JV S, F C, I B, A. F. Eating disorders-related hospitalizations in Portugal: a nationwide study from 2000 to 2014. Int J Eat Disord. 2017; 51(10):1201–6.
12. Stuhldreher N, Wild B, Konig HH, Konnopka A, Zipfel S, Herzog W. Determinants of direct and indirect costs in anorexia nervosa. Int J Eat Disord. 2015;48(1):139–46.
13. Gowers SG, Clark AF, Roberts C, Byford S, Barrett B, Griffiths A, et al. A randomised controlled multicentre trial of treatments for adloescent anorexia nervosa including assessment of cost-effectiveness and patient acceptability - the TOuCAN trial. Health Technol Assess. 2010;14(15):1.
14. Herpertz-Dahlmann B, Schwarte R, Krei M, Egberts K, Warnke A, Wewetzer C, et al. Day-patient treatment after short inpatient care versus continued inpatient treatment in adolescents with anorexia nervosa (ANDI): a multicentre, randomised, open-label, non-inferiority trial. Lancet. 2014; 383(9924):1222–9.
15. Madden S, Miskovic-Wheatley J, Wallis A, Kohn M, Lock J, Le Grange D, et al. A randomized controlled trial of in-patient treatment for anorexia nervosa in medically unstable adolescents. Psychol Med. 2015;45(2):415–27.
16. Moher D, Liberati A, Tetzlaff J, Altman DG, Group P. Preferred reporting items for systematic reviews and meta-analyses: the PRISMA statement. J Clin Epidemiol. 2009;62(10):1006–12.
17. Guyatt GH, Oxman AD, Vist G, Kunz R, Brozek J, Alonso-Coello P, et al. GRADE guidelines: 4. Rating the quality of evidence--study limitations (risk of bias). J Clin Epidemiol. 2011;64(4):407–15.
18. Anis N, Isomaa R, Kaltiala-Heino R. Adolescent psychiatric inpatients with first hospitalization due to anorexia nervosa: can rehospitalization be predcited by clinical features. Psychiatr Fenn. 2016;47:76–94.
19. Ayton A, Keen C, Lask B. Pros and cons of using the mental health act for severe eating disorders in adolescents. Eur Eat Disord Rev. 2009; 17(1):14–23.
20. Bourion-Bedes S, Baumann C, Kermarrec S, Ligier F, Feillet F, Bonnemains C, et al. Prognostic value of early therapeutic alliance in weight recovery: a prospective cohort of 108 adolescents with anorexia nervosa. J Adolesc Health. 2013;52(3):344–50.
21. Castro-Fornieles J, Casula V, Saura B, Martinez E, Lazaro L, Vila M, et al. Predictors of weight maintenance after hospital discharge in adolescent anorexia nervosa. Int J Eat Disord. 2007;40(2):129–35.
22. Goddard E, Hibbs R, Raenker S, et al. A multi-centre cohort study of short term outcomes of hospital treatment for anorexia nervosa in the UK. BMC Psychiatry. 2013;13:287:1–14. https://doi.org/10.1186/1471-244X-13-287.
23. Heinberg LJ, Haug NA, Freeman YL, Ambrose D, Guarda AS. Clinical course and short-term outcome of hospitalized adolescents with eating disorders: the success of combining adolescents and adults on an eating disorders unit. Eat Weight Disord. 2003;8(4):326–31.
24. Hetman I, Brunstein Klomek A, Goldzweig G, Hadas A, Horwitz M, Fennig S. Percentage from target weight (PFTW) predicts re-hospitalization in adolescent anorexia nervosa. Isr J Psychiatry Relat Sci. 2017;54(3):28–34.
25. Kalisvaart JL, Hergenroeder AC. Hospitalization of patients with eating disorders on adolescent medical units is threatened by current reimbursement systems. Int J Adolesc Med Health. 2007;19(2):155–65.
26. Leon GR, Lucas AR, Colligan RC, Ferdinande RJ, Kamp J. Sexual, body-image, and personality attitudes in anorexia nervosa. J Abnorm Child Psychol. 1985; 13(2):245–57.
27. Strik Lievers L, Curt F, Wallier J, Perdereau F, Rein Z, Jeammet P, et al. Predictive factors of length of inpatient treatment in anorexia nervosa. Eur Child Adolesc Psychiatry. 2009;18(2):75–84.
28. Mekori E, Halevy L, Ziv SI, Moreno A, Enoch-Levy A, Weizman A, et al. Predictors of short-term outcome variables in hospitalised female adolescents with eating disorders. Int J Psychiatry Clin Pract. 2017;21(1):41–9.
29. Nova E, Lopez-Vidriero I, Varela P, Casas J, Marcos A. Evolution of serum biochemical indicators in anorexia nervosa patients: a 1-year follow-up study. J Hum Nutr Diet. 2007;21:23–30.
30. Rothschild-Yakar L, Lacoua L, Stein D. Changes in patient measures as predictors of therapists' ratings of treatment collaboration and change in eating disorder subgroups. Assessment. 2013;20(6):752–63.
31. Roux H, Ali A, Lambert S, Radon L, Huas C, Curt F, et al. Predictive factors of dropout from inpatient treatment for anorexia nervosa. BMC Psychiatry. 2016;16(1):339.
32. Shugar G, Krueger S. Aggressive family communication, weight gain, and improved eating attitudes during systemic family therapy for anorexia nervosa. Int J Eat Disord. 1995;17(1):23–31.
33. Tasaka K, Matsubara K, Takamiya S, Ishikawa SI, Iwata A, Nigami H. Long-term follow up of hospitalized pediatric anorexia nervosa restricting type. Pediatr Int. 2017;59(4):482–9.
34. Toms DA, Crisp AH. Weight phobia in an adolescent male with stunted development. J Psychosom Res. 1972;16(4):289–95.
35. Vall E, Wade TD. Predictors and moderators of outcomes and readmission for adolescent inpatients with anorexia nervosa: a pilot study. Clin Psychol-Uk. 2017;21(2):143–52.
36. Fennig S, Brunstein Klomek A, Shahar B, Sarel-Michnik Z, Hadas A. Inpatient treatment has no impact on the core thoughts and perceptions in adolescents with anorexia nervosa. Early Interv Psychiatry. 2015;11(3):200–7.
37. Lock J, Litt I. What predicts maintenance of weight for adolescents medically hospitalized for anorexia nervosa? Eat Disord. 2003;11(1):1–7.
38. Goldfield GS, Boachie A. Delivery of family therapy in the treatment of anorexia nervosa using telehealth. Telemed J E-Health. 2003;9(1):111–4.
39. Halvorsen I, Reas DL, Nilsen JV, Ro O. Naturalistic outcome of family-based inpatient treatment for adolescents with anorexia nervosa. Eur Eat Disord Rev. 2018;26(2):141–5.

40. Matthews A, Peterson CM. Intensive family-based therapy during an acute medical admission for anorexia nervosa: a case report. Clin Case Stud. 2016; 15(4):313–25.
41. Salbach-Andrae H, Schneider N, Seifert K, Pfeiffer E, Lenz K, Lehmkuhl U, et al. Short-term outcome of anorexia nervosa in adolescents after inpatient treatment: a prospective study. Eur Child Adolesc Psychiatry. 2009;18(11): 701–4.
42. Schlegl S, Diedrich A, Neumayr C, Fumi M, Naab S, Voderholzer U. Inpatient treatment for adolescents with anorexia nervosa: clinical significance and predictors of treatment outcome. Eur Eat Disord Rev. 2016;24(3):214–22.
43. Paul P, Mehta S, Coffey BJ. Anorexia nervosa in a 14-year-old second-generation Hispanic adolescent boy. J Child Adolesc Psychopharmacol. 2013;23(4):295–9.
44. Alessi NE, Krahn D, Brehm D, Wittekindt J. Prepubertal anorexia nervosa and major depressive disorder. J Am Acad Child Adolesc Psychiatry. 1989;28(3): 380–4.
45. Blanchet-Collet C, Sider A, Gal B, Hanachi-Guidoum M, Melchior JC, Bouscary D, et al. Anorexia nervosa hyperactivity-induced ischemic colitis (ANHIC): a new cause of anaemia. Eat Weight Disord-St. 2016;21(3):507–10.
46. Blinder BJ, Freeman DM, Stunkard AJ. Behavior therapy of anorexia nervosa: effectiveness of activity as a reinforcer of weight gain. Am J Psychiatry. 1970;126(8):1093–8.
47. Cinciripini PM, Kornblith SJ, Turner SM, Hersen M. A behavioral program for the management of anorexia and bulimia. J Nerv Ment Dis. 1983;171(3): 186–9.
48. Clark DB, Munford PR. Behavioral consultation to pediatrics. Child Behavior Therapy. 1981;2(3):25–33.
49. Collins M, Hodas GR, Liebman R. Interdisciplinary model for the inpatient treatment of adolescents with anorexia nervosa. J Adolesc Health Care. 1983;4(1):3–8.
50. Garfinkel PE, Kline SA, Stancer HC. Treatment of anorexia nervosa using operant conditioning techniques. J Nerv Ment Dis. 1973;157(6):428–33.
51. Halmi KA, Powers P, Cunningham S. Treatment of anorexia nervosa with behavior modification. Effectiveness of formula feeding and isolation. Arch Gen Psychiatry. 1975;32(1):93–6.
52. Leitenberg H, Agras WS, Thomson LE. A sequential analysis of the effect of selective positive reinforcement in modifying anorexia nervosa. Behav Res Ther. 1968;6(2):211–8.
53. Nygaard JA. Anorexia nervosa. Treatment and triggering factors. Acta Psychiatr Scand Suppl. 1990;361:44–9.
54. Pertschuk M, Edwards N, Pomerleau O. A multiple-baseline approach to Behavioural intervention in anorexia nervosa. Behav Ther. 1978;9:368–76.
55. Poole AD, Sanson-Fisher RW, Young P. A behavioural programme for the management of anorexia nervosa. Aust N Z J Psychiatry. 1978;12(1):49–53.
56. Solanto MV, Jacobson MS, Heller L, Golden NH, Hertz S. Rate of weight gain of inpatients with anorexia nervosa under two behavioral contracts. Pediatrics. 1994;93(6 Pt 1):989–91.
57. Steinhausen HC. Evaluation of inpatient treatment of adolescent anorexic patients. J Psychiatr Res. 1985;19(2–3):371–5.
58. Groen JJ, Feldman-Toledano Z. Educative treatment of patients and parentsin anorexia nervosa. Br J Psychiatry. 1966;112(488):671–81.
59. Kronenberg J, Nachshoni T, Neumann M, Gaoni B. The treatment of anorexia-nervosa in a general-hospital - a case vignette of a multidisciplinary general hospital-based approach. J Adolesc. 1994;17(2): 163–71.
60. Jenkins ME. An outcome study of anorexia nervosa in an adolescent unit. J Adolesc. 1987;10(1):71–81.
61. Maxmen JS, Siberfarb PM, Ferrell RB. Anorexia nervosa. Practical initial management in a general hospital. JAMA. 1974;229(7):801–3.
62. Wockel L, Zepf FD, Koch S, Meyer-Keitel AE, Schmidt MH. Serotonin-induced decrease of intracellular ca(2+) release in platelets of bulimic patients normalizes during treatment. J Neural Transm (Vienna). 2009;116(1):89–95.
63. Spettigue W, Norris ML, Santos A, Obeid N. Treatment of children and adolescents with avoidant/restrictive food intake disorder: a case series examining the feasibility of family therapy and adjunctive treatments. J Eat Disord. 2018;6:20.
64. Singer L, Ambuel B, Wade S, Jaffe A. Cognitive-Behavioural treatment of health-impairing food phobias in children. J Am Acad Child Adolesc Psychiatry. 1992;31(5):847–52.
65. Pitt PD, Middleman AB. A focus on behavior Management of Avoidant/ restrictive food intake disorder (ARFID): a case series. Clin Pediatr (Phila). 2018;57(4):478–80.
66. Dalle Grave R, Calugi S, El Ghoch M, Conti M, Fairburn CG. Inpatient cognitive behavior therapy for adolescents with anorexia nervosa: immediate and longer-term effects. Front Psychiatry. 2014;5:14:1–7. https://doi.org/10.3389/fpsyt.2014.00014.
67. El Ghoch M, Milanese C, Calugi S, Muller MJ, Pourhassan M, Ruocco A, et al. Regional fat distribution in adolescent and adult females with anorexia nervosa: a longitudinal study. Clin Nutr. 2014;34(6):P1224–32. https://doi.org/10.1016/j.clnu.2014.12.012.
68. Hillen S, Dempfle A, Seitz J, Herpertz-Dahlmann B, Buhren K. Motivation to change and perceptions of the admission process with respect to outcome in adolescent anorexia nervosa. BMC Psychiatry. 2015;15:140.
69. Strober M, Freeman R, Lampert C, Diamond J, Teplinsky C, DeAntonio M. Are there gender differences in core symptoms, temperament, and short-term prospective outcome in anorexia nervosa? Int J Eat Disord. 2006;39(7): 570–5.
70. Treat TA, McCabe EB, Gaskill JA, Marcus MD. Treatment of anorexia nervosa in a specialty care continuum. Int J Eat Disord. 2008;41(6):564–72.
71. Asch M, Esteves J, De Hautecloque D, Bargiacchi A, Le Heuzey MF, Mouren MC, et al. Cognitive remediation therapy for children and adolescents with anorexia nervosa in France: an exploratory study. Encephale. 2014;40(3):240–6.
72. Kuge R, Lang K, Yokota A, Kodama S, Morino Y, Nakazato M, et al. Group cognitive remediation therapy for younger adolescents with anorexia nervosa: a feasibility study in a Japanese sample. BMC Res Notes. 2017;10(1):317.
73. Harrison A, Stavri P, Ormond L, McEnemy F, Akyol D, Qureshi A, et al. Cognitive remediation therapy for adolescent inpatients with severe and complex anorexia nervosa: a treatment trial. Eur Eat Disord Rev. 2018;26(3): 230–40.
74. Herbrich L, van Noort B, Pfeiffer E, Lehmkuhl U, Winter S, Kappel V. Follow-up assessment of cognitive remediation therapy in adolescent anorexia nervosa: a pilot study. Eur Eat Disord Rev. 2017;25(2):104–13.
75. Depestele L, Claes L, Dierckx E, Colman R, Schoevaerts K, Lemmens GMD. An adjunctive multi-family group intervention with or without patient participation during an inpatient treatment for adolescents with an eating disorder: a pilot study. Eur Eat Disord Rev. 2017;25(6):570–8.
76. Janas-Kozik M, Krzystanek M, Stachowicz M, Krupka-Matuszczyk I, Janas A, Rybakowski JK. Bright light treatment of depressive symptoms in patients with restrictive type of anorexia nervosa. J Affect Disord. 2011;130(3):462–5.
77. Couturier J, Mahmood A. Meal support therapy reduces the use of nasogastric feeding for adolescents hospitalized with anorexia nervosa. Eat Disord. 2009;17(4):327–32.
78. Kells M, Davidson K, Hitchko L, O'Neil K, Schubert-Bob P, McCabe M. Examining supervised meals in patients with restrictive eating disorders. Appl Nurs Res. 2013;26(2):76–9.
79. Kells M, Schubert-Bob P, Nagle K, Hitchko L, O'Neil K, Forbes P, et al. Meal supervision during medical hospitalization for eating disorders. Clin Nurs Res. 2016;26(4):525–37.
80. Leacy KA, Cane JN. Effect of non-select menus on weight and eating concern in adolescents hospitalized with anorexia nervosa. Eat Disord. 2012; 20(2):159–67.

Initial validation of a screening tool for disordered eating in adolescent athletes

Samantha F. Kennedy[1*], Jeffrey Kovan[2], Emily Werner[3], Ryley Mancine[4], Donald Gusfa[4] and Heather Kleiman[5]

Abstract

Background: Disordered eating (DE) is a growing problem among all athletes, particularly adolescents. To help prevent the progression of DE to a clinical eating disorder (ED), a brief screening tool could offer an efficient method for early identification of DE in athletes and facilitate treatment. The aim of this study is to validate a screening tool for DE that will identify male and female adolescent athletes of all sports and levels of competition who are at risk for DE. The Disordered Eating Screen for Athletes (DESA-6) consists of only 6 items and was designed for use in both male and female athlete populations.

Methods: Validation involved two phases: Phase I consisted of screening high school athletes using the Eating Attitudes Test (EAT-26) and the DESA-6; and Phase II included inviting all high school athletes categorized as "at risk" after screening, plus age- and self-reported gender- matched athletes categorized as not "at risk", to complete the same surveys a second time along with clinical interview. Validity and regression analyses were used to compare the DESA-6 to the EAT-26 and EDE 17.0D.

Results: When comparing to clinical interview, the DESA-6 had a total sensitivity of 92% and specificity of 85.96%, respectively. Upon comparison of concurrent validity, Phase II DESA-6 had a strong significant positive correlation for both males and females when compared to Phase II EDE 17.0D.

Conclusions: A brief, easy to administer screening tool for recognizing DE that can be used by physicians, psychologists, athletic trainers, registered dietitians, and other sport/healthcare staff is of utmost importance for early intervention, which can lead to improved treatment outcomes. The DESA-6 is a promising tool for risk assessment of DE in athletes.

Keywords: Anorexia nervosa, Bulimia nervosa, Sports, Disordered eating, Eating disorder, Screening tool, Desa-6

* Correspondence: fugatesa@msu.edu

DESCRIPTION: This manuscript introduces and validates the Disordered Eating Screen for Athletes (DESA-6) screening tool. This tool is currently designed to identify risk for disordered eating in adolescent athletes. Identification of disordered eating risk is very important because early intervention has been linked with improved treatment. Creation of this tool would allow athletic trainers, physicians, and concerned school nurses or administrators to quickly identify student athletes who may be at risk for disordered eating. Future research will attempt to validate the DESA-6 in adult, college, and professional athletes.

[1]Department of Psychiatry, Michigan State University, 909 Wilson Rd, Room B119, East Lansing, MI 48824, USA
Full list of author information is available at the end of the article

Plain English

Disordered eating, a subclinical spectrum of eating disorders, can potentially progress into numerous physical health complications. Disordered eating may progress to a clinical eating disorder if left untreated. If individuals with disordered eating are identified quickly, treatment outcomes may improve. Athletes are particularly susceptible to disordered eating. This manuscript attempts to introduce the Disordered Eating Screen for Athletes (DESA-6) screening tool, which aims to quickly identify both males and females who may be at risk for disordered eating. Current screening tools are generally only focused on validation in females, but the DESA-6 also aims to be validated in males. Additionally, the DESA-6 is much shorter than previous screening tools and significantly shorter than the current gold standard clinical interview. This study showed the DESA-6 have promised as a tool that athletic trainers, primary care physicians, and sport/healthcare staff may use to quickly screen a student athlete for disordered eating behaviors.

Introduction

The Diagnostic and Statistical Manual of Mental Disorders, Fifth Edition (DSM-5) defines eating disorders (EDs) as "the persistent disturbance of eating or eating-related behavior, which results in altered consumption of food and a significant impairment of physical health and/or psychosocial functioning [1]." There are two primary presentations of EDs, anorexia nervosa (AN) and bulimia nervosa (BN), both of which are characterized by an undue influence of body weight and/or shape on self-evaluation [1]. Additional EDs include binge eating disorder (BED) and other specified feeding and eating disorder (OSFED). The prevalence of EDs in the general population is estimated to be less than 1% for AN and 1–2% for BN [2].

Previous researchers have indicated that eating-related issues exist on a spectrum, with the clinically diagnosable DSM-5 EDs at the more extreme end of the spectrum [2]. Within the spectrum of eating-related issues is a condition referred to as "disordered eating" (DE), a term which has been used in research to generally describe the abnormal and potentially harmful eating behaviors that do not meet diagnostic criteria for clinical EDs [3]. Although it is believed that DE lies on the same spectrum of eating-related issues as ED, there is currently no formally accepted definition for DE. Furthermore, previously suggested definitions may not encompass the full spectrum of potential behaviors. An editorial on the continuum of DE defined DE as a variety of abnormal eating behaviors (e.g. restrictive eating, fasting, excessive eating, diet pills, laxatives/enemas, and purging [4]. This article provided a comprehensive list of potential abnormal eating behaviors; however, it did not include potential abnormal time parameter restrictions. In athletes, DE has been defined as a general term that describes the spectrum of abnormal eating behaviors with the goal of achieving or maintaining an unhealthy body weight [3]." However, not all DE behaviors in athletes are intended to achieve a lower weight. Athletes, especially male athletes, may engage in DE behaviors with the intent to increase muscle mass to improve performance [5, 6].

With the previous definitions and associated drawbacks in mind, we propose the following definition for disordered eating: intentional chronic abnormal, unhealthy eating/drinking behaviors that can lead to clinically relevant problems and do not necessarily meet DSM-5 criteria for eating disorders. This can include a number of behaviors including (but not limited to): restrictive eating (including excessive fasting or frequently skipping meals); overeating or binge eating; purging; and/or the use of weight loss supplements (e.g., diet pills, laxatives, diuretics). In an athlete population, DE is often done with the intent to alter body weight, shape, and/or athletic performance. Although eating patterns similar to those with DE can arise from a lack of nutrition knowledge by the athlete, it is important to distinguish those athletes who engage in these behaviors intentionally as having DE. Adolescent athletes in particular are susceptible to unintentional DE behavior, as they likely have little knowledge of optimal food intake and may have little access to sports dietitians or nutritional knowledge.

DE is a growing problem among all athletes, particularly adolescent athletes [3, 4]. Adolescents with a pattern of DE often results in them having low energy availability, electrolyte abnormalities and dehydration, which all negatively impact physical and mental health, as well as athletic performance [7]. DE can lead to injuries that result in more participation days lost and longer recovery periods from injuries [8]. If untreated, DE could progress to a clinical ED, putting these adolescents at an increased risk of ED-related mood, anxiety, impulse-control and substance use disorders [9]. Additionally, EDs have one of the highest mortality rates of all mental disorders [7] and are associated with many potentially life-threatening complications, including cardiac arrhythmias, bone loss, colon hypofunction and kidney failure [10]. In order to potentially prevent the progression of DE to a clinical ED, a brief screening tool could offer an efficient method for identifying DE in athletes, thus facilitating early identification and necessary treatment [11–13].

Prevalence estimates of DE/EDs among adolescent athletes vary widely due to the differing criteria and definitions between research studies; however, a number of studies have indicated the prevalence of DE and EDs is higher among adolescent athletes than in the general population [14, 15]. The National Athletic Trainers' Association (NATA), the American College of Sports Medicine (ACSM) and the International Olympic Committee (IOC) have released statements supporting regular screening for DE in athletes using a screening tool designed specifically for athletes [7, 16, 17]. However, the NATA Position Statement noted that widely used questionnaires, such as the Eating Attitudes Test (EAT-26), the Eating Disorder Inventory (EDI) and the Eating Disorder Examination Questionnaire (EDE-Q), should be used cautiously as these screening tools have not been validated in athletes [7]. The EDE-Q is a self-report questionnaire based on the Eating Disorder Examination (EDE), which is the gold standard for clinically diagnosing EDs and is currently on version 17, referred to as EDE 17.0D. For athletes, specifically, there are six ED-specific screening tools in existence, with the four most common being the Athletic Milieu Direct Questionnaire (AMDQ), Female Athlete Screening Tool (FAST), Physiologic Screening Test (PST), and the Brief Eating Disorder in Athletes Questionnaire (BEDA-Q) [11, 13, 18, 19].

A review by Knapp et al. discusses reasons the four athlete-related screeners should be used with caution [20]. Although the AMDQ was validated utilizing the EDE-16, the tool was validated only in female collegiate athletes, therefore it is unknown if the AMDQ could be generalized to non-collegiate or recreational athletes. Additionally, the AMDQ evaluates presence of menstruation, thus is cannot be used to screen male athletes [13]. The FAST exhibits a similar issue as the wording is specific to female athletes and it was validated in a population of female collegiate athletes ages 18 to 23 years [18]. Neither of these screeners would be appropriate to use in an adolescent athlete population of mixed sexes. The PST was developed specifically for DE screening [11]; however, it requires physiologic measurements (e.g., body fat percentage, parotid gland evaluation), which require specialized equipment and/or training, thus making this screener difficult to use in the field. Additionally, the PST includes a question about the regularity of menstrual cycles, so it cannot be used in male athletes. Lastly, although the BEDA-Q was validated in female adolescent athletes, it is unknown if it would be valid for all levels of competition or male adolescent athletes [19]. The BEDA-Q was developed using DSM-IV criteria, which included amenorrhea as a diagnostic criterion, so it is unclear if this screening tool could be generalized to include male athletes.

A standardized, brief, efficient screening tool for DE that could be given to a large population of both male and female athletes is necessary [10, 19]. The aim of this study is to validate a screening tool for DE that will identify male and female adolescent athletes of all sports and levels of competition who are at risk for DE. The Disordered Eating Screen for Athletes (DESA-6) consists of only 6 items and was designed specifically for use in both male and female athlete populations. We hypothesize that the DESA-6 will be an efficient screening tool to identify DE in adolescent athletes, and may help decrease the potential for progression to clinical ED.

Methods

All methods were approved by the university's Institutional Review Board, where the full protocol can be accessed. After initial generation of the DESA-6 questions, we conducted pilot testing in a population of adult athletes using the EAT-26 as a comparison to the DESA-6. After a final version of the DESA-6 was decided, the validation involved two phases: Phase I, which consisted of screening high school athletes using the EAT-26 and the DESA-6; and Phase II in which we invited all high school athletes categorized as "at risk" after screening, along with age- and self-reported gender-matched athletes categorized as not "at risk", to complete the surveys a second time with clinical interview in which we used the gold-standard EDE 17.0D for comparison. Participants were recruited from Midwestern United States high schools during the months of January through June of 2019.

Eating attitudes test (EAT-26)

The EAT-26 is a 26-item self-report instrument that utilizes a 6-point Likert scale ranging from 1 (never) to 6 (always). The EAT-26 is an abbreviated version of a 40-item scale developed by Garner et al. and is a validated psychometric measure that identifies risk for EDs in the general population [21]. The criterion validity of the EAT-26 was evaluated and found to have an overall accuracy of 0.90 [22]. Additionally, the EAT-26 has a high degree of internal reliability with an alpha coefficient of 0.79 in patients with AN and an alpha coefficient of 0.94 comparing patients with AN and normal controls [21].

Although the EAT-26 was validated in the general population and not athletes [21], it was chosen as the external validity comparison because it is a well-accepted tool for detecting EDs and is a relatively brief measure for use in the field. A score of 20 or greater on the EAT-26 indicates risk for ED [22, 23]; however, the purpose of the DESA-6 is to detect DE and not ED, so a different scoring system was needed. A study of female athletes found a mean EAT-26 score of 12.66 was associated with DE [24]; therefore, a score of 12 was chosen for this study to indicate someone being "at risk" for DE. was agreed upon with expert opinion from two sports psychiatrists.

Eating disorder examination (EDE 17.0D)

The Eating Disorder Examination is the current gold standard for diagnosing EDs [25]. It is a psychometrically validated semi-structured interview. It has been revised numerous times with the aim of maximizing reliability [26]. The EDE 17.0D is based on the diagnostic criteria outlined in the DSM-5 to evaluate for AN, BN, binge eating disorder and unspecified EDs. It consists of 62 items categorized into four subscales (Restraint, Eating Concern, Weight Concern, Shape Concern) and takes up to an hour to complete. Previous work on validity of the EDE has demonstrated the majority of the individual items are able to discriminate between patients with and without EDs [25, 26]. Additionally, inter-rater reliability of all items has been found to be high [25]. The EDE 17.0D was chosen as the Concurrent validity test because it is the current gold standard for diagnosing EDs [25] and no gold standard for DE exists.

DESA-6 question development

The DESA-6 was designed for this study by a former professional triathlete based on a previous study that surveyed over 1000 triathletes in the United States [27]. A review of literature was conducted on DE/EDs in athletes and a pool of 18 items was created. The initial pool included triathlon-specific questions and "competitive athletes" questions, which applied to all sports. Interviews were then conducted with randomly selected triathletes to assess the items. The questions, along with the EAT-26 for comparison purposes, were distributed randomly to triathletes via an online survey, which was completed by 1033 adult triathletes. The chi square test was used in that previous study to assess the statistical significance of relationships between EAT-26 scores and the "triathlon-specific" and "competitive athlete factors." Following statistical analysis, the items were narrowed down to six, which all assessed "competitive athlete factors," [27] meaning no questions were specific to triathletes, thus applicable to all sports.

Each of the final six questions were purposely designed to assess a specific facet of DE unique to athletes (see Supplemental Digital Content 1, DESA-6). As DE/EDs are associated with an increased injury rate, more frequent injuries or more severe injuries may indicate higher risk for DE [8]; therefore, question 1 was intended to assess the frequency and severity of injuries due to the increased risk for injury and increased length of recovery following injury [10]. Question 2 was intended to assess fear of weight gain but was specifically tailored to athletes by asking about periods of time when they cannot train or are not training as intensely, so fear of weight gain may be more pronounced. This reflects the DSM-5 Criteria B of AN, which is an intense fear of gaining weight and/or of becoming fat [1]. Many athletes believe that losing weight results in improved performance [28], and with DE may be unhappy with their weight even if they are normal weight or underweight; therefore, Question 3 evaluates happiness with weight and Question 4 assesses the intensity of dissatisfaction with current weight. These questions are related to the DSM-5 Criteria C of AN, which is a disturbance in the way in which one's body shape or weight is experienced [1]. Dieting is a risk factor for development of EDs in female elite athletes [16, 29], thus, Question 5 is intended to assess the presence of dieting. Because being told to lose weight by a coach/authority figure was found to be a risk factor for development of EDs [14], Question 6 is intended to evaluate the presence of this pressure. To verify that the wording was appropriate and sufficient for all athletes, the six questions and answer choices were reviewed for face validity and adjusted following interviews with athletes of different sports and experts in the field, including sports psychiatrists, sports psychologists, and registered dietitians. A positive score, which is a score of 3 or greater, on the DESA-6 is intended to indicate risk for DE.

Pilot testing

A total of 22 randomly selected adult athletes aged 18–19 years old were recruited at a local sports medicine clinic. Individuals who were recruited were selected at random from the patient list of two sports medicine providers. Inclusion criteria was self-identification as an athlete participating in a "sport", defined as an activity requiring a higher level of physical exertion and/or skill than walking. This convenience sample was used for pilot testing because it was an available, responsive population that could prove valuable for future validation of the DESA-6.

Participants completed both the DESA-6 and EAT-26. None were excluded. There were 11 female athletes and 11 male athletes. Twelve different sports were represented in this sample. Following informed consent, athletes were provided a paper survey that included demographic questions (age, a free-text gender question, sport, number of training hours per week), anthropometric questions (self-reported height and weight), the DESA-6, and the EAT-26. Identifying information of the participants was not collected in order to assure anonymity. Athletes completed the survey in a private room with a trained researcher available outside the room.

DESA-6 validation

Phase I: initial screening in adolescent athletes

Power was calculated a priori analysis using the standard alpha of 0.05, power 0.95, and effect size of 0.3, which gave a suggested sample size of 111 for phase I of research. High school student athletes (ages 12 to 19 years, defined as those participating in a high school sponsored sport) were recruited from 12 different Midwest high schools via emails to administrators and athletic trainers. Student athletes were provided with consent forms by school faculty approximately one week prior to survey administration by a member of lab personnel in order to obtain parental consent. Student athletes aged 18 to 19 years were provided adult consent forms. A convenience sample of 308 student athletes provided consent, and none were excluded. A total of 17 sports were represented, including basketball, baseball, football, etc. (see Table 3 for full list of sports). Student athletes were provided a paper survey that included demographic questions (age, a free-text gender question, sport, number of training hours per week), anthropometric questions (self-reported height and weight), the DESA-6, and the EAT-26.

Phase II: clinical interviews

Based on Phase I results, student athletes classified as "at risk" for DE based on EAT-26 scores (score ≥ 12) were invited to attend the clinical interview to determine presence of DE/EDs. A total of 77 student athletes were classified as "at risk" and all were invited to participate in Phase II. 41 of these "at risk" students consented to participate. We then invited age- and self-reported gender- matched athletes classified "not at risk" to serve as a control group. A total of 82 student athletes ($n = 41$ at risk) completed Phase II and none were excluded. A total 15 sports were represented (gymnastics and rugby were not represented versus Phase I).

Student athletes under the age of 18 years came to the interview with a parent/guardian to provide written consent and assent. Adult student athletes completed a written consent form. Prior to the clinical interview, participants completed the DESA-6 and EAT-26 again. Due to scheduling conflicts, as many athletes were actively competing, time between initial completion of the DESA-6 and the EAT-26 ranged from 3 weeks to 12 weeks. Height was verified with a stadiometer (Seca 216, Germany) and weight was verified with a scale (Detecto 758C, Welch City, MO). The private clinical interview utilized the EDE 17.0D, which is the gold standard for diagnosing EDs (2). Interviewers ($n = 5$) were trained to conduct the interviews by a board-certified child and adolescent psychiatrist with extensive experience treating DE/EDs and athletes. This board-certified child and adolescent psychiatrist then tabulated the results of the EDE 17.0D and interpreted the results of the self-administered DESA-6. The interviewers verified that each survey was completely answered before moving on with the next phase of the study, which resulted in no missing data on the DESA-6 or EDE 17.0D tests. No observed adverse effects from performing the DESA-6, EAT-26, or ED 17.0D were noted.

Statistical analyses

An EDE 17.0D with a positive score on two out of four subscales was considered positive for DE. This accommodates for the subclinical nature of DE in comparison to ED, which is measured with a score of 3 or more subscales [26]. A DESA-6 score of three or more was considered a positive screening due to its ability to achieve strong sensitivity while maintaining an acceptable specificity. As a score of three was used as a cutoff value, there were no indeterminate scores. Validity and regression analyses were used to compare the DESA-6 to the EAT-26 and EDE 17.0D. All regressions were interpreted via guidelines from "Statistics without maths for Psychology". Phase I data of the DESA-6 were compared to Phase I EAT-26 scores to show concurrent validity. Phase I data of the DESA-6 were compared to Phase II EDE 17.0D scores to show the predictive validity. Phase II data of the DESA-6 were compared to Phase II EDE 17.0D scores to show construct validity. Phases I and II data of the DESA-6 scores were compared using regression analysis to determine test-retest reliability. Receiver Operating Characteristic (ROC) Area Under the Curve (AUC) analysis was then explored to further assess correlation between Phase II EDE 17.0D and DESA-6 scores [30]. Statistics were performed with Excel Data ToolPak Version 2016, Software, SPSS version 25, and MedCalc.org [31].

Results

Pilot testing showed that the DESA-6 was written at an appropriate reading level as no participants reported confusing regarding the wording of the questions or answer choices. There were no changes made to the DESA-6 following pilot testing.

Table 1 describes the demographics of athletes recruited in Phases I and II. There were more females than males in Phase II due to more females scoring positively in Phase I. Figure 1 demonstrates the flow of recruitment for Phase I and Phase II of the study.

Table 2 describes the prevalence found in the adolescent athlete population during Phase I. More female athletes than male athletes were reported due to recruiting variance. Females (Median = 1) were shown to have a significantly higher rate of DE than males (Median = 0) with a Mann-Whitney U test for medians showing U = 7735, $p < 0.001$. This is consistent with populations of previous studies showing higher rates of DE amongst female athletes than male athletes. Total population rates were within the range of previous studies [15]. As participants were being screened for DE behaviors, a clinical spectrum of eating pathologies, other diagnoses are unlikely.

Table 1 Participant Demographics

	Phase I *N* = 308	Phase II *N* = 82
Males (n)	148 (48%)	23 (28%)
Females (n)	160 (52%)	59 (72%)
Mean Age (years)	15.96	16.17
Positive DESA-6 Screening Mean Age (years)	16.14	16.43
Negative DESA-6 Screening Mean Age (years)	15.91	16.01
Mean age and gender adjusted BMI-z score (95% CI)	0.75 (0.68, 0.82)	0.88 (0.75, 1.03)

Overview of demographics of Phase I and Phase II studies. Scores of ≥ 3 are used as a positive DESA-6 score

Table 3 describes the number of participants who screened positively in Phase I on either the DESA-6 or the Phase I EAT-26. Because athletes were selected at random from a larger population of athletes for participation, this resulted in slightly more females than males and a large discrepancy between the rate of response between each sport. We categorized by sport type, with 5 participants representing aesthetic sports, 234 participants playing ball, 56 from endurance sports, and 13 from weight-dependent sports. The highest number of positive results on either survey were from basketball athletes; however, there was a larger number of basketball athletes surveyed than any other sport.

Additionally, defining "at risk" student athletes as those with a score of 12 or greater on the EAT-26 (versus the typical positive score of 20 or greater), allowed the inclusion of athletes typically considered borderline cases. In Phase II, 41 athletes classified as "at risk" in Phase I consented to complete the EDE 17.0D, with 19 of the "at risk" group screening positive. Of the total 82 Phase II athletes, the DESA-6 screened positive for a total of 31 athletes while the EDE-17D found only 25 to have DE. Table 4 details the comparison of these scores. The DESA-6 favors a positive screen in borderline cases, screening positive for 7 (77.8%) of the borderline positive cases and 7 (75.0%) of the borderline negative cases.

Diagnostic accuracy of the DESA-6 to the EDE-17 and EAT-26

Table 5 shows the validity analyses for the DESA-6 versus the EAT-26 (Phase I) and versus the EDE 17.0D (Phase II) separated into male and female participants. Compared to the EAT-26 in the total sample analyses, the DESA-6 had a total sample sensitivity of 62.5% and a specificity of 87.7%. When comparing to the EDE 17.0D, the DESA-6 had a total sensitivity of 92% and specificity of 85.96%, respectively. Amongst males there was a sensitivity of 100% and a specificity of 85.0%. Amongst females there was a sensitivity of 90.9% and a specificity of 86.5%. The DESA-6 showed an overall accuracy of 87.80% when compared to the EDE 17.0D. Positive predictive value and negative predictive value are used to compare the rates in which positive and negative screens of the DESA-6 match the EAT-26 or EDE-17.

Figure 2 further compares Phase II DESA-6 Scores and EDE 17.0D scores using ROC Curve analysis. This is a calculation of the overall ability of a parameter can

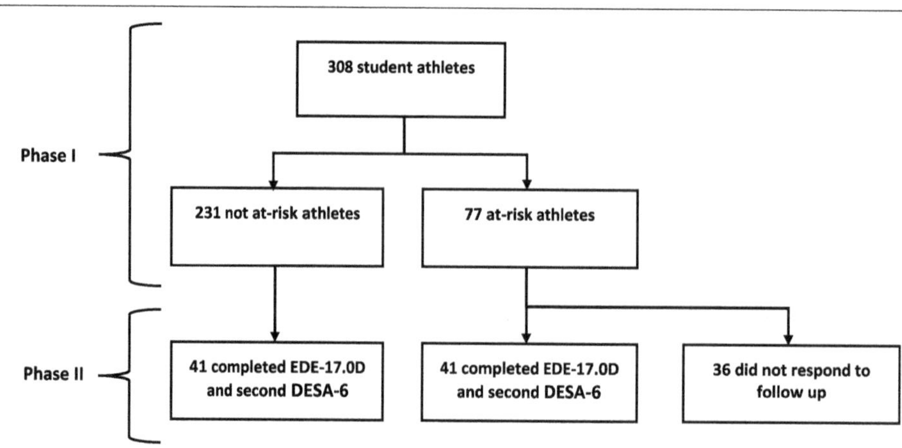

Fig. 1 Flow of Participants

Table 2 Prevalence of DE

	Phase I $N = 308$		
	Total Sample ($N = 308$)	Males ($n = 148$)	Females ($n = 160$)
Result	24.03%	12.84%	34.38%
CI (95%)	18.87, 30.16%	7.73, 20.05%	25.59, 44.74%

Prevalence of DE as found by the DESA-6. Scores of ≥ 3 are used as a positive DESA-6 score

distinguish between an experimental and control group. ROC-AUC showed a moderate approaching high correlation of 0.89 between the two measures [32].

Construct validity

Construct validity of the DESA-6 was performed via regression analysis. Upon comparison of concurrent validity, Phase II DESA-6 had a strong significant positive correlation [r (23) = .80, $p < 0.001$] for males and [r (59) = .80, $p < 0.001$] for females when compared to Phase II EDE 17.0D. Comparison of the DESA-6 to the EAT-26 showed a low to moderate significant positive correlation with scores of [r (146) = .49, $p < 0.001$] in males and a moderate to strong positive correlation of [r (160) = .63, $p < 0.001$] in females.

Reliability

Test-retest reliability comparing DESA-6 scores in Phase I to scores in Phase II showed a strong significant positive correlation [r (23) = 0.83, $p < 0.001$] in males and a significant positive correlation in females [r (59) = 0.76, $p < 0.001$].

Discussion

The aim of this study was to validate a brief screening tool to detect risk for DE in adolescent athletes. The DESA-6 showed acceptability in detecting athletes both at risk for DE and athletes without risk for DE with sensitivity of 92% and specificity of 85.96%, respectively, when compared to the gold-standard EDE 17.0D. In comparison, the AMDQ had a sensitivity of 80% and a specificity of 77% [13, 20], the PST had a sensitivity of 86.5% and specificity of 77.7% [11], and the BEDA-Q had a sensitivity of 82.1% and specificity of 84.6% (20). These three screening tools were each created specifically for female collegiate athletes (AMDQ, PST) or female elite athletes (BEDA-Q), so it is worth noting that the DESA-6 had comparable sensitivity and specificity, but in a broader athletic population.

The proportion of adolescent athletes within this study population who were at risk for DE, as determined by the DESA-6, was 30.86%. Two studies conducted in collegiate female athlete populations found 35% of the

Table 3 Number of Athletes who Screened Positive for DE & ED

Sport Category		Phase I DESA-6		
Type	Sport	Total Sample ($N = 308$)	Males ($n = 148$)	Females ($n = 160$)
Aesthetic ($n = 5$ total)	Cheer ($n = 4$)	0	0	0
	Gymnastics ($n = 1$)	1	0	1
Ball ($n = 234$ total)	Basketball ($n = 56$)	14	5	9
	Softball ($n = 15$)	4	0	4
	Soccer ($n = 31$)	9	2	7
	Baseball ($n = 15$)	2	2	0
	Volleyball ($n = 31$)	7	0	7
	Football ($n = 47$)	5	5	0
	Lacrosse ($n = 17$)	7	0	7
	Tennis ($n = 5$)	1	0	1
	Water polo ($n = 14$)	2	0	2
	Rugby ($n = 2$)	0	0	0
	Ice Hockey ($n = 1$)	0	0	0
Endurance ($n = 56$ total)	Cross Country ($n = 15$)	6	0	6
	Track ($n = 26$)	4	0	4
	Swimming ($n = 15$)	6	0	6
Weight Dependent ($n = 13$ total)	Wrestling ($n = 13$)	6	5	1

This table gives the number of athletes of each sport who scored positively on the DESA-6 during Phase I. Scores of ≥ 3 are used as a positive DESA-6 score

Table 4 Overview of DESA-6 Scores in comparison to EDE-17 Subscales

Number of Positive EDE-17 Subscales	Number with EDE-17 Score	Number Screened Positive with DESA-6 (Percent)	Average DESA-6 Score (± 95% CI)
0	49	2 (4.1%)	0.71 (0.35, 1.07)
1	8	6 (75.0%)	2.63 (1.64, 3.62)
2	9	7 (77.8%)	3.00 (1.98, 1.02)
3	9	9 (100%)	4.56 (3.88, 5.24)
4	7	7 (100%)	5.43 (7.02, 3.84)

Scores of ≥ 2 positive subscales are used as a positive EDE-17 score. Scores of ≥ 3 are used as a positive DESA-6 score

female athletes had DE [11, 13] and a study by Torstveit et al. in 2008 on adolescent and adult elite female athletes found a prevalence of DE of 32.8% [33]. These prevalence rates are slightly higher than the results of this study, which is likely because our study included both male and female athletes. Although limited research exists on the individual prevalence of DE in female versus male athletes, a study by Sundgot-Borgen and Torstveit using the EDE 16.0 to assess EDs in adolescent and adult female and male elite athletes reported EDs in 20% of female athletes and 8% of male athletes [34]. This study also found a higher prevalence of DE in female athletes with 34.4% of female athletes scoring positive and 12.8% of male athletes scoring positive. The percent of male athletes scoring positive is also similar to a study by Rosendahl et al. in 2009 which found a DE prevalence rate of 10.4% in male high school athletes using the EAT-26 [35].

Although the results of the current study align similarly with previous research, it is important to note that each used different instruments to assess the presence of DE in their population, which contributes to the wide variation in reported rates. Additionally, none of these tools are specific to athletes, which also contributes to the variation.

Previous research has indicated athletes of aesthetic sports (e.g., wrestling, gymnastics) are at higher risk for DE/EDs [34, 36, 37]. In the present study, wrestlers

Table 5 DESA-6 Diagnostic Accuracy Measures of the DESA-6 to the EDE-17

Phase II		Total Sample (n = 82)	Males (n = 23)	Females (n = 59)
		Result (95% CI)	**Result (95% CI)**	**Result (95% CI)**
DESA-6 vs. EDE-17	**Sensitivity**	92% (74.0%, 99.0%)	100% (29.24, 100%)	90.9% (70.8, 98.9%)
	Specificity	85.96% (74.2, 93.3%)	85.0% (62.1, 96.8%)	86.5% (71.2, 95.5%)
	Positive Likelihood Ratio	6.56 (3.65, 14.9)	6.7 (2.35, 18.92)	6.7 (2.95, 15.36)
	Negative Likelihood Ratio	0.09 (0.02, 0.35)	0 (0, 0)[b]	0.11 (0.03,0.40)
	Disease Prevalence[a] (EDE-17)	[a]30.5% (20.8%, 41.6%)	[a]13.0% (2.78, 33.59%)	[a]37.3% (25.04%, 50.%)
	Positive Predictive Value	74.2% (60.0%, 84.7%)	50.0% (26.05, 73.95%)	80.0% (63.66, 90.13%)
	Negative Predictive Value	96.1% (86.6%, 98.9%)	100% (N/a)[b]	94.1% (80.9, 98.4%)
	Accuracy	87.8% (78.7%, 94.0%)	87.0% (66.4, 97.2%)	88.1% (77.1, 95.1%)
Phase I		**Total Sample (n = 308)**	**Males (n = 148)**	**Females (n = 160)**
		Result (95% CI)	**Result (95% CI)**	**Result (95% CI)**
DESA-6 vs. EAT-26	**Sensitivity**	62.50% (50.30, 73.64%)	41.67% (22.11, 63.36%)	72.92% (58.15, 84.72%)
	Specificity	87.71% (82.83, 91.61%)	92.74% (86.67, 96.63%)	82.14% (73.78, 88.74%)
	Positive Likelihood Ratio	5.09 (3.46, 7.47)	5.74 (2.61, 12.62)	4.08 (2.65, 6.30)
	Negative Likelihood Ratio	0.43 (0.32, 0.58)	0.63 (0.45, 0.89)	0.33 (0.21, 0.53)
	Disease Prevalence (EDE-17)	23.38% (18.76, 28.51%)	16.22% (10.67, 23.16%)	30.00% (23.02, 37.74%)
	Positive Predictive Value	60.81% (51.36, 69.52%)	52.63% (33.58, 70.95%)	63.64% (53.16, 72.96%)
	Negative Predictive Value	88.46% (85.00, 91.20%)	89.15% (85.37, 92.04%)	87.62% (81.53, 91.90%)
	Accuracy	81.82% (77.05, 85.96%)	84.46% (77.60, 89.89%)	79.38% (72.27, 85.36%)

Overview of the DESA-6's ability to screen for DE in an athlete population. Scores of ≥ 3 were used as a positive DESA-6 Score. Scores of ≥ 12 were used as a positive EAT-26 Score. For the EDE-17, a positive DE score is defined as a positive score on the "Restraint OR Eating Concern" subscales and a positive score on the "Weight Concern OR Shape Concern" subscale. [a] Prevalence is not representative of population due to recruitment constrictions.[b] Could not be calculated due to no false negative results

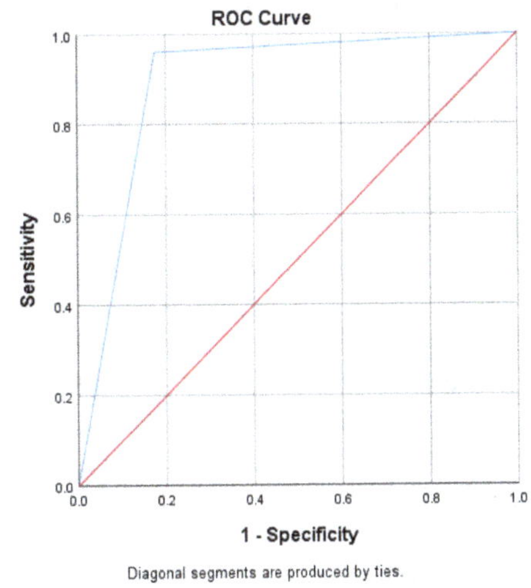

Area Under the Curve

Test Result Variable(s): Did Respondent's DESA-6 Phase TWO Score Indicate Risk for ED?

Area
.892

Fig. 2 ROC Curve Analysis of the DESA-6 in comparison to the EDE-17.0D

showed the highest prevalence of DE (46%, n = 6 of 13, scored positive). A study of DE in Division I college athletes by Engel et al. found elevated levels of drive for thinness, food restriction and purging behaviors in wrestling compared to other sports [38]. Additionally, a study by Chapman and Woodman in 2016 found wrestlers reported a greater incidence of DE [39]. The number of gymnasts in our population was too low (n = 1) for further analysis. This is due to the high schools involved in this research, as only one offered gymnastics as a school sport.

Research has also indicated endurance athletes (e.g., cross-country, swimming) are at higher risk. In the present study in Phase II, 40% (n = 6 of 15) of cross-country athletes and 40% (n = 6 of 15) of swimmers scored positive on the DESA-6. Higher-than-average rates of DE among distance runners and swimmers was expected, as previous research has indicated endurance athletes are at higher risk for DE/EDs [34]. Additionally, a study by Schtscherbyna et al. reported 44.9% of adolescent female elite swimmers had DE [36].

Research has also indicated that risk for DE/EDs is not isolated to endurance or aesthetic sports [2, 11, 13, 18]. A study by Black et al. found DE/EDs among athletes representing 10 of 12 sports studied, including swimming, tennis, track & field, volleyball, cross country, golf, gymnastics, cheer, dance and modern dance [11]. A study by McNulty et al. found female athletes with EDs in 5 different sports, including crew, cross country/track & field, lacrosse, soccer and softball [18]. In the present study, DE was detected in athletes of 14 out of 17 sports represented. The highest prevalence of DE among ball sports was lacrosse (41%, n = 7 of 17 scored positive). This above-average prevalence may be due to all lacrosse athletes assessed being female. The only sports in this study without positive DESA-6 scores were cheer, ice hockey and rugby. This is likely due to the fact that the number of athletes assessed in each of these sports was small (n = 4, 1 and 2, respectively). Thus, this result does not mean athletes in these sports are not at risk for DE as the sample size was too small for analysis.

Strengths, limitations, and future directions

Strengths of the study include the fact that the sample size includes male athletes and multiple sport types. The DESA-6 is unique because of the inclusion of male athletes in our populations, which are typically not included in samples for statistical validation of screening tools regarding DE behavior risk. Additionally, the brevity and lack of required physiological measurements makes the DESA-6 easy to administer to athletes of all types. Also, this study was able to assess validity across multiple diagnostic tools. However, this study is not without limitations. First, the DESA-6 was pilot tested in an athlete population at the higher end (ages 18 to 19 years) of the age range of the validation population (ages 12–19 years) due to convenience, thus limiting our ability to interpret results from pilot testing for applicability in the lower end of the validation population age range. Second, as data were collected through self-report surveys, the results may be susceptible to response bias. We attempted to limit response bias as much as possible by having the athletes complete the EAT-26 and DESA-6 in private and assuring the participants that results would not be shared with coaches or their school. Additional response bias could be due to only 41 of 77 "at risk" athletes consenting to complete Phase II. Multiple attempts were made to contact all of the "at risk" athletes. Third, although the DESA-6 was developed based on the DSM-5 criteria for ED and expert opinion, the lack of a universally accepted definition and diagnostic criteria for DE gives room for question of the content validity of the DESA-6. However, the similarity in results between the DESA-6 and other screeners, as well as high sensitivity and specificity based on the gold-standard EDE 17.0D give support for validity of this screener. A further limitation of this study is that current results are specific to adolescent athletes of one geographical area (Midwest USA); therefore, generalizability to athletes of other ages or geographic regions cannot be done at this time. Additionally, participants in phase II of the study were not matched to a control by sport, though they were matched by age and gender. A further limitation may be the variations in length of time between completion of Phase I and Phase II, which unfortunately was due to the complicated practice and competition schedule of the student athletes. Further research aimed at addressing these concerns is necessary, including testing validity of the DESA-6 in adult athletes (ages > 19 years) and younger athletes of different levels of competition, inclusion of genders other than male or female, as well as different regions of the United States.

Conclusions

The DESA-6 is currently the shortest screening tool for flagging risk of DE in athletes, as well as the only known screening tool that can be used for adolescent athletes aged 13 to 19 years of both genders and all sports. A screening tool which assesses DE in athletes is essential due to the high prevalence of DE/EDs in athletes versus the general population [2, 19]. As all athletes face a unique variety of struggles pertaining to eating and nutritional needs, a tool that successfully accounts for male and female athletes of all sports and all levels of competition is essential. Additionally, the use of screening tools for the early detection of DE in athletes has been recommended to help prevent long term consequences, as well as to provide benefits associated with early intervention. This necessity has been recognized by multiple previous studies, as well as the NATA, IOC, and ACSM [7, 16, 17, 20]. A shorter, more efficient screening tool for DE that could be given to a large athlete population without extensive investment of time and resources is necessary, as no current tools can quickly evaluate a large group of adolescent athletes [10, 19]. With only 6 questions, the DESA-6 can be used by physicians, athletic trainers, registered dietitians, or other sport/healthcare personnel to screen an athlete or an entire team quickly and efficiently (brief administration and scoring duration). The DESA-6 does not require psychometric expertise, an extensive time commitment, nor a large number of resources, thus making it a promising tool for risk assessment of DE in adolescent athletes. Future research investigating the validity of the DESA-6 in additional athlete populations, such as adult athletes and sports that were under-represented in this study, could further expand the generalizability of the DESA-6. This could potentially result in the ability to use the DESA-6 to assess all athletes, no matter age, gender, sport, or level of competition.

Abbreviations

DE: Disordered eating; ED: Eating disorder; AN: Anorexia nervosa; BN: Bulimia nervosa; EAT-26: Eating Attitudes Test; OSFED: Other specified feeding and eating disorder; DESA-6: Disordered Eating Screen for Athletes; DSM-5: Diagnostic and Statistical Manual of Mental Disorders, Fifth Edition; BED: Binge Eating Disorder; NATA: National Athletic Trainers' Association; ACSM: American College of Sports Medicine; IOC: International Olympic Committee; EDE-Q: Eating Disorder Examination Questionnaire; EDE: Eating Disorder Examination; AMDQ: Athletic Milieu Direct Questionnaire; FAST: Female Athlete Screening Tool; PST: Physiologic Screening Test; BEDA-Q: Brief Eating Disorder in Athletes Questionnaire

Acknowledgements

The authors would like to acknowledge Dr. Robert Norris for his assistance; Jacob Babb, Zach Bauer, Tonye Burutolu, Jackie Davis, Cailyn D'Haem, Dr. Alexander Hayek, Ali Moshrefi, Tom Porter, Moshiur Rahman, Jack Sims, Melanie Smalls, and Peter Stephan for their assistance with data collection.

Authors' contributions

SK, JK, EM, designed the study protocol. RM, DG, HK recruited/interviewed participants according to the protocol. HK helped contact and recruit local high schools and obtained administrative permission to run the study. DG formulated the Tables. SK, JK, EW, RM, DG, wrote the first draft of the manuscript. SK supervised all other authors and analyzed/revised the article critically. All authors contributed to the interpretation of data. All authors contributed to and have approved the final manuscript.

Authors' information

RM, DG, and SK have recently been accepted into JOED with the article, "Prevalence of Disordered Eating in Athletes Categorized by Emphasis on Leanness and Activity Type – A Systematic Review". RM and DG have been invited to speak regarded disordered eating and eating disorders in athletes from several organizations, including the Michigan Osteopathic Neuropsychiatric Society, for continuing medical education credit. RM and DG were awarded second place at the Michigan Osteopathic Association Scientific Research Exhibit competition, where they presented on the various types of athletes that exist in literature. RM was awarded first place at the research competition hosted by the Michigan Association of Osteopathic Family Practitioners for a similar topic. SK is a child and adolescent psychiatrist who is primarily focused on the treatment of disordered eating and eating disorders, especially those affecting athletes.

Competing interests

The authors declare that they have no competing financial interests or other conflicts of interest.

Author details

[1]Department of Psychiatry, Michigan State University, 909 Wilson Rd, Room B119, East Lansing, MI 48824, USA. [2]Department of Sports Medicine, Michigan State University, East Lansing, MI 48824, USA. [3]Department of Kinesiology, Michigan State University, East Lansing, MI 48824, USA. [4]Michigan State University College of Osteopathic Medicine, Michigan State University, East Lansing, MI 48824, USA. [5]Grand Ledge High School, Grand Ledge, MI 48837, USA.

References

1. American Psychiatric Association. Diagnostic and Statistical Manual of Mental Disorders. 5th ed. Arlington (VA): American Psychiatric Association; 2013.
2. Bryne S, McLean N. Eating disorders in athletes: a review of the literature. J Sci Med Sport. 2001;4(2):145–59.
3. Beals K. Disordered eating among athletes: a comprehensive guide for health professionals. Hum Kinet. 1st edition (April 12, 2004). 2004:4–19.
4. Sundgot-Borgen J, Torstveit MK. Aspects of disordered eating continuum in elite high-intensity sports. Scand J Med Sci Spor. 2010;20(S2):112–21.
5. Baum A. Eating disordered in the male athlete. Sports Med. 2006;36(1):1–6.
6. Mountjoy M, Sundgot-Borgen J, Burke L, et al. The IOC consensus statement: beyond the Female Athlete Triad – Relative Energy Deficiency in Sport (RED-S). Br J Sport Med. 2014;48:491–7.
7. Bonci CM, Bonci LJ, Granger LR, et al. National Athletic Trainers' Association position statement: preventing, detecting, and managing disordered eating in athletes. J Athl Train. 2008;43(1):80–108.
8. Rauh MJ, Nichols JF, Barrack MT. Relationships among injury and disordered eating, menstrual dysfunction, and low bone mineral density in high school athletes: a prospective study. J Athl Train. 2010;45(3):243–252.B.
9. Hudson JI, Hiripi E, Pope HG, Kesslet RC. The prevalence and correlates of eating disorders in the national comorbidity survey replication. Biol Psychiatry. 2007;61:348–58.
10. DePalma MT, Koszewski WM, Romani W, Chase JG, Suiderhof NJ, McCoy PM. Identifying college athletes at risk for pathogenic eating. Br J Sports Med. 2002;36:45–50.
11. Black DR, Larkin DC, Coster DC, Leverenz LJ, Abood DA. Physiologic screening test for eating disorders/disordered eating among female collegiate athletes. J Athl Train. 2003;38(4):286–97.
12. Cotton M, Ball C, Robinson P. Four simple questions can help screen for eating disorders. J Gen Intern Med. 2003;18:53–6.
13. Nagel DL, Black DR, Leverenze LJ, Coster DC. Evaluation of a screening test for female college athletes with eating disorders and disordered eating. J Athl Train. 2000;35(4):431–40.
14. Martinsen M, Sherman RT, Thompson RA, Sundgot-Borgen J. Coaches' knowledge and management of eating disorders: a randomized controlled trial. Med Sci Sports Exerc. 2015;47(5):1070–8.
15. Martinsen M, Sundgot-Borgen J. Higher prevalence of eating disorders among adolescent elite athletes than controls. Med Sci Sports Exerc. 2013;45(6):1188–97.
16. Nattiv A, Loucks AB, Manore MM, Sanborn CF, Sundgot-Borgen J, Warren MP. American College of Sports Medicine Position Statement: the female athlete triad. Med Sci Sports Exerc. 2007;39(10):1867–82.
17. Ljungqvist A, Jenoure P, Engbretsen L, et al. The International Olympic Committee (IOC) Consensus Statement on periodic health evaluation of elite athletes. Br J Sports Med. 2009;43(9):631–43.
18. McNulty KY, Adams CH, Anderson JH, Affenito SG. Development and validation of a screening tool to identify eating disorders in female athletes. J Am Diet Assoc. 2001;101(8):886–92.
19. Martinsen M, Holme I, Pensgaard AM, Torstveit MK, Sundgot-Borgen J. The development of the Brief Eating Disorder in Athletes questionnaire. Med Sci Sports Exerc. 2014;46(8):1666–75.
20. Knapp J, Aernia G, Anderson A. Eating disorders in female athletes: use of screening tools. Curr Sports Med Rep. 2014;13(4):214–8.
21. Garner DM, Garfinkel PE. The Eating Attitudes Test: an index of symptoms of anorexia nervosa. Psychol Med. 1979;9:273–9.
22. Mintz LB, O'Halloran MS. The Eating Attitudes Test: validation with DSM-IV eating disorder criteria. J Pers Assess. 2000;74(3):489–503.
23. Garfinkel PE, Newman A. The Eating Attitudes Test: twenty-five years later. Eat Weight Disord. 2001;6:1–24.
24. Haase AM. Weight perception in female athletes: associations with disordered eating correlates and behavior. Eat Behav. 2011;12:64–7.
25. Cooper Z, Fairburn CG. The Eating Disorder Examination: A semi-structured interview for the assessment of the specific psychopathology of eating disorders. Int J Eat Disord. 987;6(1):1–8. https://onlinelibrary-wiley-com.proxy2.cl.msu.edu/doi/abs/10.1002/1098-108X(198701)6:1%3C1::AID-EAT2260060102%3E3.0.CO;2-9.
26. Berg KC, Peterson CB, Frazier P, Crow SJ. Psychometric evaluation of the Eating Disorder Examination and Eating Disorder Examination-Questionnaire: a systematic review of the literature. Int J Eat Disorder. 2012;45:428–38.
27. Kennedy SF, Ley AF, Fugate BN, Hayek A. Factors associated with disordered eating behaviors among triathletes. Spartan Med Res J. 2017;2(1):1–14.
28. Ghoch ME, Soave F, Calugi S, Grave RD. Eating disorders, physical fitness and sport performance: a systematic review. Nutrients. 2013;5:5140–60.
29. Hulley AJ, Hill AJ. Eating disorders and health in elite women distance runners. Int J Eat Disord. 2001;30(3):312–7.
30. Fawcett T. An introduction to ROC analysis. Pattern Recog Letters. 2006;27: 861–74.
31. Schoonjans, F. (2020). MedCalc's Free statistical calculators. Retrieved Febuary 21, 2020, from https://www.medcalc.org/calc/
32. Steiner DL, Cairney J. What's under the ROC? AN introduction to receiver operating characteristics curves. Can J Psychiatry. 2007;52(2):121–8.
33. Torstveit MK, Rosenvinge JH, Sundgot-Borgen J. Prevalence of eating disorders and the predictive power of risk models in female elite athletes: a controlled study. Scan J Med Sci Spor. 2008;18(1):108–18.
34. Sundgot-Borgen J, Torstveit MK. Prevalence of eating disorders in elite athletes is higher than in the general population. Clin J Sport Med. 2004;14:25–32.
35. Rosendahl J, Bormann B, Aschenbrenner K, Aschenbrenner F, Strauss B. Dieting and disordered eating in German high school athletes and non-athletes. Scand J Med Sci Sports. 2009;19(5):731–9.
36. Schtscherbyna A, Soares EA, de Oliveria FP, Ribeiro BG. Female athlete triad in elite swimmers of the city of Rio de Jeneiro, Brazil. Nutrition. 2009;25(6):634–9.
37. Martinsen M, Bratland-Sanda S, Eriksson AK, Sundgot-Borgen J. Dieting to win or to be thin? A study of dieting and disordered eating among adolescent elite athletes and non-athlete controls. Br J Sports Med. 2010;44(1):70–6.
38. Engel SG, Johnson C, Powers PS, Crosby RD, Wonderluch SA, Wittrock DA, Mitchell JE. Predictors of disordered eating in a sample of elite division I college athletes. Eat Behav. 2003;4:333–43.
39. Chapman J, Woodman T. Disordered eating in male athletes: a meta-analysis. J Sports Sci. 2016;34(2):101–10.

11

Targeting maladaptive overcontrol with radically open dialectical behaviour therapy in a day programme for adolescents with restrictive eating disorders: an uncontrolled case series

Julian Baudinet*†, Mima Simic†, Helena Griffiths, Cecily Donnelly, Catherine Stewart and Elizabeth Goddard

Abstract

Background: Radically Open Dialectical Behaviour Therapy (RO-DBT) was developed to target maladaptive overcontrol, a proposed core difficulty of restrictive eating disorders. RO-DBT is now the main group treatment model at the Intensive day Treatment Programme (ITP), Maudsley Hospital. This ITP case series aimed to investigate whether overcontrol is associated with restrictive eating disorder symptoms in adolescents and to evaluate ITP outcomes since RO-DBT skills classes were introduced.

Method: Self-report measures of eating disorder symptoms and temperament, personality and social characteristics linked to overcontrol were collected at assessment and discharge from ITP for all consecutive adolescents who attended between February 2015 and January 2019 ($N = 131$). Weight change, global outcomes and treatment needs post-ITP were also recorded.

Results: Eating disorder symptoms at assessment were significantly correlated with overcontrol factors, including social connectedness ($r = -.67$), reward responsivity ($r = -.54$), and cognitive inflexibility ($r = .52$). Adolescents stayed in ITP on average 13.40 weeks. 70.8% had a Good-Intermediate outcome on Morgan-Russell scale. 4.6% did not respond and were referred to inpatient treatment from ITP. Significant improvements in drive for thinness ($d = .33$), depressive mood ($d = .41$), social connectedness ($d = .48$), and emotional expressiveness ($d = .97$) were reported at discharge. No changes were observed in perfectionism or negative temperament.

Conclusions: This study offers preliminary evidence that eating disorder symptoms are associated with overcontrol factors in adolescence and that they can improve with RO-DBT informed day programme treatment. RO-DBT is a promising treatment that offers a new way of conceptualising treatment targets and recovery for adolescent restrictive eating disorders.

Keywords: RO-DBT, Eating disorders, Anorexia nervosa, Day programme, Partial hospitalization programme

* Correspondence: Julian.Baudinet@slam.nhs.uk
†Julian Baudinet and Mima Simic contributed equally to this work.
Maudsley Centre for Child and Adolescent Eating Disorders, Maudsley Hospital, De Crespigny Park, Denmark Hill, London SE8 5AZ, UK

Plain English summary

Restrictive eating disorders have been associated with overcontrolled coping, e.g. high levels of perfectionism, inflexibility, and a tendency to inhibit emotional expression leading to loneliness and social isolation. Radically Open Dialectical Behaviour Therapy (RO–DBT) suggests that targeting this coping style will lead to improvements in eating disorder symptoms. RO-DBT proposes that overcontrol is the main difficulty, not the eating disorder symptoms themselves. This study examined the relationship between overcontrol and adolescent eating disorder symptoms. RO-DBT skills classes were included in a day programme and changes in overcontrolled coping and eating disorder symptoms at the end of treatment were measured. Results from 131 adolescents with restrictive eating disorders showed that more severe eating disorder symptoms co-occurred with more overcontrol on some measures (social connection, reward sensitivity, and flexibility). Only 4.6% did not improve during the treatment and were referred for inpatient treatment; a low proportion compared to other day programme studies. Adolescents also reported significant improvements in drive for thinness, depressed mood, social connectedness, and emotional expression at discharge. These results suggest that a day hospital programme that includes RO-DBT can have a positive impact on overcontrolled coping and the clinical outcomes of adolescent restrictive eating disorders.

Background

Outpatient family therapies for adolescents with restrictive eating disorders have moderate to good outcomes. However, it is now well established that there is a significant proportion for whom family therapy is not enough [1, 2]. Historically, this group of young people were offered inpatient treatment, which can be lengthy and costly, with poor or mixed outcomes [3, 4]. To try and better support this group of young people and their families, day programmes, or partial hospitalisation programs, have been developed as an alternative intensive treatment option.

Research investigating the efficacy of day programmes for eating disorders has predominately focused on adults [5, 6], however there is a growing body of evidence for day programmes for adolescents [7–13], including one randomised controlled trial [14]. Results demonstrate that day programme attendance leads to significant improvements in physical and psychological health [8–10, 12, 13, 15–19], which are maintained at follow up [7, 8].

Despite these promising findings, no day programme is effective for all adolescents, with some going on to require inpatient care and/or multiple day programme admission. Dancyger et al. [20] reported that 26% of adolescents left their day programme before goals were met and 15% required inpatient treatment. Similarly, Simic et al. [8] reported that 18% needed to be discharged from day programme to inpatient treatment. Clearly there is a need to continue to improve day programme treatments.

In recent years, new evidence is emerging of a distinct bio-temperamental profile for people with restrictive eating disorders [21–23]. This bio-temperamental profile is characterised by high levels of neuroticism [24], perfectionism [25], obsessionality [26], persistence [22], and low reward sensitivity [27, 28]. Socially, people with restrictive eating disorders report distant relationships and high levels of loneliness [29] as well as high suppression of negative emotions and a minimisation of their own needs in order to preserve their relationships [30]. Hempel et al. [21] propose that this cluster of traits and difficulties associated with restrictive eating disorders point to a core difficulty with maladaptive self-control, or overcontrol.

Concepts of overcontrol and undercontrol have been described in the literature in various form for some time [31–34]. The current conceptualisation of maladaptive overcontrol is defined by four core difficulties; a) low openness and tolerance of uncertainty b) cognitive and behavioural rigidity and inflexibility, c) pervasive inhibited emotional expression and emotional awareness, and d) low social connectedness and intimacy which is often manifested in aloof and distant relationships [35]. Other markers of overcontrol include low reward sensitivity, high threat sensitivity, high inhibitory control and high attention to detail [35, 36]. Conversely, undercontrol is characterised by low inhibitory control (e.g. impulsivity, disinhibition, novelty seeking, affective lability) and a more chaotic pattern of relationships [35, 36]. Overcontrol has been associated with internalising disorders, whereas undercontrol with externalising disorders [37].

Given the reconceptualization of restrictive eating disorders as primarily disorders of overcontrol [21], it has been proposed that treatments specifically targeting overcontrol may lead to improved outcomes, as they target the broader core psychopathology of eating disorders, which may also improve relapse rates, behaviours and cognitions. There is a need to examine the efficacy of treatments designed to target maladaptive overcontrol and the key bio-temperamental factors associated with overcontrol among adolescents with anorexia nervosa and restrictive eating disorders.

Radically Open Dialectical Behaviour Therapy (RO-DBT) is a new, trans-diagnostic, manualised treatment that targets psychological disorders associated with maladaptive overcontrol [35]. While traditional Dialectical Behaviour Therapy (DBT) [38] targets behaviours associated with maladaptive undercontrol, RO-DBT addresses maladaptive overcontrol via the novel change mechanism of targeting social connection and social signalling. RO-DBT posits that improving social signalling, the verbal and non-verbal cues that people constantly consciously and unconsciously send to others, will increase the closeness and quality of relationships and networks [35]. RO-DBT hypothesises that the development of closer social connections leads to improved eating disorder symptom management and reduction. Similar to standard Dialectical Behaviour Therapy, RO-DBT is offered as a combination of weekly groups (named skills classes in RO-DBT) and concurrent weekly individual therapy sessions [35]. There is emerging evidence that it is effective for adults with eating disorders [39] and the model has recently been adapted for adolescents [40].

In an attempt to improve outcomes of day programme treatment for adolescents with restrictive eating disorders, the clinical team at the Intensive Treatment Programme (ITP), a day programme at the Maudsley Centre for Child and Adolescent Eating Disorders (MCCAED), introduced RO-DBT skills classes into the programme. All ITP staff were trained in the model and RO-DBT skills classes became the main group therapy intervention offered from March 2015.

This study has two aims. Firstly, to explore whether temperament, personality and coping related to overcontrol are associated with restrictive eating disorder and the related psychopathology in adolescence. Secondly, to evaluate whether ITP with RO-DBT skills classes leads to changes in these characteristics as well as in eating disorder symptoms and psychological symptoms associated with eating disorders. Given the exploratory nature of this uncontrolled case series, no a priori hypotheses were generated.

Method

ITP Programme description

ITP is a day programme that operates Monday to Friday at The Maudsley Hospital, London, UK. Included in the therapeutic treatment programme are individual, family and group therapy, meal support and education support. ITP is a rolling open-ended programme aiming to establish a stable trajectory towards recovery and effective re-engagement with outpatient treatment. The group therapy programme is spread over 6.25 h per week, of which 2.5 h are dedicated to RO-DBT skill classes, split over 2 sessions per week. RO-DBT skill class content was modified from Lynch's original skills manuals [41] to be more adolescent appropriate and offered over 16 sessions, rather than the original 30. The content of the skill classes is repeated approximately every 8 weeks. The remaining ITP group therapy content includes cognitive behavioural therapy (CBT) (1.5 h), cognitive remediation treatment (CRT) (45 min) and art therapy (1 h).

Study design

Adolescents completed a diagnostic interview at assessment, as well as self-report questionnaires at assessment and discharge from ITP. The battery of self-report measures targeted three main domains (a) eating disorder symptoms and psychological symptoms associated with eating disorders (mental health symptomatology), (b) temperamental, personality and coping factors associated with overcontrol, and (c) relationship quality and attachment. Time one assessment measures were used to explore the relationship between these three domains and eating disorder symptoms. Changes on these measures at discharge from ITP were used to evaluate whether ITP was effective in supporting reductions in eating disorder symptoms as well as overcontrolled coping and related domains such as social connectedness. The battery of measures was changed twice with additional measures added at two different time points to better evaluate ITP outcomes and the assessment of factors associated with overcontrol. Changes in weight, menstruation status, length of treatment and treatment needs following ITP were also recorded.

Measures

Self-report measures

Measures assessing eating disorder and other mental health symptomatology Eating disorder symptoms and psychological symptoms associated with eating disorders were assessed using the Eating Disorder Inventory – 3rd Version (EDI-3) [42]. The EDI-3 consists of 91 items organised into 12 primary scales. Five composite scales and a global score can be derived from the 12 subscales, including an eating disorder risk composite. The EDI-3 is widely used, has good reliability, internal consistency and discriminate validity [42, 43] and has published adolescent norms [42].

Symptoms of depression were screened using the 33-item Moods and Feelings Questionnaire (MFQ) [44]. The MFQ is a reliable measure of depression in children and adolescents. Scores of 27 and higher indicate the presence of depression [45, 46]. The MFQ been shown to have good validity, reliability and internal consistency with adolescents [47].

At assessment all adolescents and one or both parent also completed the online version of the Development and Wellbeing Assessment (DAWBA, [48]) to assess symptoms of comorbid psychiatric diagnoses. The DAWBA is a widely used structured diagnostic assessment that can generate DSM-V [49] and ICD-10 [50] psychiatric diagnoses for two to 17-year olds [48]. The DAWBA involves two steps. Firstly, computer-generated predicted diagnoses are provided from self-report responses to an online questionnaire. These responses can then be reviewed by an expert clinical rater to confirm individual diagnoses. The computer-generated predicted diagnoses alone have been shown to be a useful tool to estimate comorbidity for children and adolescent [51], although may slightly underestimates total rates of psychiatric disorders in this group. In this study, only the predicted diagnoses are reported.

Measures assessing temperament, personality factors and coping associated with overcontrol Measures targeting factors associated with overcontrol were selected to identify temperament, personality and coping factors for adolescents with restrictive eating disorder. As overcontrol is a recently defined construct not previously investigated with adolescents, validated adolescent measures were not available for the full range of overcontrol related factors at the time of the study design. In their absence, adult measures were used.

The Negative Temperament subscale of the Schedule of Non-adaptive and Adaptive Personality for Youth (SNAPY-Y) [52] was used to assess level of maladaptive negative temperament and its stability across treatment. This subscale measures tendencies towards fear, anger, sadness, irritability and distress. Given temperament is relatively stable and likely biologically based [53], change was not expected on the SNAP-Y from baseline to discharge. The SNAP-Y has shown to be a valid measure of personality in adolescence, with good internal consistency and structural validity [52], as well as availability community and clinical norms [52, 54].

The Five Factor Obsessive Compulsive Inventory – Short Form (FFOCI-SF) [55, 56] was included to assess levels of risk aversion, cognitive flexibility, perfectionism, workaholism and punctiliousness. The FFOCI-SF has not been validated for children and adolescents, however, was included in this study in the absence of a validated measure of obsessive-compulsive personality in children and adolescence and recent developments indicating personality pathology does occur in children and adolescents [57]. The FFOCI-SF has demonstrated good discriminant validity and internal consistency with an undergraduate university sample [56].

Reward processing, as one marker of overcontrol, was measured using the Temporal Experience of Pleasures [58]. The 18-item self-report measure is based on Klein's [59] model of anhedonia and has two subscales that measure distinct facets of trait-based reward processing; namely, the anticipatory (TEPS-ANT) and consummatory (TEPS-CON) aspects. The anticipation subscale (TEPS-ANT) assesses how much someone "wants" or is motivated by pleasurable things (example item: "when something exciting is coming up in my life, I really look forward to it"). The consummatory scale assesses how much a person "likes" or is able to enjoy pleasurable things in the moment (example item: "I love the sound of rain on the windows when I'm lying in my warm bed"). Anticipatory ("wanting") aspects, as opposed to the consummatory ("liking") aspects, of reward processing have been associated with motivation, reinforcement learning and reward-based decision-making [60]. The TEPS has not been used with an adolescent sample, however has demonstrates good internal consistency, test-retest reliability, and convergent and divergent validity in undergraduate university age samples [58].

The Emotion Regulation Questionnaire (ERQ) [61] is a validated 10-item scale designed to measure emotion regulation using two separate sub-scales, the tendency to regulate emotions via cognitive reappraisal strategies or via the suppression of emotion expression. Cognitive reappraisal strategies refer to when a person changes how they think in an attempt to change their emotional experience (example item: "when I want to feel less negative emotion [such as sadness or anger], I change what I'm thinking about"). The suppression of emotion expression subscale assesses a person's attempts to inhibit the behavioural expression of their emotions (example item: "when I am feeling negative emotions, I make sure not to express them") [62]. Cognitive reappraisal scores are typically considered adaptive and associated with low psychological distress and alexithymia, whereas expressive suppression is considered less adaptive and associated with psychological distress and alexithymia [62]. The ERQ has demonstrated good reliability and validity [61], good internal consistency [62], and has been used with adolescents [63].

Measures assessing relationships quality and attachment Level of perceived social withdrawal and isolation was assessed using the 8-item Withdrawal subscale of the Youth Self-Report questionnaire (WS-YSR) [64]. The YSR is a widely used and validated self-report measure used to assess a range of problems in adolescents [64].

The 20-item Social Connectedness Scale (SCS-R) [65] was used to assess how connected one feels to others in their social environment. Low scores indicate low levels of social connection. This measure has not been validated with adolescents, however, has demonstrated good validity and internal consistency in adult samples [65].

Attachment characteristics and the quality of relationships were assessed using the 40-item attachment styles questionnaire (ASQ) [66]. The ASQ contains five subscales assessing different dimensions of attachment, including relationship confidence, need for approval, discomfort with closeness, pre-occupation and relationships as secondary. The ASQ has been used with adults and adolescents [67]. It has been shown to be valid and reliable, with good internal consistency [66, 68, 69].

Physical health and other markers of ITP outcome

Information on physical health and other markers of ITP outcome were extracted from medical records. Weight gain was used as the primary marker of treatment outcome. Weight was calculated as a percentage of median Body Mass Index (%mBMI) adjusting for age and gender. The modified Morgan-Russell Global

Outcome Assessment Schedule [70, 71] was used to classify outcome at discharge. Good outcome indicates weight greater than 85%mBMI with menstruation or premenarchal (under the age of 15 and before the onset of the first period) and no bulimic symptoms. Intermediate outcome indicates weight greater than 85%mBMI without menstruation or bulimic symptoms averaging < 1 per week over the last month. Poor outcome indicates weight below 85%mBMI without menstruation or bulimic symptoms averaging ≥1 per week over the last month. Intensity of treatment required at discharge from ITP was identified as either outpatient or inpatient (either a psychiatric or medical stabilisation admission) and was also considered a marker of treatment outcome.

Sample

The total sample comprised 131 adolescents (age 11–18 years) who consecutively attended ITP between February 2015 and January 2019. Data from the first admission to ITP was used for this study (2 admissions n = 11, 3 admissions n = 1). Nine adolescents (6.9%) attended for 5 days or less and were considered non-starters. One person had a diagnosis of bulimia nervosa and was excluded from further data analysis. No exclusions were made based on previous treatment, clinical severity, medication or comorbid diagnosis.

Analysis plan

Individual and group mean scores on all self-report measures were obtained at assessment and discharge from ITP. To analyse relationships at baseline (Aim 1) Pearson's r correlations were conducted between EDI-3 composite scales and measures assessing the biopsychosocial factors linked with maladaptive overcontrol. Due to poor internal consistency at assessment (Cronbach a < 0.70) three scales were removed and not included in further analysis. These were the FFOCI-SF Punctiliousness subscale (a = 0.68), ASQ Confidence subscale (a = 0.68) and the ERQ cognitive reappraisal subscale (a = 0.65). Paired t-tests were then conducted to analyse the mean difference in self-report measures from assessment to discharge. Due to the large number of tests, the Benjamini-Hochberg procedure (adjusted to <.05) [72] was applied to correct for multiple comparisons. Given the exploratory nature of this study both uncorrected and corrected data are reported.

As measures were introduced at different time points over a four year period in a busy clinical service, there were inconsistencies in data collection and differences in the number of measures collected at different time points. As a result, there are varying degrees of missing data for each measure included in this study, particularly for the paired EDI-3. To examine potential sampling bias, analyses were conducted to compare those who had completed each questionnaire to those who had not, across key demographic and clinical outcomes. Results showed that there were no differences between those who had completed the outcome measures at time 1 (assessment: EDI-3, SCS-R, MFQ, WS-YSR, ASQ, FFOCI-SF, SNAP-Y, ERQ, TEPS) compared to those who did not complete them on age, %mBMI at beginning of treatment or referral source (inpatient or outpatient). Further analyses were conducted to examine the impact of missing data at time 2 (discharge). There were no differences between those who completed time 2 measures and those who did not complete end of treatment measures on age, %mBMI at beginning of treatment, or referral source (outpatient or inpatient).

Results

Demographics

Demographic information including age, gender and referral source of adolescents at assessment are presented in Table 1. All participants identified as cis gendered.

Correlation analysis at assessment

Pearson's correlations between EDI-3 composites and measures assessing overcontrolled temperament, personality and the quality of relationships at assessment are presented in Table 2. Almost all correlations were moderate to strong and significantly correlated at the $p < 0.01$ level. The EDI-3 Eating Disorder Risk composite had a strong negative correlation with social connectedness (SCS-R) and moderate negative correlation with anticipation of pleasure (TEPS-ANT), reflecting that those with more eating disorder risk felt less socially connected and had reduced anticipation of pleasure. Furthermore, Eating Disorder Risk composite was moderately positively correlated with the social withdrawal subscale of the YSR and all subscales of the ASQ, indicating those with increased eating disorder risk were more socially withdrawn and had more difficulty in their attachment relationships. Both the Risk Aversion and Cognitive Inflexibility subscales were significantly moderately correlated with eating disorder risk, meaning those with increase eating disorder risk were more risk averse and cognitively inflexible.

The Perfectionism and Workaholism subscales of the FFOCI-SF, however, were not significantly correlated with Eating Disorder Risk composite. The Negative Temperament subscale of the SNAPY-Y was only significantly correlated with the Ineffectiveness composite of the EDI-3. All measures, except for the Consummatory subscale of the TEPS (TEPS-CON), were significantly correlated with the Overcontrol Composite of the EDI-3.

ITP outcomes

The mean length of stay in ITP was 13.40 weeks (sd = 5.91, range 1–30 weeks). Mean percent median BMI at assessment was 82.39% (sd = 8.46). This increased to a mean of

Table 1 Demographic Information at assessment

Age	**15.02 years (sd = 1.52, range = 11–18)**
Gender	
- Female	94.62% (*n* = 123)
- Male	5.38% (*n* = 7)
Referral Source	
- Outpatient	86.92% (*n* = 113)
- Inpatient	13.08% (*n* = 17)
- Paediatric Admission	*5.38% (n = 7)*
- Adolescent Psychiatric Unit	*3.85% (n = 5)*
- Specialist Eating Disorder Unit	*3.85% (n = 5)*
Primary diagnosis at assessment	
- Anorexia nervosa	93.13% (*n* = 122)
- Restrictive subtype	*83.84% (n = 109)*
- Binge-purge subtype	*4.61% (n = 6)*
- Atypical anorexia nervosa	*5.38% (n = 7)*
- Other Specified Feeding and Eating Disorder (OSFED)	6.15% (*n* = 8)
Comorbid diagnoses predicted at assessment	
- Major Depressive Disorder	41.54% (*n* = 54)
- OCD	10.00% (n = 13)
- Anxiety disorder (> 1 diagnosed)	46.92% (*n* = 61)
- Generalised Anxiety Disorder	*36.15% (n = 47)*
- Social Phobia	*24.62% (n = 32)*
- Separation Anxiety	*6.15% (n = 8)*
- PTSD	*1.54% (n = 2)*
- Panic Disorder	*6.92% (n = 9)*
- Specific Phobia	*13.08% (n = 17)*
- Agoraphobia	*3.85% (n = 5)*
- ASD	*0.77% (n = 1)*
- Missing	*6.92% (n = 9)*
Number of comorbidities predicted at assessment	
- 1 or more	57.69% (*n* = 75)
- 2 or more	38.46% (*n* = 50)
- 3 or more	23.85% (*n* = 31)

Abbreviations: *OCD* obsessive compulsive disorder, *PTSD* post-traumatic stress disorder, *ASD* autism spectrum disorder

89.51% (sd = 8.59) at discharge. This corresponds to a mean gain of 7.19%mBMI during ITP, at a mean rate of 0.54%mBMI per week. At discharge, more than 70% (n = 92) of adolescents had a Good or Intermediate outcome using the Morgan-Russell Global Outcome measure (Good = 53.08%, n = 69; Intermediate = 17.69%, n = 23). The remainder had a Poor outcome (28.46%, n = 37) and 1 had missing data and could not be categorized. Six people (4.62%) required inpatient treatment during or after ITP (specialist eating disorder unit = 3.08%, n = 4; general adolescent psychiatric unit = 1.54%, n = 2).

Changes in symptoms of eating disorders and depression

There was a significant reduction in self-report eating disorder and associated symptomatology on seven of the 12 subscales of the EDI-3 (see Table 3). Notably, the drive for thinness subscale reduced from the typical clinical to low clinical range, while most others remained within the typical clinical range [42]. Adolescents reported a significant reduction in symptoms of depression on the MFQ with medium effect size (d = .41) over the course of ITP. Individuals scoring above the cut-off indicating the likely presence of depression (total score > 27) [45] reduced from 71.4% at assessment to 62.8% at discharge. After adjusting for multiple comparisons using

Table 2 Pearson's r correlation matrix for self-report measures at assessment

	EDI-3 Composites					
	Eating Disorder Risk	**Ineffectiveness**	**Interpersonal Problems**	**Affective Problems**	**Overcontrol**	**Global Psychological Maladjustment**
Relationship quality and attachment						
SCS-R	−.67[a]	−.79[a]	−.79[a]	−.74[a]	−.57[a]	−.84[a]
ASQ Discomfort	.54[a]	.71[a]	.74[a]	.63[a]	.54[a]	.76[a]
ASQ Preoccupation	.47[a]	.50[a]	.36[a]	.39[a]	.46[a]	.52[a]
ASQ Relationships as secondary	.44[a]	.37[a]	.49[a]	.45[a]	.53[a]	.53[a]
ASQ Need for approval	.57[a]	.66[a]	.51[a]	.48[a]	.55[a]	.66[a]
YSR Withdrawal subscale	.52[a]	.66[a]	.71[a]	.63[a]	.44[a]	.71[a]
Overcontrolled temperament, personality and coping						
FFOCI-SF Risk aversion	.48[a]	.49[a]	.39[a]	.33[a]	.39[a]	.53[a]
FFOCI-SF Inflexible	.52[a]	.52[a]	.40[a]	.41[a]	.49[a]	.59[a]
FFOCI-SF Perfectionism	.17	.12	−.02	−.08	.30[b]	.10
FFOCI-SF Workaholism	.06	−.02	−.01	−.03	.26[b]	.04
SNAP-Y Negative Temperament	.12	.24[b]	.01	.14	.24	.18
TEPS-ANT	−.54[a]	−.53[a]	−.59[a]	−.54[a]	−.38[a]	−.57[a]
TEPS-CON	−.25[b]	−.23[b]	−.28[a]	−.22[b]	−.18	−.26[b]
ERQ Emotional Suppression	.36[a]	.30	.44[a]	.38[a]	.41[a]	.46[a]

Abbreviations: *EDI-3* Eating Disorder Ineventory-3, *SCS-R* Social Connectedness Scale-Revised, *ASQ* Attachment Style Questionnaire, *YSR* Youth Self Report, *FFOCI-SF* Five Factor Obsessive Compulsive Inventory-Short Form, *SNAP-Y* Schedule for Nonadaptive and Adaptive Personality for Youth, *TEPS-ANT* Temporal Experience of Pleasure Scale-Anticipatory, *TEPS-CON* Temporal Experience of Pleasure Scale-Consummatory, *ERQ* Emotion Regulation Questionnaire
[a]correlation significant at .01 level; [b]correlation significance at .05 level

the Benjamini-Hochberg procedure (adjusted to <.05) changes on the MFQ, EDI-drive for thinness subscale, EDI-personal alienation subscale and the EDI-interoceptive deficits subscale remained significant.

Changes in Overcontrolled temperament, personality and coping

On the Emotion Regulation Questionnaire (ERQ) there was a significant reduction in the suppression of emotional expression as an emotion regulation strategy with large effect size (d = .97). There was also a significant decrease in cognitive inflexibility with a small effect size (d = .34) on the FFOCI-SF, however no changes were observed on any other subscale of the FFOCI-SF. Similarly, there was no significant difference between assessment and discharge in self report of negative treatment (SNAP-Y). Finally, analysis revealed significant differences between assessment and discharge on both subscales of the TEPS, reflecting an increase in reward responsiveness (TEPS-ANT; d = .42) and the consumption of pleasure (TEPS-CON; d = .51). All observed significant changes remained significant after correction for multiple comparisons using the Benjamini-Hochberg procedure (adjusted to <.05).

Changes in relationship quality and attachment

There was a significant increase in means scores on the SCS-R with medium effect size (d = .48), indicating improved social connectedness by the end of ITP. Mean scores on the WS-YSR significantly reduced with medium effect size (d = .54), representing a reduction in self-report level of perceived isolation and social withdrawal. Similarly, on the ASQ there was a significant reduction with small to medium effect size in adolescents' level of discomfort in close relationships (d = .43), as well as an increase in their preoccupation with relationships (d = .22) and a reduction in relationships being seen as secondary (d = .32). No significant change was observed on the need for approval subscale of the ASQ. After adjusting for multiple comparisons using the Benjamini-Hochberg procedure (adjusted to <.05) all significant changes remained significant, except for the ASQ-Preoccupation subscale.

Discussion

This is the first study to explore whether the RO-DBT concept of overcontrol is applicable to adolescents with restrictive eating disorders. This exploratory study provides preliminary evidence that temperament, personality

Table 3 Mean scores at assessment and discharge from the Intensive Treatment Programme (ITP) on self-report measures

Measure (n attendees whilst measure in use)	Assessment mean (sd)	Discharge mean (sd)	Test statistic (paired n)	Effect size	*Cronbach alpha*	
					Pre ITP	*Post ITP*
Eating disorder and mental health symptomatology						
EDI-3 ($n = 105$)						
- Drive for Thinness raw score	18.31[c] (8.45)	15.16[b] (8.92)	$p = 0.01^{*,a}$ ($n = 62$)	$d = 0.33$	.91	.93
- Bulimia raw score	2.63[b] (2.91)	2.84[b] (4.15)	$p = 0.71$ ($n = 62$)	$d = 0.05$	.78	.83
- Body dissatisfaction raw score	27.60[c] (11.95)	24.34[c] (11.72)	$p = 0.051$ ($n = 62$)	$d = 0.25$	.94	.93
- Low self-esteem raw score	14.50[c] (6.93)	12.63[c] (6.88)	$p = 0.04^{*}$ ($n = 62$)	$d = 0.26$	.91	.90
- Personal Alienation raw score	14.28[c] (7.24)	11.44[c] (6.93)	$p = 0.003^{**}$ ($n = 61$)	$d = 0.39$	.88	.85
- Interpersonal insecurity raw score	12.21[c] (7.19)	10.60[c] (8.04)	$p = 0.048^{*}$ ($n = 62$)	$d = 0.26$	.87	.86
- Interpersonal alienation raw score	10.19[c] (6.46)	8.45[c] (6.60)	$p = 0.014^{*}$ ($n = 62$)	$d = 0.32$	.86	.85
- Interceptive deficits raw score	14.82[c] (8.76)	11.74[c] (9.00)	$p = 0.004^{**}$ ($n = 62$)	$d = 0.38$	.90	.89
- Emotional dysregulation raw score	8.71[c] (5.88)	7.97[c] (6.96)	$p = 0.43$ ($n = 62$)	$d = 0.10$	.82	.75
- Perfectionism raw score	11.85[c] (6.22)	11.19[c] (6.14)	$p = 0.37$ ($n = 48$)	$d = 0.13$	.76	.82
- Ascetism raw score	11.81[c] (7.05)	9.81[c] (7.50)	$p = 0.027^{*}$ ($n = 59$)	$d = 0.29$	.84	.86
- Maturity Fears raw score	15.76[d] (7.78)	14.71[d] (8.52)	$p = 0.19$ ($n = 59$)	$d = 0.17$	.88	.90
MFQ ($n = 51$)	38.05[e] (15.62)	30.84[e] (18.47)	$p = 0.01^{*,a}$ ($n = 43$)	$d = 0.41$	.94	.98
Relationship quality and attachment						
SCS-R ($n = 81$)	67.97 (21.43)	75.51 (22.98)	$p < 0.001^{***,a}$ ($n = 67$)	$d = 0.48$	.95	.97
ASQ ($n = 101$)						
- Discomfort	42.32 (10.99)	38.65 (11.60)	$p < 0.001^{***,a}$ ($n = 81$)	$d = 0.43$	.82	.93
- Preoccupation	30.02 (7.53)	31.44 (7.67)	$p = 0.048^{*}$ ($n = 81$)	$d = 0.22$	.80	.78
- Relationships as secondary	20.23 (6.31)	18.46 (7.54)	$p = 0.006^{**,a}$ ($n = 81$)	$d = 0.32$	.80	.87
- Need for approval	32.48 (6.66)	31.69 (7.16)	$p = 0.24$ ($n = 81$)	$d = 0.13$	.84	.86
YSR Withdrawal subscale ($n = 101$)	8.75[g] (4.24)	6.48[f] (4.60)	$p < 0.001^{***,a}$ ($n = 81$)	$d = 0.54$	.89	.90
Overcontrolled temperament, personality and coping						
FFOCI-SF ($n = 81$)						
- Risk aversion	12.12 (4.20)	12.15 (10.93)	$p = 0.98$ ($n = 65$)	$d < 0.01$	.85	.88
- Inflexible	11.91 (3.64)	10.83 (3.83)	$p = 0.007^{**,a}$ ($n = 65$)	$d = 0.34$	.82	.89
- Perfectionism	15.02 (3.30)	14.91 (3.45)	$p = 0.75$ ($n = 65$)	$d = 0.04$	.78	.85
- Workaholism	12.32 (3.83)	12.25 (4.08)	$p = 0.83$ ($n = 65$)	$d = 0.03$	.87	.89
SNAP-Y Negative Temperament ($n = 81$)	30.47 (10.11)	30.08 (11.43)	$p = 0.67$ ($n = 62$)	$d = 0.05$	.86	.87
TEPS ($n = 113$)						
- Anticipatory (TEPS-ANT)	32.79 (8.93)	36.79 (9.92)	$p < 0.001^{***,a}$ ($n = 96$)	$d = 0.42$	.80	.71
- Consummatory (TEPS-CON)	32.18 (7.03)	35.19 (7.54)	$p < 0.001^{***,a}$ ($n = 96$)	$d = 0.51$	.71	.74
ERQ Expressive Suppression ($n = 51$)	19.50 (6.82)	14.02 (7.41)	$p < 0.001^{***,a}$ ($n = 42$)	$d = 0.97$	.87	.93

n for each measure provided in table indicates the number of young people who attended ITP while that measure was being administered

Abbreviations: *EDI-3* Eating Disorder Inveentory-3, *SCS-R* Social Connectedness Scale-Revised, *ASQ* Attachment Style Questionnaire, *YSR* Youth Self Report, *FFOCI-SF* Five Factor Obsessive Compulsive Inventory-Short Form, *SNAP-Y* Schedule for Nonadaptive and Adaptive Personality for Youth, *TEPS-ANT* Temporal Experience of Pleasure Scale-Anticipatory, *TEPS-CON* Temporal Experience of Pleasure Scale-Consummatory, *ERQ* Emotion Regulation Questionnaire, *sd* standard deviation

*significant at $p < 0.05$ level; **significance at $p < 0.01$ level; ***significance at $p < 0.001$ level

[a]significant after Benjamini-Hochberg adjustment (<.05) for multiple comparisons

[b]Low clinical range; [c]typical clinical range; [d]elevated clinical range (Garner, 2004)

[e]above clinical cut off for depression (total score > 27; Wood, et al., 1995)

[f]one standard deviation above community norms (mean = 3.1, sd = 2.5; Achenbach & Rescorla, 2001)

[g]two standard deviation above community norms (mean = 3.1, sd = 2.5; Achenbach & Rescorla, 2001)

and social factors related to overcontrol may be associated with restrictive eating disorder and related psychopathology in adolescence. The results also indicate that a RO-DBT informed day programme may lead to improvements in eating disorder symptoms and several factors associated with overcontrol.

Adolescents in this study reported high levels of both eating disorder symptoms and other difficulties associated with maladaptive overcontrol. At assessments the majority of adolescents attending ITP presented with eating disorder and associated psychological symptoms on the EDI-3 within the typical clinical range with the exception of maturity fears subscale, which was in the elevated clinical range, and the bulimia subscale, which was in the low clinical range [42]. Comorbidity for this group was the norm, with more than half (57.69%) predicted to have one or more comorbid diagnosis and almost one quarter (23.85%) with three or more at assessment. Seventy percent of the adolescents scored above the cut-off indicative of depression on the MFQ at assessment [45], indicating low mood, irrespective of a diagnosis, was also common for this group. Perceived social withdrawal and tendencies towards negative temperament were also both very high with mean scores more than two standard deviations above adolescent community norms on the WS-YSR [64] and SNAP-Y [52] respectively.

Correlation analysis of self-report measures at assessment confirmed significant moderate to strong associations between eating disorder symptom severity and overcontrol factors. These findings imply an interplay between eating disorder symptoms, sense of isolation and withdrawal, use of emotional suppression in coping and quality of attachment relationships. Furthermore, they show the association between eating disorder symptoms and cognitive rigidity, risk aversion and reduced capacity of adolescents to anticipate or experience pleasure. Together this suggests that adolescents with restrictive eating disorders struggle with a broad range of difficulties, many of which impact upon quality of life and the capacity to build relationships. Positive relationships, self-adaptability and positive affect have all been identified as important criteria for a full recovery beyond eating disorder symptom abatement [73], highlighting the importance of identifying and targeting these difficulties in treatment.

Negative temperament on the SNAP-Y was not significantly correlated with the eating disorder risk or the overcontrol composites of the EDI-3, despite mean scores for all three being high. This lack of association in the current study, particularly between the SNAP-Y and the EDI-3 overcontrol composite, suggests a general tendency towards negative affectivity may be a co-occurring but distinct factor to eating disorder and related psychopathology. The only EDI-3 composite significantly associated with negative temperament was the Ineffectiveness composite, which combines the low self-esteem and personal alienation scales. These findings may, in part, be due to the very broad nature of what the SNAP-Y negative temperament subscale is measuring. It assesses tendencies towards a wide range of general negative affectivity and distress which may be too non-specific to correlate with overcontrol as measured on the EDI-3. Further research is needed to understand the relationship between the broad concept of negative temperament, symptoms of restrictive eating disorders and other overcontrol related factors.

The observed relationship between overcontrol factors and eating disorder symptomatology also needs to be considered in the context of the specific group of adolescents in the current study. All participants in this study were diagnosed with a restrictive eating disorder, meaning generalisability of the findings to other types of eating disorders cannot be made from the current study. Given the differences in temperament and personality profiles (see Atiye et al. for review, 22), as well as differences in emotion regulation difficulties [74], across different eating disorders, it is possible that the observed relationship is specific to restrictive eating disorder presentations only. Further investigation is required.

The second aim of the study was to determine whether ITP with RO-DBT skills classes could lead to improvements in eating disorder symptoms, overcontrol related factors and the quality of relationships. The results described above indicate that ITP with RO-DBT skills classes led to significant improvements in physical health, eating disorder symptoms, and mood, with correction for multiple comparisons using the Benjamini-Hochberg procedure [72]. The programme also led to significant improvement in overcontrol factors like cognitive flexibility, reward responsiveness, emotional expression and openness to new pleasurable experiences. The results further indicate that adolescents experienced significant improvements in their relationship quality, reporting that they felt more comfortable in their relationships, prioritised them more, felt more connected to others and were less socially withdrawn.

The results also showed that temperament and obsessional traits remained largely unchanged. This is an expected finding given emerging evidence that personality traits and temperament show moderate to high stability from childhood and adolescence onwards [52, 75–78] and that temperament is presumably largely biologically based [53]. What does appear to be changeable is how the adolescents in this study coped with this. The pattern of results suggest ITP with RO-DBT may be providing adolescents the skills to manage temperamental overcontrol traits in more adaptive ways through the increased expression of their emotions, improved relationships and processing of rewards. All of which occurred alongside improvements in physical health and psychological symptoms linked with eating disorders.

The largest change observed in this study was on the suppression of emotional expression subscale of the emotion regulation questionnaire (ERQ-suppression; large effect size). This finding indicates that adolescents considered themselves to be less reliant on inhibiting their emotional expression to manage their emotions and more emotionally expressive by the end of treatment. Being more emotionally expressive in relationships is a core treatment target in RO-DBT and is hypothesised to be one of the main treatment mechanisms via which social connection and psychiatric symptomatology improves [35]. This finding suggests that the treatment may lead to changes in the domains RO-DBT directly intends to target.

Medium effect size changes were observed for level of social withdrawal and perceived improvements in the experience of pleasure, while the changes in eating disorder symptoms were only small. Similarly, changes of only small effect size were observed in depressive symptoms, attachment and relationship quality. It is possible that this may simply reflect ITP's design and its brevity. ITP only aims to support adolescents and their families to reach a stage whereby further outpatient treatment can be sufficient and effective. ITP is not designed to support adolescents to reach a full recovery. Full recovery from a restrictive eating disorder is not expected within a programme with a mean duration of 13.4 weeks. Similarly, large changes in attachment and relationship quality are expected to take much longer than the duration of ITP. Future studies are needed to determine whether changes of the magnitude observed in this study are sufficient for the resumption of an effective and less costly outpatient treatment.

After correcting for multiple comparisons using the Benjamini-Hochberg procedure [72] the pattern of results remained largely unchanged. All significant changes observed in this study remained significant except for four subscales of the EDI-3, none of which were related to core eating disorder symptomatology (interpersonal alienation, asceticism, low self-esteem, interpersonal insecurity), and the Preoccupation subscale of the ASQ. After correction, significant changes were observed in the level of relationship quality (connectedness, withdrawal, comfort in and importance of attachment relationships), emotional expressiveness, reward sensitivity and flexibility; all characteristics targeted by RO-DBT.

Together these findings suggest that individuals enrolled in ITP with RO-DBT skills classes demonstrate significant improvements over a relatively short duration (mean duration 13.4 weeks) in both eating disorder and related symptoms as well as overcontrol characteristics. More than 70% of adolescents in this study, all of whom had not responded to or been appropriate for outpatient treatments, had a good or intermediate outcome at the end of ITP. Nevertheless, it is unclear whether symptom change was truly due to the RO-DBT components of the ITP programme, specifically, or other aspects of the programme. This will be an important focus of future research.

This study also shows that ITP can support severely ill adolescents with restrictive eating disorder to remain at home with very few requiring inpatient treatment either during or after ITP (4.6%). Rates of transfer and discharge to inpatient care can be difficult to compare across day programmes as they are likely influenced by individual programme factors, such as intensity, duration and staffing. However, rates of inpatient admissions in the current study are low compared to other published day programme studies which report between 13 and 35% of young people require an inpatient admission either during or after day programme treatment [8, 9, 20]. Prior to the introduction of RO-DBT into ITP, Simic et al. [8] published a case series of 105 adolescents who attended ITP between 2010 and 2015 with similar characteristics (mean age 15.5 years, range 11–18; 95.2% with AN; 95% female). They reported that 18% ($n = 19$) were referred for an inpatient admission during day programme treatment. This 2010–2015 case series evaluation [8] was completed before RO-DBT classes replaced Dialectical Behaviour Therapy groups in the programme, however no changes were made to the inpatient admission criteria across both study periods. The content of the remaining manualised therapy groups was identical in both case series. While this large reduction cannot be solely attributed to the introduction of RO-DBT skills classes, it was the only intentional change made to the programme. It would be useful for future research to determine whether specific treatment models are more effective than others in a day programme context.

This study has several important limitations. First, this was an uncontrolled case series making it difficult to draw conclusions about the specific contribution of RO-DBT to the outcomes. The design of the current study does not allow for any investigation into how different factors interact during day programme treatment or whether improvements in overcontrol coping lead to or are the result of improvement in other areas. As all measures used in this study were self-report, there is also potential that shared method bias is impacting the high level of correlations amongst variables. Future research studies are needed to replicate the current findings and explore effectiveness of specific components and mechanisms of change within day programme treatments.

Second, this was not a study of either pure RO-DBT or of all RO-DBT components. RO-DBT in its original form covers 30 skills classes plus individual sessions.

Given the mean length of attendance was 13.4 weeks, even with two RO-DBT skills classes per week, it is possible that not enough time passed to practice skills and observe more meaningful changes. Adolescents also did not receive individual RO-DBT sessions and they received a range of other therapeutic interventions that are likely to have contributed to treatment outcomes.

Third, being a case series in a clinical service, there were inconsistencies in data collection and missing data. Additionally, some of the measures used were not validated with adolescents and were included in the absence of such measures being available (e.g. FFOCI). It is also important to note that some improvements observed in this study, have not been measured before in adolescent eating disorder population, leaving open for consideration that these changes could occur following any day programme if the same factors were measured.

Additional limitations include the limited generalizability of the findings to more diverse groups, people with less severe eating disorder symptoms, across different treatment settings and different treatment format (individual, family, group etc). In addition, when considering the clinical impact of ITP with RO-DBT, an important future direction would include efforts to obtain post-treatment follow-up data to determine the extent to which the reported symptom improvements persist after treatment. Improvements while in treatment are promising; however, the longer-term efficacy of interventions would provide further support for this intervention approach.

Conclusions

This case series of a sizeable sample of all consecutive admissions to a day programme over four years, offers preliminary support for the effectiveness of RO-DBT informed day programme treatment for restrictive eating disorders. The results also provide tentative support for an alternate way of conceptualising treatment and recovery from restrictive eating disorders for adolescents in a day programme setting. This study evaluates outcomes with a different lens in a field that struggles to find consensus on defining recovery beyond weight gain and eating disorder symptom reduction [73, 79]. By showing that a day programme that includes RO-DBT classes can facilitate significant changes in the quality of relationships and the way bio-temperamental factors are managed, the current findings may have important and meaningful implications when considering broader psychological wellbeing, functioning and quality of life; all factors that require much more focus when considering recovery from an eating disorder.

Abbreviations

AN: Anorexia Nervosa; ASQ: Attachment Styles Questionnaire; CBT: Cognitive Behavioural Therapy; CRT: Cognitive Remediation Therapy; DBT: Dialectical Behaviour Therapy; EDI-3: Eating Disorder Inventory – 3rd Edition; ERQ: Emotion Regulation Questionnaire; FFOCI-SF: Five Factor Obsessive Compulsive Inventory – Short Form; ITP: Intensive Treatment Programme; MFQ: Moods and Feelings Questionnaire; MCCAED: Maudsley Centre for Child and Adolescent Eating Disorders; RO-DBT: Radically Open Dialectical Behaviour Therapy; SCS-R: Social Connectedness Scale – Revised; SNAP-Y : Schedule of Non-Adaptive and Adaptive Personality for Youth; TEPS: Temporal Experience of Pleasure; TEPS-CON: Temporal Experience of Pleasure – Consummatory; TEPS-ANT: Temporal Experience of Pleasure – Anticipatory subscale; WS-YSR: Youth Self Report – Withdrawal subscale; %mBMI: Percentage of median body mass index

Acknowledgements

The authors would like to thank the adolescents in this study. The authors are also thankful to Dr. Katrina Hunt, Dr. Sam Bottrill, Dr. Charlotte Watson, Dr. Rebecca Dixey and all of the ITP and MCCAED team for their work providing RO-DBT and on this project.

Authors' contributions

JB and MS contributed equally to this work. Both were significantly involved in all aspects of data collection, analysis and manuscript preparation. EG and CS contributed by assisting with study design, data analysis and manuscript preparation. HC and DC contributed by collecting and analysing data. The author(s) read and approved the final manuscript.

Competing interests

The authors declare they have no competing interests.

References

1. Jewell T, Blessitt E, Stewart C, Simic M, Eisler I. Family therapy for child and adolescent eating disorders: a critical review. Fam Process. 2016;55(3):577–94.
2. Lock J. An update on evidence-based psychosocial treatments for eating disorders in children and adolescents. J Clin Child Adolesc Psychol. 2015; 44(5):707–21.
3. Lay B, Jennen-Steinmetz C, Reinhard I, Schmidt MH. Characteristics of inpatient weight gain in adolescent anorexia nervosa: relation to speed of relapse and re-admission. Eur Eat Disord Rev. 2002;10(1):22–40.
4. Gowers SG, An JW, Shore A, Hossain F, Elvins R. Impact of hospitalisation on the outcome of adolescent anorexia nervosa. Br J Psychiatry. 2000;176(2): 138–41.
5. Abbate-Daga G, Gramaglia C, Preda S, Comba E, Brustolin A, Fassino S. Day hospital programmes for eating disorders: a review of the similarities, differences and goals. Eat Weight Disord - Stud Anorex Bulim Obes. 2009; 14(2–3):e31–41.
6. Zipfel S, Reas DL, Thornton C, Olmsted MP, Williamson DA, Gerlinghoff M, et al. Day hospitalization programs for eating disorders: a systematic review of the literature. Int J Eat Disord. 2002;31(2):105–17.
7. Bryson AE, Scipioni AM, Essayli JH, Mahoney JR, Ornstein RM. Outcomes of low-weight patients with avoidant/restrictive food intake disorder and anorexia nervosa at long-term follow-up after treatment in a partial hospitalization program for eating disorders. Int J Eat Disord. 2018;51(5): 470–4.
8. Simic M, Stewart CS, Eisler I, Baudinet J, Hunt K, O'Brien J, et al. Intensive treatment program (ITP): a case series service evaluation of the effectiveness of day patient treatment for adolescents with a restrictive eating disorder. Int J Eat Disord. 2018;51(11):1261–9.
9. Goldstein M, Peters L, Baillie A, McVeagh P, Minshall G, Fitzjames D. The effectiveness of a day program for the treatment of adolescent anorexia nervosa. Int J Eat Disord. 2011;44(1):29–38.
10. Hoste RR. Incorporating family-based therapy principles into a partial hospitalization programme for adolescents with anorexia nervosa: challenges and considerations: FBT principles for anorexia nervosa. J Fam Ther. 2015;37(1):41–60.
11. Johnston JAY, O'Gara JSX, Koman SL, Baker CW, Anderson DA. A pilot study of Maudsley family therapy with group dialectical behavior therapy skills training in an intensive outpatient program for adolescent eating disorders. J Clin Psychol. 2015;71(6):527–43.

12. Ornstein RM, Lane-Loney SE, Hollenbeak CS. Clinical outcomes of a novel, family-centered partial hospitalization program for young patients with eating disorders. Eat Weight Disord - Stud Anorex Bulim Obes. 2012;17(3):8.
13. Ornstein RM, Essayli JH, Nicely TA, Masciulli E, Lane-Loney S. Treatment of avoidant/restrictive food intake disorder in a cohort of young patients in a partial hospitalization program for eating disorders. Int J Eat Disord. 2017; 50(9):1067–74.
14. Herpertz-Dahlmann B, Schwarte R, Krei M, Egberts K, Warnke A, Wewetzer C, et al. Day-patient treatment after short inpatient care versus continued inpatient treatment in adolescents with anorexia nervosa (ANDI): a multicentre, randomised, open-label, non-inferiority trial. Lancet. 2014; 383(9924):1222–9.
15. Girz L, Lafrance Robinson A, Foroughe M, Jasper K, Boachie A. Adapting family-based therapy to a day hospital programme for adolescents with eating disorders: preliminary outcomes and trajectories of change: adapting family-based therapy. J Fam Ther. 2013 Apr;35:102–20.
16. Green J, Melvin GA, Newman L, Jones M, Taffe J, Gordon M. Day program for young people with anorexia nervosa. Australas Psychiatry. 2015;23(3):249–53.
17. Grewal S, Jasper K, Steinegger C, Yu E, Boachie A. Factors associated with successful completion in an adolescent-only day hospital program for eating disorders. Eat Disord. 2014;22(2):152–62.
18. Henderson K, Buchholz A, Obeid N, Mossiere A, Maras D, Norris M, et al. A family-based eating disorder day treatment program for youth: examining the clinical and statistical significance of short-term treatment outcomes. Eat Disord. 2014;22(1):1–18.
19. Hepburn ZM, Clark-Stone S. The short term effectiveness of day treatment for eating disorders in reducing psychosocial impairment: utilizing the clinical impairment assessment in routine practice. Ment Health Rev J. 2016; 21(1):11–22.
20. Dancyger I, Fornari V, Schneider M, Fisher M, Frank S, Goodman B, et al. Adolescents and eating disorders: An examination of a day treatment program. Eat Weight Disord - Stud Anorex Bulim Obes. 2003;8(3):242–8.
21. Hempel R, Vanderbleek E, Lynch TR. Radically open DBT: targeting emotional loneliness in anorexia nervosa. Eat Disord. 2018;26(1):92–104.
22. Atiye M, Miettunen J, Raevuori-Helkamaa A. A meta-analysis of temperament in eating disorders: temperament in eating disorders. Eur Eat Disord Rev. 2015;23(2):89–99.
23. Treasure J, Schmidt U. The cognitive-interpersonal maintenance model of anorexia nervosa revisited: a summary of the evidence for cognitive, socio-emotional and interpersonal predisposing and perpetuating factors. J Eat Disord. 2013;1(1):13.
24. Bulik CM, Sullivan PF, Tozzi F, Furberg H, Lichtenstein P, Pedersen NL. Prevalence, heritability, and prospective risk factors for anorexia nervosa. Arch Gen Psychiatry. 2006;63(3):305.
25. Fairburn CG, Cooper Z, Doll HA, Welch SL. Risk factors for anorexia nervosa: three integrated case-control comparisons. Arch Gen Psychiatry. 1999;56(5):468–76.
26. Pollice C, Kaye WH, Greeno CG, Weltzin TE. Relationship of depression, anxiety, and obsessionality to state of illness in anorexia nervosa. Int J Eat Disord. 1997 May 1;21(4):367–76.
27. Harrison A, O'Brien N, Lopez C, Treasure J. Sensitivity to reward and punishment in eating disorders. Psychiatry Res. 2010;177(1–2):1–11.
28. Haynos AF, Lavender JM, Nelson J, Crow SJ, Peterson CB. Moving towards specificity: a systematic review of cue features associated with reward and punishment in anorexia nervosa. Clin Psychol Rev. 2020;79:101872.
29. Levine MP. Loneliness and eating disorders. Aust J Psychol. 2012;146(1–2): 243–57.
30. Geller J, Cockell SJ, Hewitt PL, Goldner EM, Flett GL. Inhibited expression of negative emotions and interpersonal orientation in anorexia nervosa. Int J Eat Disord. 2000;28(1):8–19.
31. Hempel RJ, Rushbrook SC, O'Mahen H, Lynch TR. How to Differentiate Overcontrol From Undercontrol: Findings From the RefraMED Study and Guidelines From Clinical Practice, vol. 12; 2018.
32. Asendorpf JB, van Aken MAG. Resilient, overcontrolled, and undercontroleed personality prototypes in childhood: Replicability, predictive power, and the trait-type issue. J Pers Soc Psychol. 1999;77(4):815–32.
33. Huey SJ, Weisz JR. Ego Control, Ego Resiliency, and the Five-Factor Model as Predictors of Behavioral and Emotional Problems in Clinic-Referred Children and Adolescents. J Abnorm Psychol. 1997;106(3):404–15.
34. Donnellan MB, Robins RW. Resilient, Overcontrolled, and Undercontrolled personality types: issues and controversies: personality types. Soc Personal Psychol Compass. 2010;4(11):1070–83.
35. Lynch TR. Radically open dialectical behavior therapy: Theory and practice for treating disorders of overcontrol. Oakland: Context Press/New Harbinger Publications; 2018. xii, 504 p. (Radically open dialectical behavior therapy: Theory and practice for treating disorders of overcontrol.).
36. Gilbert K, Hall K, Codd RT. Radically open dialectical behavior therapy: social signaling, Transdiagnostic utility and current evidence. Psychol Res Behav Manag. 2020;13:19–28.
37. Lynch TR, Hempel RJ, Clark LA. Promoting radical openness and flexible control. In: Integrated treatment for personality disorder: a modular approach. New York: The Guilford Press; 2016. p. 325–44.
38. Linehan MM. Skills training manual for treating borderline personality disorder. New York: Guilford Press; 1993. xii, 180 p. (Skills training manual for treating borderline personality disorder.).
39. Chen EY, Segal K, Weissman J, Zeffiro TA, Gallop R, Linehan MM, et al. Adapting dialectical behavior therapy for outpatient adult anorexia nervosa-a pilot study: adapting DBT for Outpatent adult anorexia. Int J Eat Disord. 2015 Jan;48(1):123–32.
40. Simic M, Baudinet J, Ellis G. When too much control becomes the issue: radically open dialectical behaviour therapy (RO-DBT) for adolescents with restrictive eating disorders when family therapy is not enough [conference workshop]. London: In QEII Centre; 2019.
41. Lynch TR. The skills training manual for radically open dialectical behavior therapy: a Clinician's guide for treating disorders of Overcontrol. Oakland: Context Press/New Harbinger Publications; 2018.
42. Garner DM. Eating disorder Inventory-3. Professional manual. Lutz: Psychological Assessment Resources, Inc; 2004.
43. Clausen L, Rosenvinge JH, Friborg O, Rokkedal K. Validating the eating disorder Inventory-3 (EDI-3): a comparison between 561 female eating disorders patients and 878 females from the general population. J Psychopathol Behav Assess. 2011;33(1):101–10.
44. Angold A, Costello EJ, Messer SC, Pickles A, Winder F, Silver D. The development of a short questionnaire for use in epidemiological studies of depression in children and adolescents. Int J Methods Psychiatr Res. 1995;5: 237–49.
45. Wood A, Kroll L, Moore A, Harrington R. Properties of the mood and feelings questionnaire in adolescent psychiatric outpatients: a research note. Child Psychol Psychiatry Allied Discip. 1995;36(2):327–34.
46. Daviss WB, Birmaher B, Melhem NA, Axelson DA, Michaels SM, Brent DA. Criterion validity of the mood and feelings questionnaire for depressive episodes in clinic and non-clinic subjects: criterion validity of mood and feelings questionnaire. J Child Psychol Psychiatry. 2006;47(9):927–34.
47. Thabrew H, Stasiak K, Bavin L, Frampton C, Merry S, et al. Int J Methods Psychiatr Res. 2018;27(3) Available from: https://onlinelibrary.wiley.com/doi/abs/10.1002/mpr.1610. Cited 2020 Aug 7.
48. Goodman R, Ford T, Richards H, Gatward R, Meltzer H. The development and well-being assessment: description and initial validation of an integrated assessment of child and adolescent psychopathology. J Child Psychol Psychiatry. 2000;41(5):645–55.
49. American Psychiatric Association, editor. Diagnostic and statistical manual of mental disorders: DSM-5. 5th ed. Washington, D.C: American Psychiatric Association; 2013. p. 947.
50. World Health Organization, editor. International statistical classification of diseases and related health problems (ICD-10). 10th revision, 2nd edition. Geneva: World Health Organization; 2004. p. 3.
51. Goodman A, Heiervang E, Collishaw S, Goodman R. The 'DAWBA bands' as an ordered-categorical measure of child mental health: description and validation in British and Norwegian samples. Soc Psychiatry Psychiatr Epidemiol. 2011;46(6):521–32.
52. Linde JA, Stringer D, Simms LJ, Clark LA. The schedule for nonadaptive and adaptive personality for youth (SNAP-Y): a new measure for assessing adolescent personality and personality pathology. Assessment. 2013;20(4):387–404.
53. De Pauw S. In: Widiger TA, editor. Childhood Personality and Temperament, vol. 1: Oxford University Press; 2016. Available from: http://oxfordhandbooks.com/view/10.1093/oxfordhb/9780199352487.001.0001/oxfordhb-9780199352487-e-21. Cited 2020 Jun 17.
54. Kushner SC, Tackett JL, De Clercq B. The joint hierarchical structure of adolescent personality pathology: converging evidence from two approaches to measurement. J Can Acad Child Adolesc Psychiatry J Acad Can Psychiatr Enfant Adolesc. 2013;22(3):199–205.

55. Samuel DB, Riddell ADB, Lynam DR, Miller JD, Widiger TA. A five-factor measure of obsessive–compulsive personality traits. J Pers Assess. 2012;94(5):456–65.
56. Griffin SA, Suzuki T, Lynam DR, Crego C, Widiger TA, Miller JD, et al. Development and examination of the five-factor obsessive-compulsive inventory–short form. Assessment. 2016;25(1):56–68.
57. Shiner RL, Tackett JL. Personality disorders in children and adolescents. In: Child psychopathology. 3rd ed. New York: The Guilford Press; 2014. p. 848–96.
58. Gard DE, Gard MG, Kring AM, John OP. Anticipatory and consummatory components of the experience of pleasure: a scale development study. J Res Pers. 2006;40(6):1086–102.
59. Klein DN. Depression and anhedonia. In: Clark DC, Fawcett J, editors. Anhedonia and affect deficit states. New York: PMA Publishing; 1984. p. 1–34.
60. Whitton AE, Treadway MT, Pizzagalli DA. Reward processing dysfunction in major depression, bipolar disorder and schizophrenia. Curr Opin Psychiatry. 2015;28(1):7–12.
61. Gross JJ, John OP. Individual differences in two emotion regulation processes: implications for affect, relationships, and well-being. J Pers Soc Psychol. 2003;85(2):348–62.
62. Preece DA, Becerra R, Robinson K, Gross JJ. The emotion regulation questionnaire: psychometric properties in general community samples. J Pers Assess. 2020;102(3):348–56.
63. Gómez-Ortiz O, Romera EM, Ortega-Ruiz R, Cabello R, Fernández-Berrocal P. Analysis of Emotion Regulation in Spanish Adolescents: Validation of the Emotion Regulation Questionnaire. Front Psychol. 2016;6 Available from: http://journal.frontiersin.org/Article/10.3389/fpsyg.2015.01959/abstract. Cited 2020 Apr 17.
64. Achenbach TM, Rescorla L. Manual for the ASEBA school-age forms & profiles: An integrated system of multi-informant assessment. Burlington: Aseba; 2001.
65. Lee RM, Draper M, Lee S. Social connectedness, dysfunctional interpersonal behaviors, and psychological distress: testing a mediator model. J Couns Psychol. 2001;48(3):310–8.
66. Feeney J, Noller P, Hanrahan M. Assessing adult attachment. In: Sperling MB, Berman WH, editors. Attachment in adults. New York: The Guilford Press; 1994. p. 128–51.
67. Jewell T, Gardner T, Susi K, Watchorn K, Coopey E, Simic M, et al. Attachment measures in middle childhood and adolescence: a systematic review of measurement properties. Clin Psychol Rev. 2019;68:71–82.
68. Axfors C, Sylvén S, Skalkidou A, Ramklint M. Psychometric properties of the attachment style questionnaire in Swedish pregnant women: short and full versions. J Reprod Infant Psychol. 2017;35(5):450–61.
69. Iwanaga K, Blake J, Yaghmaian R, Umucu E, Chan F, Brooks JM, et al. Preliminary validation of a short-form version of the *Attachment Style Questionnaire* for use in clinical rehabilitation counseling research and practice. Rehabil Couns Bull. 2018;61(4):205–16.
70. Russell GFM, Szmukler GI, Dare C, Eisler I. An evaluation of family therapy in anorexia nervosa and bulimia nervosa. Arch Gen Psychiatry. 1987;44(12):1047.
71. Morgan HG, Russell GFM. Value of family background and clinical features as predictors of long-term outcome in anorexia nervosa: four-year follow-up study of 41 patients. Psychol Med. 1975;5(4):355–71 2009/07/09 ed.
72. Benjamini Y, Hochberg Y. Controlling the false discovery rate: a practical and powerful approach to multiple testing. J R Stat Soc Ser B Methodol. 1995;57(1):289–300.
73. de Vos JA, LaMarre A, Radstaak M, Bijkerk CA, Bohlmeijer ET, Westerhof GJ. Identifying fundamental criteria for eating disorder recovery: a systematic review and qualitative meta-analysis. J Eat Disord. 2017;5(1):34.
74. Weinbach N, Sher H, Bohon C. Differences in emotion regulation difficulties across types of eating disorders during adolescence. J Abnorm Child Psychol. 2018;46(6):1351–8.
75. De Fruyt F, Bartels M, Van Leeuwen KG, De Clercq B, Decuyper M, Mervielde I. Five types of personality continuity in childhood and adolescence. J Pers Soc Psychol. 2006;91(3):538–52.
76. Goldsmith HH, Lemery KS, Aksan N, Buss KA. Temperamental substrates of personality. In: Temperament and personality development across the life span. Mahwah: Lawrence Erlbaum Associates Publishers; 2000. p. 1–32.
77. Rothbart MK, Ahadi SA, Evans DE. Temperament and personality: origins and outcomes. J Pers Soc Psychol. 2000;78(1):122–35.
78. Kopala-Sibley DC, Olino T, Durbin E, Dyson MW, Klein DN. The stability of temperament from early childhood to early adolescence:a multi-method, multi-informant examination: stability of temperament. Van Zalk M, editor. Eur J Personal. 2018;32(2):128–45.
79. Bardone-Cone AM, Hunt RA, Watson HJ. An overview of conceptualizations of eating disorder recovery, recent findings, and future directions. Curr Psychiatry Rep. 2018;20(9):79.

12

Prevalence, features and health impacts of eating disorders amongst First-Australian Yiramarang (adolescents) and in comparison with other Australian adolescents

Adam Burt[1], Deborah Mitchison[2,3*], Elizabeth Dale[4], Kay Bussey[5], Nora Trompeter[5], Alexandra Lonergan[5] and Phillipa Hay[2,6]

Abstract

Background: This study aimed to support previous research conducted with First-Australians (FA) by establishing the prevalence of eating disorders, and their demographic distribution and burden in adolescent First-Australians compared to other-Australians (OA).

Methods: Data were used from the baseline survey of the EveryBODY Study, a longitudinal investigation of eating disorders among Australian adolescents. Of the 5068 participants included, 402 (8%) identified as FA, 4586 (90.5%) identified as OA. Diagnosis of eating disorders was based on the Diagnostic and Statistical Manual version 5. Socioeconomic status and measures of impairment were assessed using validated instruments. Body mass index was calculated based on self-reported weight and height. Statistical analyses used data weighted to the distribution of gender in adolescents in New South Wales in the 2016 Australian Census. Chi-square tests were performed to determine prevalence of eating disorders amongst FA and to compare to OA. ANOVA and logistic regression analyses where conducted to examine the moderation effect of sociodemographic status, measures of impairment and FA status on the distribution of eating disorders.

Results: The prevalence rates for eating disorder diagnoses where similar for FA and OA with the exception of Night eating Syndrome (OSFED-NES), which occurred in 7.14% (95%CI 4.81–10.49) of FA vs. 3.72% (95%CI 3.17–4.36) in OA. The greater prevalence of OSFED-NES in FA was largely explained by poorer psychosocial quality of life amongst FA.

(Continued on next page)

* Correspondence: deborah.mitchison@westernsydney.edu.au
[2]Translational Health Research Institute (THRI), School of Medicine, Western Sydney University, Sydney, Campbelltown, Australia
[3]Centre for Emotional Health, Department of Psychology, Macquarie University, North Ryde, New South Wales, Australia
Full list of author information is available at the end of the article

(Continued from previous page)

Conclusion: Eating disorders are common amongst First-Australian adolescents and are associated with poor psychosocial quality of life. These findings are consistent with previous research conducted with First-Australian adults. There is a need to screen for eating disorders amongst First-Australian adolescent girls and boys.

Keywords: Feeding and eating disorders, Adolescents, Prevalence, Oceanic ancestry, Group, Aboriginal and Torres Strait islander

Plain English summary

This study aimed to support previous research conducted with First Australian adults by establishing the prevalence, distribution and burden of eating disorders amongst First Australian adolescents, and compare this to other Australian adolescents. Data were used from the EveryBODY study, a survey of eating disorders amongst Australian adolescents. Of 5068 adolescents who completed the survey, 8% (402) were First Australians. All participants answered questions on basic demographic information, eating disorders, and impairment. The prevalence of eating disorders amongst First Australian adolescents was 28.62%, which was significantly greater than among other-Australian adolescents (21.68%). The greater prevalence of eating disorders amongst First Australians was largely driven by the higher prevalence of Night Eating Syndrome (7.14% amongst Fist Australians vs. 3.72% amongst other Austalians) and poorer psychosocial quality of life.

Background

First-Australians have poorer physical and mental health than other-Australians in all age groups, including adolescents [1, 2]. First-Australian adolescents have a two-fold greater all-cause mortality rate than other-Australian adolescents, mostly due to suicide and road traffic injuries. Eighty percent of this mortality has been reported as potentially avoidable within the current Australian healthcare system [2]. First-Australian adolescents also have a greater burden of non-fatal disease [1]. Approximately 20% of First-Australian adolescents are obese and 40% are either obese or overweight, amongst the highest rates for adolescents in the world [2]. First-Australian adolescents aged 18–24 years suffer twice the rate of high to very high psychological distress of other-Australian adolescents [2], not surprisingly First-Australian adolescents also have a significantly greater burden of mental disorders including: conduct disorder, intentional self-harm, anxiety disorders, depressive disorders and alcohol use disorders [1]. Hospital separations for psychosis, alcohol and other substance use disorders are three-fold higher in First-Australian adolescents compared to other-Australian adolescents [2]. These statistics are alarming, as First-Australians are on average younger than other-Australians (21.8 years vs. 37.6 years). First-Australian adolescents also make up a greater proportion of their respective population compared to other-Australian adolescents (37.7% vs. 20.4%) [1, 2].

Adolescence is an important developmental period characterised by a range of physical, cognitive and psychosocial changes, [3] it is also the time when eating disorders are most likely to emerge [4]. Evidence from an Australian prospective cohort study suggests that the prevalence of eating disorders amongst Australian adolescents is 6.2% for one of the three major eating disorders (i.e., anorexia nervosa, bulimia nervosa, binge eating disorder) and as high as 22.2% when including atypical and subthreshold eating disorders [5]. Yet the prevalence of eating disorders amongst First-Australian adolescents remains unknown.

There is a lack of good quality research into mental disorders amongst First-Australians generally, [6, 7] but especially so in regards to eating disorders. A systematic review into the prevalence of mental disorders amongst First-Australians did not identify any studies that assessed eating disorders [7]. A systematic synthesis of First-Australian Adolescent health population data resorted to the use of hospital separation data in order to measure the prevalence of eating disorders, as well as other mental disorders, as there were insufficient data available from surveys. The latter study did not describe the prevalence of individual eating disorders [2]. The research that is available on eating disorders amongst First-Australians is conflicting. An example of this was seen in the previously mentioned systematic synthesis of First-Australian adolescent health population data, which suggested that eating disorders are more common amongst other-Australian compared to First-Australian adolescents and are more common amongst urban compared to rural First-Australian adolescents [2]. These data conflict with research suggesting eating disorders occur at similar rates across urbanicity and socioeconomic status [8, 9]. Further to this, emerging research indicates that eating disorders are actually more common amongst First-Australian compared to other-Australian adults and are associated with high levels of overvaluation of weight and shape concerns. The same study found the higher prevalence of eating disorders amongst First-Australians' was largely associated with the younger age, higher BMI and poorer mental health of First-Australians [10].

In support of this, previous Australian population health and body image research has also suggested that these explanatory variables (younger age, higher BMI and mental health impairment), as well as physical health impairment and body image disturbance are also greater amongst First-Australian compared to other-Australian adolescents. This line of research thus indicates the potential of elevated risk of eating disorders among First-Australian adolescents. For example, an Australian study into media influences on body image and disordered eating among First-Australian adolescents found that First-Australian adolescents were more dissatisfied with their weight and engaged in more activity to change their weight and shape compared to other-Australian adolescents. First-Australian adolescents in this study were also more sensitive to media messaging to lose weight, despite receiving fewer media messages [11]. It should be noted however that this study was conducted in the early 2000s and newer research is needed to determine the impacts of today's widespread personalised and multimedia messaging on First-Australian adolescents' perceptions.

Based on the recent research findings into eating disorders amongst First-Australian adults, we suspect that the relatively larger pool of young people in the First-Australian community, burdened with other risk factors such as body image disturbance, poorer mental and physical health and higher rates of overweight and obesity may place them at greater risk of eating disorders.

Gap and aim

It is important to investigate the prevalence of eating disorders amongst First-Australian adolescents, especially given the sparse evidence available and the evidence to date suggesting a potentially elevated risk of eating disorders among this group. Further, this line of research forms a priority area for the Australian Government. The National Aboriginal and Torres Strait Islander Health plan 2013–2023 recognises evidence-based practice as important to guide the health care of First-Australians and asserts a need for more high quality research conducted in partnership with First-Australian communities to achieve this. The plan highlights adolescent, youth and mental health as specific priority areas for research and improvements [12, 13]. Thus this study aimed to support previous research conducted with First-Australians by establishing the prevalence of eating disorders, and their demographic distribution and burden in adolescent First-Australians compared to other-Australians.

Methods

Procedures and participants

Data were used from the baseline survey of the Every-BODY Study. The EveryBODY study is a longitudinal investigation of eating disorders among Australian adolescents. Sampling procedures have been detailed elsewhere [5, 14]. In brief, four independent and nine government schools, from a broad range of socioeconomic advantage, participated. All parents and students received information about the study over a period of four weeks using multiple methods of dissemination, and a passive parental consent procedure was used, whereby parents could opt out their child from the study. Students who provided consent were given the online survey to complete at school. Participants were offered the chance to enter a prize draw to win one of ten gift vouchers, and the schools received a general wellbeing report based on their students' data.

Of the 5280 students who commenced the survey, n = 123 were excluded due to: completion of < 10% of the survey ($n = 39$), non-serious responses to open-ended questions ($n = 79$), incorrect coding ($n = 4$) and withdrawn consent ($n = 1$). Of the remaining participants, $n = 402$ (8%) identified as First Australian ($n = 355$ of Aboriginal origin, $n = 28$ of Torres Strait Islander origin and 19 of both Aboriginal and Torres Strait Islander origin), $n = 4586$ (90.5%) identified as other-Australian, and $n = 80$ (1.6%) declined to provide a response to the question regarding Indigenous status.

Diagnostic status and measures

Sociodemographic questions

A socio-economic index for area (SEIFA) score was calculated based on the residential postcode of participants. A SEIFA score is an Australian Bureau of Statistics (ABS) product used to rank areas in Australia based on relative socioeconomic advantage or disadvantage [15]. Other demographic information collected included age, school grade, gender, sex, and country of birth.

Eating disorder diagnoses

The operationalisation of the eating disorder diagnoses that were assessed in this study has been published previously [5], and an adapted Table of this operationalisation is included in the Supplementary material. Diagnoses assessed included the three major eating disorders (anorexia nervosa, bulimia nervosa, binge eating disorder), the five Other Specified Feeding and Eating Disorders (OSFED; atypical anorexia nervosa, subthreshold bulimia nervosa, subthreshold binge eating disorder, purging disorder, night eating syndrome) and Unspecified Feeding and Eating Disorder (UFED). Most symptoms were captured by items of the Eating Disorder Examination Questionnaire (EDE-Q), which assesses the presence and severity of cognitive and behavioural eating disorder symptoms and features [16]. This questionnaire has previously been validated in Australian adolescent boys and girls and demonstrates sound reliability [17]. Items used in this study included the behavioural frequency items (self-induced vomiting, laxative misuse, driven exercise, and binge eating), and the Likert-type items that comprise the combined weight and shape concern subscales. As the frequency of behaviours were only assessed over the past 1 month (not the 3 months duration required for bulimia nervosa and binge eating disorder), we use the term "probable" for these diagnoses. Cronbach's alpha for the combined weight and shape concern subscale in the present study was 0.96 for both First-Australian and other-Australian adolescents.

Participant's self-reported current weight and height, which was converted to age and gender adjusted body mass index (BMI) percentiles for children and adolescents. A BMI percentile < 10 was used for the underweight criterion of anorexia nervosa, as this cut-off has most frequently been used in adolescent epidemiological studies of DSM-5 anorexia nervosa [18–21]. Three items from the Night Eating Questionnaire (NEQ) [22] were used to assess symptoms of night eating syndrome, including proportion of daily food intake consumed following supper, nocturnal eating (eating after going to bed), and awareness during nocturnal eating. The NEQ has been validated in adolescents and is superior to parent report [23].

Several additional questions were developed by the researchers to capture frequency of additional extreme weight control behaviours (fasting, strict dieting, detoxes, insulin misuse, other drug use for weight loss), distress associated with binge eating, and additional diagnostic binge eating disorder features (e.g., eating faster than usual, eating alone due to embarrassment). Participants were also asked about any recent weight loss in the past 4 weeks to assess atypical anorexia nervosa.

Quality of life impairment

Scores from the Paediatric Quality of Life Scale (PedsQL) SF15 [24, 25] were used to measure quality of life impairment. The 12 items from the physical functioning, emotional functioning, and social functioning subscales were included in the survey. Items ask participants to indicate on a Likert type scale how true a series of statements are of them in the past 4 weeks. Scores are reversed and transformed on a 0–100 scale, such that higher scores indicate higher functioning. Subscale scores are derived as the mean of the items for that scale. For the purposes of this study we combined the emotional and social functioning scales to create a psychosocial subscale. The PedsQL SF15 has evidence of good reliability and validity in previous studies of adolescents [25]. Cronbach's alphas in the current study sample for the physical functioning subscale was 0.89 and 0.84 for First Australian and other-Australian adolescents respectively, and for the psychosocial functioning subscale was 0.91 and 0.90 for First-Australian and other-Australian adolescents respectively.

Statistical analysis

Analyses used data weighted to the distribution of gender in adolescents in New South Wales in the 2016 Australian Census. A series of Chi-square tests were performed to determine the prevalence of eating disorders among First-Australian adolescents and to compare this to other-Australian adolescents. This was followed by 2 × 2 ANOVAs and logistic regression analyses to examine the moderation effect of First-Australian status on the sociodemographic (dependent variables: age, sex, SEIFA score, BMI percentile) distribution of eating disorders. Additional 2 × 2 ANOVAs and logistic regressions were employed to test the moderation effect of First-Australian status on the association between eating disorders and specific symptoms (dependent variables: weight and shape concerns, binge eating, self-induced vomiting, laxative use, dietary fasting, driven exercise) and impairment (psychosocial quality of life and physical quality of life impairment). Finally, four logistic regressions were performed with current eating disorder status as the outcome. In regression one, First-Australian status was the only predictor in the model; in regression two, sociodemographic variables (age, gender, SEIFA score, and BMI percentile) were added to the model; in regression three, eating disorder symptom variables (weight and shape concerns, binge eating, self-induced vomiting, laxative use, fasting, driven exercise) were added to the model; in regression four, impairment variables (psychosocial and physical quality of life impairment) were added to the model. The intention of these analyses was to examine the extent to which First-Australian status remained independently associated with the likelihood to meet criteria for a current eating disorder in the presence of other known correlates. In these analyses, SEIFA score was divided by 100 (the normed SD), BMI percentile was divided by 10, and weight/shape concerns and psychosocial and physical quality of life impairment scores were standardised, to allow more meaningful interpretation of the adjusted odds ratios.

Results

Prevalence of eating disorders amongst first-Australian adolescents

Overall, the prevalence of any eating disorder (i.e., major eating disorder, OSFED or UFED) was higher among First-Australian adolescents (28.6%) compared to other Australian adolescents (21.7%). Of note, eating disorder prevalence was also very high among adolescents who chose not to specify their First-Australian status (32.8%), however possibly due to reduced power in this smaller sub-group, this proportion did not differ statistically from either the First Australian or other-Australian groups. Further analyses excluded participants who did not disclose their First-Australian status. Table 1 displays the point prevalence for each eating disorder, separated by First-Australian status. As can be seen, there was a higher prevalence of any eating disorder and OSFED in First-Australian adolescents compared to other adolescents. This seemed to be largely explained by a higher prevalence of night eating syndrome (7.1% vs 3.7%, respectively) and purging disorder (5.1% vs 3.1%, respectively), although the latter neared but did not reach statistical significance. Other specific eating disorder diagnoses also trended to be more prevalent among First-Australian adolescents however these differences did not reach or come close to statistical significance.

Demographic distribution of eating disorders as moderated by first-Australian status

As can be seen in Table 2, although the sex distribution was similar in First-Australian and other-Australian adolescents in this sample, on average First-Australian adolescents were slightly younger, from lower socioeconomic backgrounds, and had a higher BMI percentile than other-Australian adolescents. Adolescents with eating disorders in general were more likely to be female, slightly older, and have a higher BMI percentile. Analyses of the interaction between First-Australian status and eating disorder status revealed that First-Australian status was not a significant moderator of the relationship between current eating disorder and age, sex, socioeconomic status, or BMI. These findings indicate that First-Australian and other-Australian adolescents with an eating disorder have similar sociodemographic distributions.

Clinical correlates of eating disorders and moderation by first-Australian status

As can be seen in Table 2, First-Australian adolescents in general reported greater physical quality of life impairment and more frequent self-induced vomiting but similar levels of other eating disorder symptoms and psychosocial quality of life. As expected, adolescents with eating disorders in general reported more eating disorder symptoms and greater impairment in quality of life than adolescents without an eating disorder. No moderating effects of First-Australian status were found, indicating that First-Australian and other-Australian adolescents with eating disorders report similar symptom profiles and impairment.

Multivariate model of eating disorder correlates

As can be seen in Table 3, First-Australian status was a significant univariate correlate of current eating disorder status, with First-Australian adolescents around 1.5 times more likely to meet criteria for a current eating disorder compared to other-Australian adolescents. This effect remained significant even when the model accounted for sociodemographic variables and for behavioural and cognitive eating disorder symptoms. However, when measures of impairment were added to the model, First-Australian status was no longer independently associated

Table 1 One-month prevalence of eating disorders in First-Australian (FA) and other-Australian (OA) adolescents

	First-Australian Adolescents	Other-Australian Adolescents	
	% (95% CI)	% (95% CI)	χ^2 (1), *p*
Any Eating Disorder (Major, OSFED, UFED)	28.62 (23.83–33.94)	21.68 (20.38–23.03)	**7.84, .005**
Major Eating Disorder	7.53 (5.15–10.88)	6.07 (5.38–6.85)	.13, .288
Anorexia Nervosa (AN)	.89 (.30–2.59)	.66 (.45–.96)	0.49, .401†
Probable Bulimia Nervosa (BN)	5.11 (3.21–8.02)	4.45 (3.86–5.13)	.31, .579
Probable Binge Eating Disorder (BED)	1.80 (.83–3.87)	.96 (.70–1.31)	2.16, .142
Other Specified Feeding and Eating Disorders (OSFED)	15.22 (11.71–19.55)	10.77 (9.83–11.78)	**5.97, .015**
Atypical Anorexia Nervosa (OSFED-AAN)	3.92 (2.30–6.58)	2.69 (2.23–3.23)	1.71, .191
Subthreshold Bulimia Nervosa (OSFED-SBN)	1.50 (.64–3.47)	2.21 (1.8–2.71)	.74, .390
Subthreshold Binge Eating Disorder (OSFED-SBED)	.30 (.05–1.68)	.32 (.19–.55)	<.01, .952
Purging Disorder (OSFED-PD)	5.11 (3.21–8.02)	3.12 (2.63–3.7)	3.82, .051
Night Eating Syndrome (OSFED-NES)	7.14 (4.81–10.49)	3.72 (3.17–4.36)	**9.12, .003**
Unspecified Feeding or Eating Disorder (UFED)	5.32 (3.30–8.46)	4.47 (3.85–5.19)	.46, .500

Note. Significant effects are highlighted in bold text. Based on weighted data. † based on Fishers Exact test due to low cell numbers. Total N for prevalence analyses varied for each diagnosis, dependent on the missingness of diagnostic data (AN: $N = 4425$; BN: $N = 4401$; BED/PD: $N = 4399$; AAN: $N = 4388$; sBN/sBED = 4398; NES: $N = 4220$; UFED: $N = 3989$; Major ED: $N = 4401$; OSFED: $N = 4223$; Any ED: $N = 4036$). The proportions of each diagnosis do not add up to the totals, except for the other-Australian category of Major eating disorders because where the DSM-5 allows it there is comorbidity (for instance between the OSFED diagnoses) – this is why the major eating disorder category proportion total is closer to the summation of the individual diagnoses within that category (the DSM-5 does not allow concurrent diagnosis between AN, BN and BED). The chi-square analyses are weighted, which slightly alters cell numbers

Table 2 Univariate associations between demographic and clinical correlates and First Australian (FA) and eating disorder (ED) status, and their interaction

	First Australian		Other Australian					
	ED	No ED	ED	No ED		Main Effect FA Status	Main Effect ED Status	Interaction Effect
	M (SD)				*df*	F, η_p^2, p		
Age	15.0 (1.3)	14.4 (1.5)	15.2 (1.4)	14.7 (1.4)	1, 4045	**7.35, .007, .002**	**25.40, .006, < .001**	.19, .66, < .001
Socioeconomic status	975.0 (42.4)	965.1 (42.1)	987.4 (40.9)	988.3 (42.3)	1, 3984	**40.11, < .001, .010**	2.53, .001, .112	3.64, .057, .001
BMI percentile	69.2 (27.6)	55.7 (31.7)	61.6 (29.7)	50.7 (30.7)	1, 4045	**9.95, .002, .002**	**36.69, .009, < .001**	.41, .521, < .001
Weight and Shape Concerns	4.0 (1.8)	0.9 (1.2)	4.0 (1.6)	1.0 (1.2)	1, 4045	.60, .440, < .001	**1235.15, .234, < .001**	.02, .893, < .001
Psychosocial quality of life impairment	55.7 (27.2)	79.8 (20.4)	58.5 (25.2)	82.3 (19.0)	1, 3972	3.65, .056, .001	**295.51, .069, < .001**	.02, .896, < .001
Physical quality of life impairment	72.6 (25.6)	85.4 (22.9)	77.6 (23.4)	89.0 (15.5)	1, 3972	**12.63, < .001, .003**	**101.16, .025, < .001**	.35, .555, < .001
	n (%)					OR (95% CI) FA adolescent	OR (95% CI) Current ED	β (s.e.), *p*
Female Sex	59 (67.8)	84 (38.5)	593 (73.3)	1329 (45.5)		1.32 (0.81, 2.81)	**3.30 (2.77, 3.93)**	0.01 (0.29), .965
Objective binge eating	27 (31.0)	11 (5.0)	273 (33.7)	147 (5.0)		1.00 (0.54, 1.88)	**9.54 (7.67, 11.87)**	−0.12 (0.40), .766
Fasting	24 (27.6)	13 (6.0)	249 (30.9)	129 (4.4)		1.38 (0.77, 2.49)	**9.68 (7.70, 12.17)**	−0.47 (0.39), .225
Self-induced vomiting	15 (17.4)	5 (2.3)	90 (11.1)	25 (0.9)		**2.88 (1.09, 7.61)**	**15.00 (9.51, 23.67)**	−0.49 (0.58), .394
Laxative use	6 (7.0)	4 (1.8)	45 (5.6)	22 (0.8)		2.62 (0.89, 7.70)	**7.80 (4.62, 13.17)**	−0.72 (0.71), .311
Driven exercise	8 (9.2)	7 (3.2)	123 (15.2)	95 (3.2)		1.01 (0.46, 2.21)	**5.40 (4.08, 7.13)**	−0.61 (0.55), .266

Note. Socioeconomic status measured by SEIFA score; weight and shape concerns measured with the Eating Disorder Examination Questionnaire combined Weight and Shape Concern subscales score; quality of life impairment measured with the Pediatric Quality of Life Scale; objective binge eating, fasting, self-induced vomiting and laxative use defined as ≥ 4 episodes in the past 28 days; driven exercise defined as ≥ 20 episodes in the past 28 days. *BMI* body mass index

Table 3 Multivariate associations between First Australian status, demographic and clinical correlates and eating disorder status

	Step 1	Step 2	Step 3	Step 4
	None	Socio-demographic	Socio-demographic + eating disorder symptoms	Socio-demographic + eating disorder symptoms + impairment
Variable	(Adjusted) Odds Ratio (95% CI)			
First Australian status	**1.44 (1.11, 1.87)**	**1.59 (1.20, 2.11)**	**1.55 (1.02, 2.35)**	1.49 (0.97, 2.29)
Age		**1.22 (1.16, 1.29)**	**1.08 (1.00, 1.17)**	1.01 (0.93, 1.10)
Female sex		**3.60 (3.03, 4.27)**	**0.67 (0.51, 0.86)**	**0.75 (0.57, 0.98)**
SES		1.02 (0.85, 1.23)	0.95 (0.73, 1.25)	1.05 (0.80, 1.38)
BMI-percentile		**1.14 (1.11, 1.17)**	0.98 (0.94, 1.02)	0.99 (0.95, 1.03)
Weight/shape concerns			**6.98 (6.04, 8.05)**	**6.18 (5.31, 7.20)**
Objective binge eating			**3.03 (2.25, 4.08)**	**2.95 (2.17, 3.99)**
Self-induced vomiting			**3.85 (2.01, 7.39)**	**2.48 (1.27, 4.86)**
Laxative use			**2.37 (1.03, 5.45)**	**2.89 (1.24, 6.78)**
Fasting			**2.03 (1.48, 2.79)**	**1.96 (1.41, 2.72)**
Driven exercise			1.37 (0.91, 2.07)	**1.55 (1.02, 2.37)**
Psychosocial quality of life impairment				**0.75 (0.65, 0.86)**
Physical quality of life impairment				0.93 (0.82, 1.06)

Note. Significant AORs are in bold text
Reference categories for categorical variables: other-Australian status, male sex, < 4 episodes of objective binge eating/self-induced vomiting/laxative use/fasting, < 20 episodes of driven exercise
Scale for continuous variables: years (age), standard deviation unity (SES, weight/shape concerns, psychosocial quality of life impairment, physical quality of life impairment), deciles (BMI percentile)

with odds for current eating disorder, and this appeared to be largely explained by psychosocial quality of life impairment. Other factors that remained independently associated with meeting criteria for an eating disorder in the full multivariate model included all eating disorder symptoms and male sex.

Discussion

This study is the first to our knowledge to estimate the prevalence of eating disorders amongst First-Australian adolescents and supports previous research amongst First-Australian adults. Eating disorders are common amongst First-Australian adolescents. While overall, eating disorders were more common among First-Australian adolescents, the only specific diagnosis where First-Australian adolescents were statistically more likely to meet the diagnostic criteria was OSFED-NES, with other disorders being equally prevalent among First-Australian and other-Australian adolescents alike. The greater prevalence of eating disorders amongst First-Australian adolescents was largely explained by poorer psychosocial quality of life experienced more generally by First-Australian adolescents. This finding is in-line with eating disorder research suggesting poor quality of life is associated with eating disorders, and more specifically, recent research conducted with First-Australian adults indicating that mental health related quality of life impairment partly explained the higher prevalence of eating disorders among First-Australian adults. Eating disorders are well known to be associated with quality of life impairment [26]. There is evidence also that the link is bi-directional, in that while eating disorders impair quality of life, quality of life impairment in itself also increases the risk for developing eating disorders [27]. Thus, the poorer general quality of life among First-Australian adolescents may explain the greater prevalence of current eating disorders. First-Australians in this study also had lower socioeconomic status, which was also an explanatory variable for eating disorders.

As previously stated, there is a relatively larger pool of younger people in the First-Australian population compared to the other-Australian population, who are more socioeconomically disadvantaged and psychologically distressed, with poorer mental and physical health generally. In view of the similarity in findings of recent research conducted with First-Australian adults and adolescents, we suggest the higher prevalence of eating disorders amongst First-Australian adolescents and adults may be result of a relatively larger pool of people more vulnerable to mental disorders, including eating disorders. Given the differences between First-Australian groups culturally and the lack of research evidence, it is unclear whether specific cultural differences form part of the differences in eating disorder prevalence between First-Australians and other-Australians. It is unclear why OSFED-NES is specifically more common amongst

First-Australian adolescents, whereas other eating disorders are not. One potential mechanism may be a greater prevalence of sleep problems among First-Australian children [28]. OSFED-NES is linked to insomnia and the belief that one needs to eat to initiate or maintain sleep [29]. Clearly further research is required to confirm and to understand these potential, and other, explanations for the differences found.

Eating disorders amongst First-Australian adolescents were associated with weight and shape concerns. However, unlike research amongst First-Australian adults, these concerns were not markedly greater than in the other-Australians group in univariate analysis. A possible explanation for this is that unlike previous research, this study focused on adolescents, which is the peak period for body image concerns, with all youth at heightened risk. Combining the current findings with previous findings in adults, it could be the case that the decline in weight and shape concerns typically found following the adolescent risky period either does not occur, or occurs to a lesser extent among First-Australian youth (i.e., they experience a prolonged period of risk compared to their other-Australians counterparts).

In the multivariate analyses (Table 3) the findings of the step 3 model were the reverse of what was found in the step 2 model, which included just sociodemographic variables, and where female sex was associated with greater odds for current eating disorder. However, when eating disorder symptoms and impairment were added to the model, it appears that female sex may be associated with eating disorder status due to the higher rates of eating disorder symptoms and impairment among girls. These results suggest that when boys experience disordered eating, weight/shape concerns or impairment their likelihood of meeting criteria for an eating disorder is actually greater than that for girls. These data suggest that overvaluation may be a more benign phenomenon in girls, however, when experienced by boys, in particular when it is experienced by boys with mental health vulnerabilities, they are at increased risk of eating disorders.

Unless a patient presents underweight, eating disorders are easily overlooked as a cause of illness in the primary care setting, and given the high prevalence of eating disorders amongst First-Australians, there is a need to screen for eating disorders amongst First-Australians. An opportunity for this may be during Medicare Health Assessments for Aboriginal and Torres Strait Islander People (Medicare Benefits Schedule item 715), which are often conducted in Aboriginal Community Controlled Health Services (ACCHS) by General Practitioners. These are structured health assessments funded by the Australian Government's universal health scheme, known as Medicare. The cultural and language differences between First-Australians and other-Australians, even amongst those in English-speaking communities suggests the need for a free-to-use, validated and culturally-specific instrument to assist clinicians in screening for eating disorders during these assessments. To our knowledge no such tool has been developed or validated for First-Australians. We suggest such a tool should be developed with First-Australian researchers and communities, similar to the development of the adapted Patient Health Questionnaire (aPHQ-9), a validated and culturally-specific screening tool for depression in First-Australians [29]. Finally, there is currently no evidence describing the uptake of eating disorder treatment for First-Australians. The introduction of Medicare Benefits Schedule items for eating disorders has also highlighted the need for education on eating disorders amongst stakeholders, such as General Practitioners, Nurses, Allied Health personnel and Aboriginal Health Workers, who are most likely to encounter undiagnosed eating disorders. Moreover, we suggest there should be increased awareness of eating disorders amongst school teachers, as they are also likely to encounter students with eating disorders.

This study had several strengths. It was based on data from the EveryBODY study, which was conducted over a broad geographical area including areas with sizable First-Australian populations and differing levels of socio-economic advantage. The main limitation of this study was that the original data was not gathered with a deliberate intent to investigate eating disorders among First-Australians and not in consultation or collaboration with First-Australian community members or researchers. As such a culturally-informed approach to considering how eating disorders may present in First-Australians was not adopted at the design or data collection phases. On the other hand this specific study utilising the generated data has involved leadership and collaboration from First-Australian researchers (AB, LD), which has allowed for more cultural sensitivity in the interpretation of the existing literature and current findings. As stated above, of major importance in future research in this area would be the development of studies involving First-Australian researchers, that are also grounded within a First-Australian research paradigm as well as methodologies, such as yarning and community-based participation.

Conclusions

Based on our findings, eating disorders are common amongst First-Australian adolescents, and are associated with poor psychosocial quality of life. These findings are consistent with previous research conducted with First-Australian adults. Given eating disorders occur in the context of poor psychosocial quality of life, which may increase the risk of mental disorders generally, we suggest there is a need to screen for eating disorders in

First-Australians. This process may be aided by the development of a validated, culturally specific screening tool for eating disorders in First-Australians. Finally, given the introduction of new MBS items for eating disorders, we suggest there is a need to increase education around the diagnosis and management of eating disorders, especially amongst First-Australians.

Abbreviations

χ^2: Chi Squared test; AAN: Atypical Anorexia Nervosa; ABS: Australian Bureau of Statistics; ACCHS: Aboriginal Community Controlled Health Service; AMS: Aboriginal Medical Service; AN-B: Anorexia Nervosa Broad; aPHQ-9: Adapted Patient Health Questionnaire; ARFID: Avoidant Restrictive Food Intake Disorder; BED: Binge Eating Disorder; BMI: Body Mass Index; BN: Bulimia Nervosa; CI: Confidence Interval; df: Degrees of freedom; DSM-5: Diagnostic and Statistical Manual of Mental Disorders 5th edition; ED: Eating Disorder; EDE-Q: Eating Disorder Examination Questionnaire; FA: First Australian; HOS: Health Omnibus Survey; ICD-11: International Classification of Disease 11th revision; MBS: Medicare Benefits Schedule; MWU: Mann Whitney U test; n: Number of participants; NES: Night Eating Syndrome; OR: Odds Ratio; OSFED: Other Specified Feeding or Eating Disorder; PD: Purging Disorder; PedsQL: Pediatric Quality of Life Scale; SBED: Subthreshold Binge Eating Disorder; SD: Standard Deviation; SEIFA: Socio-Economic Indexes For Areas; UFED: Unspecified Feeding or Eating Disorder; YLD: Years Lived with Disability

Authors' contributions

AB is a Wiradjuri (First-Australian) member of the research team, conceived the study, developed the research questions and was main author of the paper. DM conceived of the study with AB, conducted statistical analyses, and drafted the manuscript with AB. LD is a Worimi (First-Australian) member of the research team, assisted in drafting of the manuscript and data interpretation. PH conceived the study with AB, assisted with drafting the manuscript and data interpretation. KB, NT and AL assisted with drafting the manuscript and data interpretation. DM, KB, AL and NT collected and cleaned the data. All authors read and approved the final manuscript.

Competing interests

Professor Hay receives/has received sessional fees and lecture fees from the Australian Medical Council, Therapeutic Guidelines publication, and New South Wales Institute of Psychiatry and royalties/honoraria from Hogrefe and Huber, McGraw Hill Education, and Blackwell Scientific Publications, Biomed Central and PlosMedicine and she has received research grants from the NHMRC and ARC. She is Chair of the National Eating Disorders Collaboration Steering Committee in Australia (2012-) and Member of the ICD-11 Working Group for Eating Disorders (2012–2018) and was Chair Clinical Practice Guidelines Project Working Group (Eating Disorders) of RANZCP (2012–2015). In the past 5 years she has prepared a report under contract for Shire Pharmaceuticals) and received honoraria for education of psychiatrists from Shire Pharmaceuticals (Takeda group). All views in this paper are her own.

Author details

[1]School of Medicine, Western Sydney University, Sydney, Campbelltown, Australia. [2]Translational Health Research Institute (THRI), School of Medicine, Western Sydney University, Sydney, Campbelltown, Australia. [3]Centre for Emotional Health, Department of Psychology, Macquarie University, North Ryde, New South Wales, Australia. [4]Ngarruwan Ngadju First Peoples Health and Wellbeing Research Centre, Australian Health Services Research Institute and Illawarra Health and Medical Research Institute, School of Psychology, University of Wollongong, Wollongong, New South Wales, Australia. [5]Centre for Emotional Health, Department of Psychology, Macquarie University, Sydney, Australia. [6]Campbelltown Hospital, SWSLHD, Sydney, Campbelltown, Australia.

References

1. Al-Yaman F. Australian Burden of Disease Study: impact and causes of illness and death in Aboriginal and Torres Strait Islander people, 2011. Public Health Res Pract. 2017;27(4):56–67.
2. Azzopardi PS, Sawyer SM, Carlin JB, Degenhardt L, Brown N, Brown AD, et al. Health and wellbeing of indigenous adolescents in Australia: a systematic synthesis of population data. Lancet. 2018;391(10122):766–82.
3. Sanders RA. Adolescent psychosocial, social, and cognitive development. Pediatr Rev. 2013;34(8):354–8 quiz 8-9.
4. Volpe U, Tortorella A, Manchia M, Monteleone AM, Albert U, Monteleone P. Eating disorders: what age at onset? Psychiatry Res. 2016;238:225–7.
5. Mitchison D, Mond J, Bussey K, Griffiths S, Trompeter N, Lonergan A, et al. DSM-5 full syndrome, other specified, and unspecified eating disorders in Australian adolescents: prevalence and clinical significance. Psychol Med. 2019:1–10.
6. Azzopardi PS, Kennedy EC, Patton GC, Power R, Roseby RD, Sawyer SM, et al. The quality of health research for young indigenous Australians: systematic review. Med J Aust. 2013;199(1):57–63.
7. Black EB, Ranmuthugala G, Kondalsamy-Chennakesavan S, Toombs MR, Nicholson GC, Kisely S. A systematic review: identifying the prevalence rates of psychiatric disorder in Australia's indigenous populations. Aust N Z J Psychiatry. 2015;49(5):412–29.
8. Hay P, Girosi F, Mond J. Prevalence and sociodemographic correlates of DSM-5 eating disorders in the Australian population. J Eat Disord. 2015;3:19.
9. Mulders-Jones B, Mitchison D, Girosi F, Hay P. Socioeconomic correlates of eating disorder symptoms in an Australian population-based sample. PLoS One. 2017;12(1):e0170603.
10. Burt AMJ, Mannan H, Touyz S, Hay P. Prevalence and features of eating disorders amongst aboriginal and torres strait islander peoples. Adelaide: Australia and New Zealand Academy for Eating Disorders (ANZAED) conference 2019; 2019.
11. McCabe MP, Ricciardelli L, Mellor D, Ball K. Media influences on body image and disordered eating among indigenous adolescent Australians. Adolescence. 2005;40(157):115–27.
12. The L. Indigenous health in Australia—moves in the right direction. Lancet. 2013;382(9890):367.
13. Department of Health. National Aboriginal and Torres Strait Islander health plan 2013–2023. Canberra: Canberra Australian Government; 2013.
14. Trompeter N, Bussey K, Hay P, Mond J, Murray SB, Lonergan A, et al. Fear of negative evaluation and weight/shape concerns among adolescents: The moderating effects of gender and weight status. J Youth Adolesc. 2018; 47(7):1398–408.
15. Census of Population and Housing: Socio-Economic Indexes for Areas (SEIFA), Australia, 2016. Canberra, ACT, Australia: Australian Bureau of Statistics 2018 [Available from: https://www.abs.gov.au/ausstats/abs@.nsf/mf/2033.0.55.001.
16. Fairburn C, Beglin S. Eating disorder examination questionnaire (EDE-Q 6.0). Cognitive behavior therapy and eating disorders; 2008. p. 309–13.
17. Mond J, Hall A, Bentley C, Harrison C, Gratwick-Sarll K, Lewis V. Eating-disordered behavior in adolescent boys: eating disorder examination questionnaire norms. Int J Eat Disord. 2014;47(4):335–41.
18. Nagl M, Jacobi C, Paul M, Beesdo-Baum K, Hofler M, Lieb R, et al. Prevalence, incidence, and natural course of anorexia and bulimia nervosa among adolescents and young adults. Eur Child Adolesc Psychiatry. 2016;25(8):903–18.
19. Rojo-Moreno L, Arribas P, Plumed J, Gimeno N, García-Blanco A, Vaz-Leal F, et al. Prevalence and comorbidity of eating disorders among a community sample of adolescents: 2-year follow-up. Psychiatry Res. 2015;227(1):52–7.
20. Allen KL, Byrne SM, Oddy WH, Crosby RD. DSM-IV-TR and DSM-5 eating disorders in adolescents: prevalence, stability, and psychosocial correlates in a population-based sample of male and female adolescents. J Abnorm Psychol. 2013;122(3):720–32.
21. Hammerle F, Huss M, Ernst V, Burger A. Thinking dimensional: prevalence of DSM-5 early adolescent full syndrome, partial and subthreshold eating disorders in a cross-sectional survey in German schools. BMJ Open. 2016; 6(5):e010843.
22. Allison KC, Lundgren JD, O'Reardon JP, Martino NS, Sarwer DB, Wadden TA, et al. The night eating questionnaire (NEQ): psychometric properties of a measure of severity of the night eating syndrome. Eat Behav. 2008;9(1):62–72.
23. Gallant AR, Lundgren J, Allison K, Stunkard AJ, Lambert M, O'Loughlin J, et al. Validity of the night eating questionnaire in children. Int J Eat Disord. 2012;45(7):861–5.

24. Varni JW, Seid M, Kurtin PS. PedsQL 4.0: reliability and validity of the pediatric quality of life inventory version 4.0 generic core scales in healthy and patient populations. Med Care. 2001;39(8):800–12.
25. Varni JW, Burwinkle TM, Seid M, Skarr D. The PedsQL 4.0 as a pediatric population health measure: feasibility, reliability, and validity. Ambul Pediatr. 2003;3(6):329–41.
26. Mitchison D, Morin A, Mond J, Slewa-Younan S, Hay P. The bidirectional relationship between quality of life and eating disorder symptoms: a 9-year community-based study of Australian women. PLoS One. 2015;10(3): e0120591.
27. Blunden S, Chervin RD. Sleep, performance and behaviour in Australian indigenous and non-indigenous children: an exploratory comparison. J Paediatr Child Health. 2010;46(1–2):10–6.
28. Allison KC, Lundgren JD, O'Reardon JP, Geliebter A, Gluck ME, Vinai P, et al. Proposed diagnostic criteria for night eating syndrome. Int J Eat Disord. 2010;43(3):241–7.
29. Getting it Right Collaborative G. Getting it right: validating a culturally specific screening tool for depression (aPHQ-9) in aboriginal and Torres Strait islander Australians. Med J Aust. 2019;211(1):24–30.

13

When clean eating isn't as faultless: the dangerous obsession with healthy eating and the relationship between Orthorexia nervosa and eating disorders in Mexican University students

Alicia Parra Carriedo[1], Antonio Tena-Suck[1*], Miriam Wendolyn Barajas-Márquez[2], Gladys María Bilbao y Morcelle[1], Mary Carmen Díaz Gutiérrez[1], Isabel Flores Galicia[1] and Alejandra Ruiz-Shuayre[1]

Resumen

Introducción: La ortorexia nervosa es un trastorno de la conducta alimentaria que ha sido poco estudiado, tanto en sus características, causas y síntomas, como en sus consecuencias y en la relación con otros trastornos de la conducta alimentaria. El presente estudio tuvo como objetivo analizar dicha relación e indagar si es posible predecir la aparición de un trastorno de la conducta alimentaria a partir de la presencia de ortorexia nervosa, además de analizar diferencias por sexo en estudiantes universitarios mexicanos.

Método: Participaron en el estudio 911 estudiantes universitarios (65.4% fueron mujeres y el 34.6% hombres), en un rango de edades entre 18 y 28 años (M = 21 y DE = 1.9) que respondieron dos cuestionarios que son: ORTO-14MX, una versión del instrumento ORTO-15 previamente validada en estudiantes mexicanos y el EDE-Q en su versión corta, además de proporcionar algunos datos sociodemográficos de interés para este estudio.

Resultados: El análisis de correlación de Pearson reveló relaciones estadísticas significativas de leves a moderadas entre los factores que componen ambas escalas, mientras que el análisis de regresión lineal mostró un que un 40% de la varianza es explicada a partir de los factores que componen la escala ORTO-14MX en la muestra de estudio. Adicionalmente se encontraron diferencias estadísticamente significativas entre hombres y mujeres con respecto a todas las subescalas de los instrumentos que midieron ortorexia y trastornos de la conducta alimentaria.

Conclusiones: Estos resultados mostraron un grado de predicción moderada que sí bien es prometedora, no resulta totalmente concluyente. Asimismo, se confirmó que las mujeres siguen siendo más vulnerables a padecer ortorexia o un TCA. Se concluye la necesidad de continuar estudiando la relación entre la ortorexia y los TCAs, en muestras latinoamericanas con otras características socio demográficas y en población clínica.

Palabras clave: ORTO-14 MX, ortorexia nervosa, trastornos de la conducta alimentaria, población mexicana, instrumentos de tamizaje

* Correspondence: antonio.tena@ibero.mx
[1]Universidad Iberoamericana CDMX, México, Mexico
Full list of author information is available at the end of the article

Abstract

Background: Orthorexia Nervosa is an eating disorder that has been scarcely studied in characteristics, causes and symptoms, as well as in consequences and the relationship with other eating disorders. The present study had as its main objective the analysis of said relationship and inquisition of the possibility of predicting the development of an eating disorder from the presence of orthorexia nervosa. Also, it analyzed the differences by sex in Mexican university students.

Methods: The sample consisted of 911 university students (65.4% women and 34.6% men), between an age range of 18 to 28 years old (M = 21 and SD = 1.9). Two questionnaires were responded: the ORTO14MX, a version of the ORTO-15 instrument previously validated in Mexican students, and the EDE-Q in its short version. Besides, sociodemographic data of interest was obtained and used for this study.

Results: The Pearson's correlation analysis demonstrated statistically significant relations, from mild to moderate, between the factors that make up both scales, while the linear regression analysis demonstrated that 40% of the variance is explained with the factors from the ORTO-14MX scale in the overall sample for the study. Additionally, statistically significant differences were found between men and women regarding all the subscales conforming the instruments that measured orthorexia and eating disorders.

Conclusion: These results show a moderate predictive degree, that as promising as it is, isn't conclusive. Likewise, it was confirmed that women are still more vulnerable to develop orthorexia or another eating disorder. It can be concluded that there's a vast necessity for more studies measuring the relationship between orthorexia nervosa and eating disorders, in Latinamerican samples with diverse characteristics in sociocultural backgrounds, and clinical samples.

Keywords: ORTO-14MX, Orthorexia nervosa, Eating disorders, Mexican population, Screening instrument

Plain English summary

The present article explores various aspects regarding orthorexia and eating disorders in Mexican university students. The relationship between both is explored, as well as social and cultural variables that could describe their appearance and development. The ORTO-14MX scale and EDE-Q in its short version were used to grade diverse proneness and traits to both phenomena, and to find out if there was a connection between them, and if ORTO-14MX could predict EDE-Q. Also, there were differences found from men and women, with women being more susceptible to develop orthorexia, or any other eating disorder. In conclusion, psychosocial factors, as well as age and culture, influence eating habits. More studies are definitely needed to understand the experience of having disordered eating habits, particularly for Latinamerican samples.

Background

In recent years, the term "Orthorexia Nervosa" (ON) has shown an increase in literature. The word "orthorexia" comes from the Greek "orthos" ("correct"), and "orexia" ("appetite", "nutrition"), meaning overall "correct nutrition". The term was first described by Steven Bratman in 1997 as "having a pathological obsession in pursuit of a healthy diet" [1]. This concept indicates a possible new eating disorder (ED). Its main symptom is an obsessive and pathological approach to eating what is perceived as "healthy" [2].

The inclination to eat healthily is perceived as a desirable behavior in general. However, when it acquires obsessive traits and prevents the person from leading a healthy life, it is a risky behavior, and can even lead to malnutrition [3, 4]. This is why these orthorexic behaviors can be confused with anorexic behaviors (for example), or even be ignored, encouraged, or praised as a way of taking care of themselves and their body. Thus, the relation between ON and ED is complex and unequivocal; and still far from being completely understood.

Some of the shared traits between ON and ED's that have been previously reported are: a cognitive fixation on nutrition, perfectionism, high anxiety levels, the need to keep everything under control, feeling guilty if they had transgressions with their diet, self-discipline actions in direct proportion to adherence to the diet, cognitive rigidity, and denial of the functional deficiencies associated to the disorder [5]. However, ON does not include the primary symptoms of anorexia nervosa (AN) and bulimia nervosa (BN), which are fear of gaining weight, an excessive obsession with being slim, and a distorted perception of the body [3]. Varga et al., point out that even if the difference between ON and EDs resides effectively in the final motivation (weight loss for EDs, and "feeling healthy" for ON), the social and psychological consequences are similar [6].

It has been proposed that ON could precede the development of an ED, or could as well present itself as the evolution of an ED on remission and rehabilitation, allowing an individual with a previously diagnosed ED, to feel accepted by society again. Hence, this would serve as an approved way to maintain control over the body and food [7]. Barthels et al. [8] believe that eating behaviors consistent with ON's symptomatology can be associated with a certain level of recovery eating disorders and what he considers can be a shift to "less grave" ED behaviors. This suggests that ON could be a way for people with AN to recover [9]. In a study led by Segura-Garcia et al., it was observed that 28% of patients with AN and BN showed tendencies of ON. Additionally, they observed that the proportion of patients with ON tendencies increased up to a 53% by the termination of treatment for an ED [7]. Another study carried out demonstrated that 67% of the professionals in charge of treating patients with ED observed ON behaviors in their clinical practice, and 69% considered that ON as a disorder deserves, and requires, more attention [9].

Despite its similarities with AN, ON is not yet recognized as an eating disorder in the DSM-5 (Diagnostic and Statistical Manual of Mental Disorders), nor in the ICD-10 (International Classification of Diseases) [2, 10]. Therefore, there is no consensus to date, neither in the diagnostic criteria nor in the evaluation procedures for ON.

There are various attempts by a couple of authors to try to establish the diagnostic criteria of ON. There authors are: Setnick et al. [11], Moroze et al. [3], Barthels et al. [8], and Dunn and Bratman [12], amongst others. Out of the proposed criteria, two main characteristics must be included:

a) An obsessive approach to food and eating practices, to promote optimal well-being through a diet considered as healthy (but is inflexible and shows persistent and recurring concern over food).
b) Significant clinical deterioration, which may include medical, nutritional, and/or psychological complications, high levels of distress, and/or decline in important areas of social functioning [2].

As for the evaluation procedures, ON has been measured with the Bratman's Orthorexia Test (BOT) [1] and the ORTO-15 [13], the latter based on the former. Both instruments have been translated into several languages and applied in clinical samples and according to personal convenience. The limited existing literature on the prevalence of ON has been primarily written based on the ORTO-15, reporting a prevalence ranging from 6.9% [14] up to 57.6% [4]. Currently, there is little to no research with representative samples studying the prevalence of ON in the general mexican population. Besides, most studies have been conducted with high-risk groups [6], mainly university students [9, 15, 16].

The teen and college-aged population is a particularly vulnerable group from a nutritional point of view, since they're individuals who are starting to take responsibility over their own eating habits. Because of this, this time becomes a critical period in the consolidation of habits and eating behaviors, as well as the development of their body image [17, 18]. If it is considered that most of the behaviors established during the teenage years persist throughout development, this period represents a valuable opportunity to evaluate predictors and risk factors for the development of an ED [19]. It is because of this that most studies that have taken place, on ON and on the validation of the tools used for its detection, have been on college students [20]. Within the group of college students there have even been subgroups described, which would be considered even more at risk, such as Nutrition, Medicine and Sport Sciences students [21–25]. They present a higher risk because these students have more awareness and information on healthy eating [24, 26–28]. Other groups with higher risks would be people who give great importance to body image, such as actors, dancers, and athletes [29–31], and people who previously had an ED [32].

Previous studies that have analyzed the appearance and symptoms of ON have mainly focused on the eating behaviors, evaluating ON's tendency in groups of people who follow a special diet. In a study led by Plichta et al., it was observed that the risk of showing a tendency toward ON and symptoms of an ED was less in students who did not follow a diet previously or at the time of the study (OR: 0.34 and 0.26 respectively), in comparison to students who had followed a diet previously or at the time of the study. This suggests that the use of diets in the past or present must be considered as well as an important predictor of the presence of tendencies toward ON [33].

In another study also conducted by Plichta et al., where 1120 university students from Poland were evaluated (546 students from health-related careers and 573 students from other areas), it was observed that 46.7% of the population had a score in the ORTO-15 ranging between 35 and 40, regardless of their degree (indicative of ON). However, within this percentage range, there were more students from health-related degrees than students from other areas [34].

In another study carried out by Malmborg et al., the incidence of ON was evaluated in university students in Sweden. These students belonged to health-related careers (exercise physiology, nutrition, and health), and students from business-related areas (finance, marketing, and accounting). The authors reported that 76.6% of the full population presented scores lower than 40 (< 40) in the ORTO-15, an indicative of ON. Consistently with other studies and data in literature, higher prevalence was observed in students from health-related careers than in students from business-related areas (84.5% vs. 65.5%) [25].

It is important to emphasize that there are rather few studies that have tested for ON in the general population [6]; therefore, more studies are required to better comprehend what the possible implications of ON are for them.

Eating behaviors are profoundly molded by the context in which the person lives, including the cultural, social, and ecological environments [35]. The interaction between the sociocultural context and ON has been scarcely studied, too. Most studies done on ON have been tried on European, Turkish, or American populations [36]. There are few studies which have been developed with Brazilian or Latinamerican populations [37] Partly, the observed differences in prevalence in studies done in different countries could be explained by the relation between the sociocultural factors and the eating habits of each country [38, 39].

It would be of great interest to understand the differences in the cultural backdrop that exist in terms of what the students consider to be a healthy lifestyle and how to achieve it. It was observed in a study led by Gramaglia et al., in which a transcultural comparison was made between university students in Spain, Italy and Poland, that a greater prevalence of ON existed in the Polish sample, in contrast to the Spanish and Italian ones. One of the proposed explanations for the findings is that Polish students believe that a healthy diet is the best way to improve their health, consequently having good consumption practices and control over the composition of their products. In contrast, Spanish and Italian people have a wine and food culture based on a Mediterranean diet, and value more the social aspects of having a meal [40].

Thus, the objective of this study in its first stance, was to analyze the existing relationship between the composing factors of the ORTO-14MX and the factors from the Eating Disorders Questionnaire (EDE-Q) in its short version, to later find out if these factors that indicate orthorexia nervosa (ON) accurately predict eating disorders in university students from Mexico City. Additionally, we tested for differences in these same variables between men and women, according to these same variables.

Method

Type of study

This non-experimental cross-sectional study was conducted during Summer 2018. Specifically, the dates in which the study was carried out were May 15 to July 15.

Participants

The sample consisted of 911 university students (65.4% women and 34.6% men), between an age range of 18 to 28 years old (M = 21 and SD = 1.9). These students belonged to different majors at bachelor and specialty levels. Out of these, 27.8% studied Nutrition, 20.5% Social Sciences, 16.9% Arts and Humanities, 15.6% Engineering, 9.9% Economic-Administrative careers, and 9.4% Health Sciences. These students were taking Summer classes from May to July in 2018.

The average BMI in women was 21.8 (SD = 3.08), while in men the average was 23.4 (SD = 3.41); this can be seen in Table 1 (IMC = [kg]/ [m^2]).

All participants completed the questionnaires used for the study. Yet, there were some that did not answer all the questions; thus, these were discarded. Data was recollected randomly, seeing as specific classes from each building on campus were selected. Professors were asked for a specific time span during class- either at the beginning or at the end-, for voluntary students to sign the Informed Consent letter, and answer the two instruments. Those students who were not willing to participate in the study, left the room. Six internship students from the Nutrition Clinic available on campus aided in visiting each classroom, handing out, and applying all the questionnaires. Hence, the applications were not administered directly by the researchers conducting the study.

Instruments

The ORTO-14MX $_{[TSEA2]}$ Questionnaire $_{[TSEA1]}$, adapted to Mexican university students, was used to measure ON (Annex 1). The objective of the instrument is to examine obsessive behaviors in a person regarding the selection of food, its preparation and consumption habits, and attitudes towards food considered "healthy". It is important to add that the original instrument for the Orthorexia Nervosa (ORTO-15) was previously validated in Spanish [9]. The ORTO-14MX consists of 14 questions, measured in 4 points on a Likert-type scale that goes from "always" to "never". A score of 40 points or less means that there is a pathological behavior characterized by a strong concern for healthy eating. However, the score does not imply having a mental health disorder. The items as a group evaluate the obsessive attitude of people to choose, buy, prepare, and eat food that they consider healthy. A cut point of less than 35 has been implemented to increase specificity, and improve diagnostic trends [4, 13].

For the present research, a shorter version of the original instrument (ORTO-15) was used; its factorial structure was previously validated, precisely, in Mexican university students by Parra and her collaborators. As a result of this analysis, four factors that measure thoughts, emotions and behaviors related to food were

Table 1 Anthropometric data of the sample in men and women

	Women (*N* = 598)		Men (*N* = 313)	
Age (years)	M = 21.02 years	SD = 1.99 years	M = 21.24 years	SD = 1.71 years
Weight (kgs)	M = 57.58 kgs	SD = 9.16 kgs	M = 72.83 kgs	SD = 12.35 kgs
Height (meters)	M = 1.62 m	SD = 0.70 m	M = 1.75 m	SD = 0.70 m

obtained. This version contains 14 of the 15 original test items of the ORTO-15 in its original version. The overall Cronbach's Alpha value was equal to 0.78 with 52.4% of the total variance explained. The factors [41] are:

Factor 1, called "Obsessive Cognition", corresponds to test items 3, 4 and 7. They refer to thoughts and attitudes that generate excessive concern, and because of its duration and intensity, it's difficult to control on a daily basis. This causes emotional discomfort and a need to stay healthy and eat "correctly." These thoughts are hypervigilant and can be used as a coping strategy, particularly for stress.

Factor 2 was named "Rational Cognition". It contains test items 6, 10, 11, 12 and 14. It refers to a mental and rational construction that generates logical thoughts in order to evaluate, understand and take action in what is seen as a "healthy lifestyle". It indicates a great need to be accepted for one's appearance, levels of self-confidence, and the desire of approval of others.

Factor 3, "Emotional Regulation", was composed of test items 1, 2 and 13. It is a factor that measures the influence of emotions on the individual, and how he or she experiences and expresses them. In this sense, food has a strong motivational component for the individual in terms of their biological and social adaptation.

Finally, factor 4, "Normative Social", contains test items 8, 9 and 15. It measures compliance with social rules accepted by the group they belong to and that people must follow to have a healthy coexistence with food.

In the process of validating instrument in Mexican university students, a Principal Component analysis with a Varimax rotation was run. Also, the anti-image matrix was obtained with the purpose of identifying if any item could be reducing the total explained variance. In consequence, item number 5 (For you, is the taste of food the principal criteria to determine its quality?) reduced the total explained variance from 52.5 to 49.9%.

Additionally, an analysis was run to verify if by eliminating said item, Cronbach's Alpha decreased. There was no significative change in the Alpha value; therefore, the decision was made to only keep 14 items.

On the other hand, the detection of eating disorders was executed using the Eating Disorder Questionnaire (EDE-Q) in its short version. It was designed by Grilo, Reas, Hopwood and Crosby [42] as a measure of specific psychopathology found in eating disorders. The EDE-Q evaluates aspects such as: weight, shape, eating concerns, and food restriction. The Questionnaire uses a grading system in points: the higher the score in the questionnaire, the greater the severity of the disorder It is composed of 7 questions divided into 3 sub scales: restriction, concern for one's shape and weight, and dissatisfaction with these two (Annex 2). They are evaluated on a scale from 0 to 6, where a higher score reflects a higher pathology symptomatology. Lastly, the Questionnaire ought to be answered considering the 28 days prior to the application; this way, frequencies are measured according to the amount of days in which disordered behaviors are present.

Despite the unusual structure of the Questionnaire, which consists of very few items that do make up factors, this version has been analyzed and validated, as well as published, and is therefore accepted as a trustworthy methodological instrument. Actually, it's considered a viable alternative to the EDE and has shown high internal consistency [43, 44]. For example, Luce and Crowther found excellent reliability in this test [44]. Likewise, Unikel et al. [45] recently validated the instrument in Mexican women (revise Annex 1).

Procedure

The study consisted of applying both, the EDE-Q in its short version, and the ORTO-14MX Questionnaire in its validated version for Mexican population [TSEA3]. The instruments were administered on a sample of university students from Mexico City. Participants were approached trhough non-probabilistic convenience, seeing as professors from indiscriminate classes were to invite their students to voluntarily participate in the study. The Questionnaires were self-administered. Those questionnaires which were not answered in their totality, were discarded from the study. For ethical reasons, the participants did not receive any financial compensation in exchange for their participation in the study.

To protect the confidentiality of all participants, they were informed that their answers would be treated anonymously and only for statistical purposes. They were asked to respond with the answer considered most appropriate to their attitude and behaviors. The Research Ethics Committee of the University approved this study, and it is in accordance with the General Health Law in México regarding research procedures. Therefore, participants signed a Consent Informed letter, included in Annex 3.

Data analysis

The SPSS software version 25 was used to perform data analysis. Descriptive analyses were done using frequency and percentages for categorical variables, such as mean and standard deviation, for continuous measures. Furthermore, it was intended to investigate if, just like in previous studies, statistically significant differences were found between men and women regarding the total obtained scores both in the ON scale and in the Specific Symptomatology one (ED). A Student T-Test for independent simples was run for each factor that compose both scales.

To achieve the objective of this investigation, which main purpose was to analyze if the factors from the ORTO-14MX instrument managed to predict accurately and trustworthily the apparition of specific symptomatology of eating disorders, statistical analyses were run. First, a Pearson's Correlation was used between the ORTO-14MX factors, and the total points obtained with the EDE-Q in its short version. Furthermore, a linear regression analysis by steps was applied to obtain which specific factors from the ORTO-14MX can precisely predict the probability to develop an eating disorder.

Results

In the first place, the total scores from the scale measuring orthorexia in the sample were obtained; 61.8% of the total sample obtained scores equal or lower to 40, and 34.3% of that percentage obtained scores equal or lower to 35. Both scores are indicators of orthorexia; however, considering a cut point lower than 35 has proven higher specificity and better diagnostic tendencies. When analyzing this same percentage in women from the sample, it increases to 65.7% considering the cut point at scores equal or lower to 40, and 38.1% considering the cut point at scores equal or lower to 35. Regarding men, the initial percentage decreased to 54.7 and 27.4%, respectively. In relation to the prevalence found in Nutrition students, 75.7% scored with 40 or less in the questionnaire that measures orthorexia.

Respecting the average obtained was 12.02 for the whole sample (SD = 8.95), with a minimum score of 0 and a maximum of 42. For the sample constructed entirely of women the average calculated is 13.46 (SD = 9.32), with the same minimum and maximum scores for the whole sample. In contrast, the men's average value is 9.36 (SD = 7.48), with a minimum of 0 and a maximum of 34 points.

Concerning the ORTO-14MX, every single factor had higher marks in men than in women. Consistently, these grades indicate higher risks of developing orthorexia in women, while a greater score from women in the EDE-Q demonstrates greater liability in specific symptomatology of ED. In relation to the comparison between men and women's samples, statistically significant differences were found in factors 1, 2 and 3 of the scale that measures ON, as well as in every subscale from de EDE-Q; these are shown in Table 2.

A Pearson's correlation analysis was conducted to analyze the relationship between the subscales that make up the variable of ON, and the subscales on the EDE-Q scale in its short version. As it can be seen in Table 3, statistically significant and inversely proportional relationships were found between the three EDE-Q factors and the four factors of the ORTO-14MX. Although the correlations ranged from mild to moderate, a relationship between the presence of orthorexia and the specific symptomatology of an ED is identified. It is feasible to test the hypothesis of a possible prediction (see Table 3).

Eating disorder prediction from the factors composing the variable of orthorexia nervosa

The purpose of this paragraph is to get to know the influence that the different components of ON have over the global score obtained in the EDE-Q in university students in Mexico. Step- wise linear regression was analyzed. The results are presented in Table 4.

The dependent variable used in the regression analysis corresponds to the global score from the EDE-Q in its short version. Specific symptomatology of an eating disorder was predicted in four steps in the following order. The first step involved the subscale "Obsessive Cognition" ($F = 433.85$, $p = .000$). The second step involved subscale "Emotional Dysregulation" ($F = 249.42$, $p = .000$). The third step involved factor "Rational Cognition" ($F = 170.71$, $p = .000$). The fourth and last step involved factor "Social Normative" ($F = 133.12$, $p = .000$). This can be observed in Fig. 1.

Discussion

The present study's main objective was to analyze if there was a possible relationship and predictive value between the factors that measure if someone has orthorexia, and the overall score from the EDE-Q, and determine if this relationship could indicate a specific's eating disorder symptomatology amongst university students in Mexico. Additionally, the sample's prevalence in these values was obtained, and the differences between men and women regarding these variables.

Firstly, a significant prevalence of orthorexia was found in the sample, seeing as out of the 100, 68.1% obtained scores equal or lower to 40, which is an indicator of the presence of certain pathological behavior characterized by the strong worry and desire to eat healthily. Out of this 68.1, 34.3% obtained a score equal or lower to 35. Just as it was found in the sample and its results in the present study, various authors have found higher psychosocial vulnerability in adolescent and university

Table 2 Descriptive statistics and differences between men and women regarding orthorexia nervosa and specific symptomatology of an ED in Mexican university students

	Women		Men			
	M	SD	M	SD	t	p
ORTO-14 MX						
Obsessive Cognition	8.78	2.33	9.35	2.10	−3.74	.00**
Rational Cognition	7.69	2.35	8.07	2.60	−2.15	.03*
Emotional Regulation	8.96	2.24	9.67	1.96	−4.91	.00**
Normative Social	7.91	1.88	8.20	1.98	−2.15	.03*
Total	35.45	6.70	37.59	6.88	−4.48	.00**
EDE-Q						
Restriction	4.50	4.39	3.56	4.00	3.24	.00**
Concern for one's shape and weight	3.98	3.18	2.59	2.40	7.43	.00**
Dissatisfaction	4.99	3.50	3.21	3.21	7.44	.00**
Total	13.46	9.33	9.36	7.49	7.13	.00**

*$P \leq .05$ **$P \leq .01$

population, regarding eating disorder behavior. This is a critical period in which this age-group consolidates and strengthens their own behavioral and eating habits, as well as a major importance in the development of body image [22, 23]. Besides, within university students, sub-groups have been described as even in higher risk, such as students form nutrition, medicine, and sport's science [6].

However, the authors from the present study consider it especially important to put forward two contrasting situations. On one hand, students are immersed in fast-paced lifestyles, and they lack the possibility of investing enough time and money in controlling what they eat; hence, health becomes a secondary concern. On the other, students with high obsessive cognition can be found. Due to the concern over eating "healthy", "clean", and "correct", most of their personal and economic resources are invested in what is perceived that aids in keeping eating habits under control. Thus, this group of people are deprived of time and space to perform other personal, social, and integration activities because of focus on what is being consumed.

After analyzing prevalence by sex, it was found that percentages were higher in women than in men, which is consistent with what other authors have found in their own studies. It has been detected that there is a higher prevalence of eating disorders, and pathological or disordered eating in the female population. The same results could be observed for global scores obtained in the EDE-Q: women had an average score higher than men. With results in agreement with what is mentioned before, statistically significant differences were found when comparing each one of the factors that make up instruments used in women and in men. Adding on, the factors from the ORTO14-MX instrument were also statistically significant, and lower for women, whilst the factors from the EDE-Q scale in its short version showed statistically significant averages, higher in women.

Now, regarding the relationship between orthorexia nervosa and eating disorders, it can be said that researchers are still far from understanding it clearly, seeing as ON hasn't even been included as a pathology in the DSM-5, and health professionals don't have much information on it. This hinders even more its

Table 3 Relationship between orthorexia nervosa and eating disorder specific symptomatology in university students in Mexico

	OC	RC	ER	NS	EDE-Q1	EDE-Q2	EDE-Q3
Obsessive Cognition (OC)		.450**	.466**	.287**	−.530**	−.494**	−.437**
Rational Cognition (RC)			.307**	.302**	−.335**	−.307**	−.251**
Emotional Regulation (ER)				.267**	−.429**	−.347**	−.315**
Normative Social (NS)					−.208**	−.266**	−.267**
Restriction (EDE-Q1)						.506**	.461**
Concern for one's shape and weight (EDE-Q2)							.638**
Dissatisfaction (EDE-Q3)							

Note: *$p \leq .05$, **$p \leq .01$

Table 4 Linear regression by steps analysis summary to predict EDE-Q total final scores from the factors that make up the ORTO-14MX scale

Step and predictive variable	B	SD B	β	R^2	Δ R^2
Step 1: Obsessive Cognition	−5.17	.37	−.43	.34	.349
Step 2: Emotional Dysregulation	−2.35	.37	−.19	.38	.037
Step 3: Rational Cognition	−1.38	.39	−.09	.39	.011
Step 4: Social Normative	−1.16	.43	−.08	.40	.005

exploration and possible description. Actually, studies that have been published so far have precisely found that it's those healthcare professionals who exhibit more frequently these disordered behaviors. One hypothesis as to why this happens is that more knowledge directed over healthy eating is acquired in their studies. But there's a thin line that separates this knowledge from pathological behavior, making it quite difficult to perceive the difference. In fact, in the sample used for this study, 75.7% of students that were majoring in Nutrition obtained scores equal or lower to 40 in the instrument that measures orthorexia, which is consistent with other studies who have obtained similar prevalence values in dietitians and nutrition students. For example, Tremeling et al. found that out of 2, 500 dietitian in the United States, 49.5% were at risk of developing orthorexia, and 12% in risk of developing a diagnosed eating disorder; also noting that those at risk for ON had lower BMI values, and 8.2% self-reported having been previously in treatment for an eating disorder. These authors argued that the relationship between ON and an ED associates not only in disordered eating behaviors, but also in concern about body size and image [46].

Regarding the ability to predict an eating disorder based on the presence of orthorexia, it's necessary to mention that a promising score was obtained, but it wasn't conclusive, given that the obtained correlations between factors were significant with a mild to moderate magnitude, while the determination coefficient obtained from the linear multiple regression indicates that the percentage of explained variance reached a percentage of 40%, which is considered acceptable as a predictor for eating disorders when orthorexia is detected. This finding is overly valuable as a predictor (but isn't sufficient), because this is a psychosocial study in a poorly studied Latin sample.

When the factors' order was analyzed (obtained from the linear regression analysis), the objective was to explain specific symptomatology from eating disorders. "Obsessive cognition" was found to be the first factor in the model, also explaining most of the variance's score, followed by "emotional dysregulation", "rational cognition", and "social normative" last.

Obsessive cognition is conformed by a series of persistent and involuntary thoughts, as well as high levels of concern for at least 3 hours daily over what will be eaten, through the past 3 months. Said concern is moved by the need to be physically "healthy", regardless of concern over weight and body image. There's also a constant search and attempt to "keep clean", "eat clean and correctly", and maintain control of surroundings. Along this line, diverse studies performed with patients diagnosed with different types of eating disorders, show

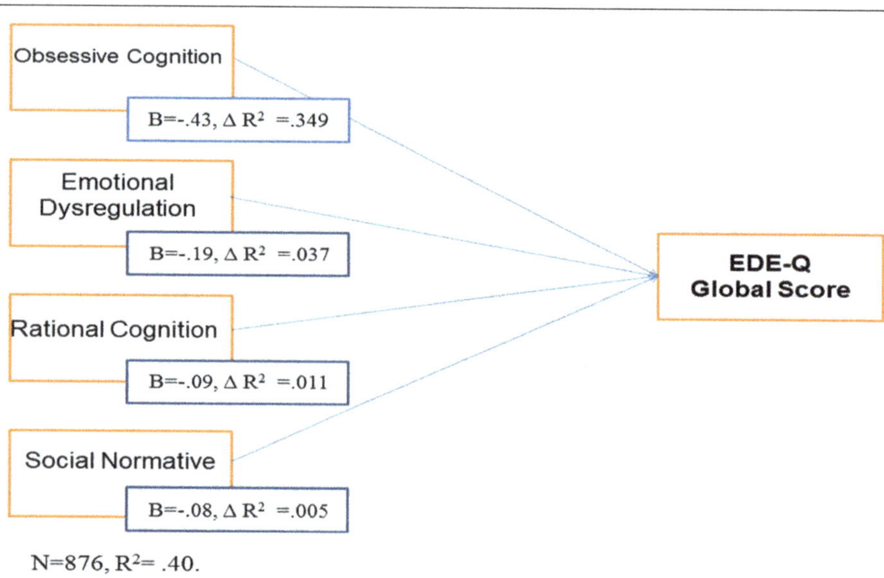

Fig. 1 Linear regression analysis for the EDE-Q

obsessive traits in 27 to 61% of cases; shyness and dependent characteristics in 21 to 48%, and anxiety in 51 to 64% of cases. Earlier research on this topic agrees that the prevailing personality type to develop an eating disorder combines obsessive, inhibition, and conformism traits [47]. Therefore, there is a relationship between thought rumination, and obsessive personality traits.

The second factor, "emotional dysregulation", is composed by the presence of confusion, anxiety and preoccupation, and the difficulty to stay calm in situations where the person doesn't have control partially or wholly. Congruently, the Minnesota Multiphasic Personality Inventory (MMPI) has provided relevant information about general characteristics found in affective states (sadness, pessimism, euphoria, etc.), the quality of interpersonal relationships (difficulty in establishing deep affective compromise), and excessive demanding and expressing characteristics of affection in patients with an eating disorder (or at risk of developing one). Lastly, people with an ED usually have trouble with impulse control and tolerating frustration. As a matter of fact, it is esteemed that around 53 to 93% of patients with an eating disorder have personality alterations [48]. Likewise, the simultaneous manifestation of more than one personality disorder in said samples, especially in patients diagnosed with bulimia nervosa and previous story of anorexia nervosa, has been documented [49, 50].

In what refers to the "rational cognition" and "social normative" factor, it can be said that despite their inclusion in the model, the variance's percentage explained through them is quite low. In this case, it is hypothesized that the presence of both obeys socioeconomic and cultural characteristics, rather than individual ones. These 2 factors include items related to spending more money to eat more healthily, or the perception of types of foods sold at local markets and supermarkets. About this, it's relevant to explain that in Mexico "healthy" or "wholesome" food is considerably more expensive than fast food or "garnachas", which are also more easily found to buy. Additionally, Mexican population consists of a collectivist culture. This means that it's almost compulsory to eat accompanied by other members of endogroups, or interact in every context associated with food, despite individual personality traits [51, 52].

In conclusion, the cultural factor permeates every psychosocial behavior, such as eating. Although eating is an act of survival biologically determined, it is also immersed in society. In this sense, eating behaviors are profoundly shaped by the person's context, involving cultural, social, and environmental contexts [35]. The interaction found between sociocultural context and ON has been scarcely studied in Mexican population; most studies of this type have been made with European, Turkish, and American samples [36].

Ergo, it's necessary to consider the importance given to food as an interaction ritual in Mexico, besides being used as a tool to unite people. Mexican gastronomy is loaded with collective emotions because of the country's history and endoculturation found inside families. Consequently, it's not a simple task to compare the findings of this study with those obtained in nations considered individualistic. Plus, Mexican people have rather high levels of social desirability. In turn, this becomes a potential source of internal invalidation in every research that uses instruments such as interviews and self-reports [53].

Conclusions

In conclusion, the objectives of this investigation were achieved. This study analyzes the existing relationship between the composing factors of the ORTO-14MX and the factors from the Eating Disorders Questionnaire (EDE-Q) in its short version. It was later found that these factors that indicate orthorexia nervosa (ON) accurately predict to some degree eating disorders in university students from Mexico City. Additionally, it analyzed statistical differences found between men and women, according to these same variables.

The factors from the ORTO-14MX and the EDE-Q don't have a 100% predictive capacity. However, it does have a significant enough capacity to be said that it is very valuable as an initial screening instrument that manages to give quick and reliable information on the mental state of the person regarding eating habits (which is a very complex phenomena). If the fact that most of the habits acquired during adolescent and early-adulthood years is taken in consideration, this period is of utmost importance and gives a worthwhile opportunity to evaluate predictive factors, and risk factors to develop eating disorders.

Given that there are not enough elements to stablish a definite cut-point, a score equal to 32 based on the value that marks the superior limit in the first quarter 32 ≥ is tentatively proposed. However, this value will be corroborated or adjusted according to other researchers and their usage of the ORTO14-MX in clinical and non-clinical samples.

It is necessary to consider taking into account these traits from orthorexia grave and important enough to offer integral treatment since this moment, and not wait until a full-on eating disorder has developed to offer help or even seek for help. For this to happen, there must be more information accessible for sanitary professions in general: Nutrition is one of the most in need, but also students and practitioners from Medicine, Nursing, Social Work, and Psychology, amongst others. The more interdisciplinary the knowledge, the more tailored evaluation and intervention strategies can be.

Regarding the differences in the frequency of ON found among the Italian, Polish and Spanish samples, we cannot exclude that a role is played by gastronomic culture, Mediterranean diet, convivial and social value attributed to eating and main approaches aimed at improving one's health typical of each socio-cultural context. Disordered eating behavior rarely has to do completely with losing weight or being healthy; it's a priority for researchers in this field to study and integrate the relevance of society and different systems in how a person views eating, and the purpose of their eating habits. That is, after all, what makes the study of eating disorders so complex and arduous: family, friends, school, workplaces, and general socio-economic markets will inevitably influence how food, health, and the body is viewed.

Limitations and suggestions

The results obtained in this research highlight the long path that is still to be travelled by the scientific community, for orthorexia to be considered a new eating disorder that can be included in the diagnostic manuals. The relationship between eating disorders and orthorexia is, undoubtedly, intricate, and is far from being understood. Additional studies are needed to describe specific behaviors from people with orthorexia (its etiology, diagnosis, treatment, and prevention). In order to convincingly affirm predictions between orthorexia and specific symptomatology of eating disorders, comparisons must be made with clinical samples. The sample used in this subject was taken from university students, and it was not a heterogeneous nor generalizable sample. However, using a non-clinical sample can help generalize results to more people, therefore being a possible strength. Also, other confirming instruments, rather than screening or self-report instruments, could be used to confirm a presumed diagnostic, both for ON and for ED. Likewise, this study was only applied in a specific socioeconomic background. More studies comparing scores from other backgrounds would be quite useful, particularly done with low social classes, students from public universities, and students from different geographical regions of the country.

Abbreviations

ON: Orthorexia Nervosa; AN: Anorexia Nervosa; ED: Eating Disorder; DSM-5: Diagnostic and Statistical Manual of Mental Disorders; ICD-10: International Classification of Diseases; BOT: Bratman's Orthorexia Test; EDE: Eating Disorder Examination; EDE-Q: Eating Disorder Examination Questionnaire

Acknowledgements

This research was conducted at the Iberoamericana University. We thank our colleagues from different university departments for their valuable expertise and support provided for this research project and all the students that participated in it. The authors thank the students who took part in this study and generously granted us their time.

Special thanks to Dra. Claudia Unikel S., Ms. Paulina Villarreal P. and Dra. Sarah Gordon F.

Informed consent

Informed consent was obtained from all individual participants included in the study.

Authors' contributions

All authors meet all four criteria for authorship:1.- Study conception and design: APC, ATS, GMBM, MBM: 2.- Data collection: APC, GMBM, MBM, MCDG, IFG: 3.- Substantial contributions to the conception or design of the work, the acquisition, analysis and interpretation of data for the work: APC, ATS, GMBM; MBM, MCDG, IFG: 4.- Statistical expertise, analysis and interpretation of data: APC, ATS, MBM, ARS: 5.- Drafting the work or revising it critically for important intellectual content; APC, ATS, GMBM; MBM, MCDG, IFG, ARS: 6.- Final approval of the version to be published; APC, ATS, GMBM; MBM, MCDG, IFG, ARS: 7.- Agreement to be accountable for all aspects of the work in ensuring that questions related to the accuracy or integrity of any part of the work are appropriately investigated and resolved. APC, ATS, GMBM; MBM, MCDG, IFG, ARS. The authors read and approved the final manuscript.

Competing interests

The authors declare that they have no conflict of interest.

Author details

Universidad Iberoamericana CDMX, México, Mexico. [2]Universidad Nacional Autónoma de México, Mexico, Mexico.

References

1. Bratman S, Knight D. Health food junkies: Orthorexia nervosa: overcoming the obsession with healthful eating. New York: Broadway; 2001.
2. Cena H, Barthels F, Cuzzolaro M, Bratman S, Brytek-Matera A, Dunn T, et al. Definition and diagnostic criteria for orthorexia nervosa: a narrative review of the literature. Eat Weight Disord. 2018;24(2):209–46. https://doi.org/10.1007/s40519-018-0606 [Epub ahead of print].
3. Brytek-Matera A. Orthorexia nervosa –an eating disorder, obsessive-compulsive disorder or disturbed eating habit? Arch Psychiatry Psychother. 2012;1:55–60.
4. Ramacciotti C, Perrone P, Coli E, Burgalassi A, Conversano C, Massimeetti G, et al. Orthorexia nervosa in the general population: a preliminary screening using a self-administered questionnaire (ORTO-15). Eat Weight Disord. 2011; 16(2):e127–30.
5. Moroze RM, Dunn TM, Holland JC, Yager J, Weintraub P. Microthinking about micronutrients: a case of transition from obsession about healthy eating to near-fatal "orthorexia nervosa" and proposed diagnostic criteria. Psychosomatics. 2014;56:397–403.
6. Varga M, Dukay-Szabó S, Túry F, van Furth EF, van Furth Eric F. Evidence and gaps in the literature on orthorexia nervosa. Eat Weight Disord. 2013;18: 103–11. https://doi.org/10.1007/s40519-013-0026-y.
7. Segura-García C, Ramacciotti C, Rania M, Aloi M, Caroleo M, Bruni A, et al. The prevalence of orthorexia nervosa among eating disorder patients after treatment. Eat Weight Disord. 2015;20(2):161–6. https://doi.org/10.1007/s40519-014-0171-y.
8. Barthels F, Meyer F, Pietrowsky R. Orthorexic eating behavior. A new type of disordered eating. Ernahrungs Umschau. 2015;62(10):156–61. https://doi.org/10.4455/eu.2015.029.
9. Parra-Fernandez ML, Rodríguez-Cano T, Onieva-Zafra MD, Perez-Haro MJ, Casero-Alonso V, Muñoz Camargo JC, et al. Adaptation and validation of the Spanish version of the ORTO-15 questionnaire for the diagnosis of orthorexia nervosa. PLoS One. 2018;13(1):1–14 [cited 2020 May 22]. Available from: http://search.ebscohost.com/login.aspx?direct=true&db=a9h&AN=127214876&lang=es&site=ehost-live.
10. Roncero M, Barrada J, Perpiñá C. Measuring Orthorexia nervosa: psychometric limitations for the ORTO-15. Span J Psychol. 2017;20:eXX. https://doi.org/10.1017/sjp.2017.36.
11. Setnick J. The eating disorders clinical pocket guide, second edition: quick reference for healthcare providers. Dallas: Understanding Nutrition; 2013.
12. Dunn T, Bratman S. On orthorexia nervosa: a review of the literature and proposed diagnostic criteria. Eat Behav. 2016;21:11–7. https://doi.org/10.1016/j.eatbeh.2015.12.006

13. Donini L, Marsili D, Graziani MP, Imbriale M, Cannella C. Orthorexia nervosa: validation of a diagnosis questionnaire. Eat Weight Disord. 2005;10(2):e28–32. https://doi.org/10.1007/bf03327537.
14. Donini L, Marsili D, Graziani MP, Imbriale M, Cannella C. Orthorexia nervosa: a preliminary study with a proposal for diagnosis and an attempt to measure the dimension of the phenomenon. Eat Weight Disord. 2004;9(2): 151–7. https://doi.org/10.1007/bf03325060.
15. Bundros J, Clifford D, Silliman K, Neyman M. Prevalence of Orthorexia nervosa among college students based on Bratman's test and associated tendencies. Appetite. 2016;101:86–94. https://doi.org/10.1016/j.appet.2016.02.144.
16. Poínhos R, Alves D, Vieira E, Pinhao S, Oliveira B. Eating behaviour among undergraduate students. Comparing nutrition students with other courses. Appetite. 2015;84:28–33. https://doi.org/10.1016/j.appet.2014.09.011.
17. Sánchez Socarrás V, Aguilar Martínez A. Food habits and health-related behaviors in a university population. Nutr Hosp. 2014;31:449–57. https://doi.org/10.3305/nh.2015.31.1.7412.
18. Nelson MC, Story M, Larson NI, Neumark-Sztainer D, Lytle LA. Emerging adulthood and college-aged youth: an overlooked age for weight-related behavior change. Obesity. 2008;16:2205–11. https://doi.org/10.1038/oby.2008.365.
19. Parra-Fernández ML, Rodríguez-Cano T, Onieva-Zafra MD, et al. Prevalence of orthorexia nervosa in university students and its relationship with psychopathological aspects of eating behaviour disorders. BMC Psychiatry. 2018;18(1):364Published 2018 Nov 13. https://doi.org/10.1186/s12888-018-1943-0.
20. Parra-Fernández ML, Onieva-Zafra MD, Fernández-Martínez E, Abreu-Sánchez A, Fernández-Muñoz JJ. Assessing the prevalence of Orthorexia nervosa in a sample of university students using two different self-report measures. Int J Environ Res Public Health. 2019;16(14):2459Published 2019 Jul 11. https://doi.org/10.3390/ijerph16142459.
21. Fidan T, Ertekin V, Işikay S, Kirpinar I. Prevalence of orthorexia among medical students in Erzurum. Turkey Compr Psychiatry. 2010;51(1):49–54.
22. Kinzl JF, Hauer K, Traweger C, Kiefer I. Orthorexia nervosa in dieticians. Psychother Psychosom. 2006;75(6):395–6.
23. Bo S, Zoccali R, Ponzo V, Soldati L, De Carli L, Benso A, et al. University courses, eating problems and muscle dysmorphia: are there any associations? J Transl Med. 2014;12:221.
24. Bağci Bosi AT, Camur D, Güler C. Prevalence of orthorexia nervosa in resident medical doctors in the faculty of medicine (Ankara, Turkey). Appetite. 2007 Nov;49(3):661–6. https://doi.org/10.1186/s12967-014-0221-2.
25. Malmborg J, Bremander A, Olsson MC, Bergman S. Health status, physical activity, and orthorexia nervosa: a comparison between exercise science students and business students. Appetite. 2017;109:137–43.
26. Alvarenga MS, Martins M, Sato K, Vargas S, Philippi S, Scagliusi FB. Orthorexia nervosa behavior in a sample of Brazilian dietitians assessed by the Portuguese version of Orto-15. Eat Weight Disord. 2012;17:e29–35. https://doi.org/10.1007/bf03325325.
27. Asil E, Saip M. Orthorexia nervosa in Turkish dietitians. Ecol Food Nutr. 2015; 54(4):303–13. https://doi.org/10.1080/03670244.2014.987920.
28. Karakus B, Hidiroglu S, Keskin N, Karavus M. Orthorexia nervosa tendency among students of the department of nutrition and dietetics at a university in Istanbul. North Clin Istanb. 2017;4(2):117–23. https://doi.org/10.14744/nci.2017.20082.
29. Aksoydan E, Camci N. Prevalence of orthorexia nervosa among Turkish performance artists. Eat Weight Disord. 2009;14(1):33–7. https://doi.org/10.1007/bf03327792.
30. Almeida C, Vieira V, Santos L. Orthorexia nervosa in a sample of Portuguese fitness participants. Eat Weight Disord. 2018;23:443. https://doi.org/10.1007/s40519-018-0517-y.
31. Clifford T, Blyth C. A pilot study comparing the prevalence of orthorexia nervosa in regular students and those in university sports teams. Eat Weight Disord. 2019;24:473–80. https://doi.org/10.1007/s40519-018-0584-0.
32. Volpe U, Atti AR, Cimino M, Monteleone AM, De Ronchi D, Fernández-Aranda F, et al. Beyond anorexia and bulimia nervosa: What's "new" in eating disorders? J Psychopathol. 2015;21(4):415–23.
33. Plichta M, Jezewska-Zychowicz M. Orthorexic tendency and eating disorders symptoms in polish students: examining differences in eating behaviors. Nutrients. 2020;12(1):218Published 2020 Jan 15. https://doi.org/10.3390/nu12010218
34. Plichta M, Jezewska-Zychowicz M. Eating behaviors, attitudes toward health and eating and symptoms of orthorexia nervosa among students. Appetite. 2019;137:114–23. https://doi.org/10.1016/j.appet.2019.02.022.
35. Healy D. In: Vandereycken W, van Deth R, editors. From fasting saints to anorexic girls: the history of self-starvation. London: Athlone Press; 1994. Irish Journal of Psychological Medicine. Cambridge University Press; 1995; 12(1): 41–2.
36. Scarff JR. Orthorexia nervosa: an obsession with healthy eating. Fed Pract. 2017;34(6):36–9.
37. Barcelos Pontes J, Montagner MI, Montagner MA. Orthorexia nervosa: cultural adaptation of ortho-15. DEMETRA: Food Nutr Health. 2014;9(2):533–48. https://doi.org/10.12957/demetra.2014.8576.
38. Arusoğlu G, Kabakçi E, Köksal G, Merdol TK. Orthorexia nervosa and adaptation of ORTO-11 into Turkish. Turk Psikiyatri Derg. 2008;19:283–91 Available. http://www.ncbi.nlm.nih.gov/pubmed/18791881.
39. Varga M, Dukay-Szabo S, Túry F. Orthorexia nervosa and its background factors. Ideggyogy Sz. Available. 2013;66:220–7 http://www.ncbi.nlm.nih.gov/pubmed/23971352.
40. Gramaglia C, Gambaro E, Delicato C, et al. Orthorexia nervosa, eating patterns and personality traits: a cross-cultural comparison of Italian, polish and Spanish university students. BMC Psychiatry. 2019;19:235. https://doi.org/10.1186/s12888-019-2208-2.
41. Tena SA, Parra CA, Barajas MW, Bilbao GM, Díaz GM, Flores GI, et al. When eating "correctly" is not so healthy: factor analysis of the ORTO-15 in university students from Mexico City. Rev Mex de Trastornos alimenticios. 2020.
42. Grilo CM, Reas DL, Hopwood CJ, Crosby RD. Factor structure and construct validity of the eating disorder examination-questionnaire in college students: further support for a modified brief version. Int J Eat Disord. 2015; 48(3):284–9. https://doi.org/10.1002/eat.22358.
43. Berg K, Peterson C, Frazier P, Crow S. Psychometric evaluation of the eating disorder examination and eating disorder examination-questionnaire: a systematic review of the literature. Int J Eat Disord. 2012;45(3):428–38. https://doi.org/10.1002/eat.20931.
44. Luce K, Crowther J. The reliability of the eating disorder examination—self-report questionnaire version (EDE-Q). Int J Eat Disord. 1999;25(3):349–51. https://doi.org/10.1002/(sici)1098-108x(199904)25:3<349::aid-eat15>3.3.co;2-d.
45. Unikel C, Bojórquez I, Díaz de León C, Vázquez V, Rivera J, Galván G, et al. Validation of eating disorders examination questionnaire in Mexican women. Int J Eat Disord. 2018:1–9. https://doi.org/10.1002/eat.22819.
46. Tremelling K, Sandon L, Vega GL, Mc Adams CJ. Orthorexia nervosa and eating disorder symptoms in registered dietitian nutritionists in the United States. J Acad Nutr Diet. 2017;117(10):1612–7. https://doi.org/10.1016/j.jand.2017.05.001.
47. Vitousek KY, Manke F. Personality variables and disorders in anorexia nervosa and bulimia nervosa. J Abnorm Psychol. 1994;103(1):137–47.
48. Garner DM. Pathogenesis of anorexia nervosa. Lancet. 1993;341:1631–5.
49. Braun DL, Sunday SR, Halmi KA. Psychiatric comorbidity in patients with eating disorders. Psychol Med. 1994;24:859–67.
50. Herzog DB, Keller MB, Lavori PW, Kenny GM, Sacks NR. The prevalence of personality disorders in 210 women with eating disorders. J Clin Psychiatry. 1992;53(5):147–52.
51. León S, Jiménez B, López A, Barrera K. Ideas sobre las causas de la obesidad en estudiantes universitarios mexicanos y españoles. Enseñanza e Investigación en Psicología. 2013;18(1):95–110 [citado 22 mayo 2020]. Disponible en: https://www.redalyc.org/articulo.oa?id=29228948007.
52. Díaz GR. Bajo las Garras de la Cultura: Psicología del mexicano 2. México: Trillas; 2003.
53. Vizcarra-Zamora I. Factores psicológicos, psicosociales y socioculturales en el desarrollo del sobrepeso y la obesidad Como problemas de salud pública en México. Dissertation [BS Th]. México: UNAM; 2010.

14

ERP and oscillatory differences in overweight/obese and normal-weight adolescents in response to food stimuli

Stefanie C. Biehl[1,2*], Julian Keil[3], Eva Naumann[1] and Jennifer Svaldi[1]

Abstract

Background: Findings are mixed regarding the association of electroencephalographic (EEG) attentional bias measures and body weight, with few studies measuring food craving or intake and no study reporting oscillatory measures.

Methods: EEG data were collected while 28 satiated adolescents (14 overweight/obese) viewed pictures of neutral, low-calorie food, and high-calorie food stimuli and rated their desire to eat, before having access to high-calorie snacks.

Results: Unlike normal-weight adolescents, overweight/obese participants showed similar P300 amplitudes for high- and low-calorie food, and strongest event-related alpha band desynchronization for low-calorie stimuli. P300 amplitudes and state craving for low-calorie food furthermore predicted snack intake in this group.

Conclusions: The current research focus in overweight/obesity might need to be extended to include low-calorie food. While all participants showed an attentional bias for high-calorie food, it was the processing of low-calorie food which distinguished the two weight groups on measures of neural activity and which was associated with snack food intake in the overweight/obese group.

Keywords: Overweight, Obesity, Adolescents, Food stimuli, Event-related potentials, Alpha band oscillations

Plain English summary

This study tried to find out if the way the brain directs attention to food pictures is related to a person's body weight. We therefore looked at different brain waves that indicate attention in 28 adolescents (14 were overweight or obese) while they viewed pictures of low-calorie and high-calorie food. In addition, we checked how much they craved and actually ate high-calorie food afterwards. We found that the brains of overweight/obese adolescents reacted similarly to low-calorie and high-calorie food. This was different from the normal-weight adolescents, who reacted more strongly to high-calorie food. The reaction to low-calorie food in overweight/obese adolescents was also related to the amount of snacks they ate afterwards. We think that the brain's increased attention to low-calorie food in overweight/obese adolescents might be caused by their social environment, which constantly reminds them to watch their weight and eat low-calorie food. More studies should therefore investigate how low-calorie food is perceived and how this is related to weight and eating behaviour.

* Correspondence: stefanie.biehl@psychologie.uni-regensburg.de
[1]Department of Clinical Psychology and Psychotherapy, University of Tuebingen, Schleichstrasse 4, 72076 Tuebingen, Germany
[2]Department of Clinical Psychology and Psychotherapy, University of Regensburg, Universitaetsstrasse 31, 93053 Regensburg, Germany
Full list of author information is available at the end of the article

Background

Overweight and obesity in childhood and adolescence have been recognized as a severe problem of global extent, with approximately 20 % of children and adolescents in developed countries currently classified as overweight or obese [1]. Although recent studies suggest no further increase in the rates of overweight and obesity in Western Europe and North America, numbers stagnate at a very high level with rates in Eastern Europe still increasing [2]. One of the issues frequently addressed in this context is the omnipresence of highly palatable food. In fact, experimental studies show that the mere presence of food increases food intake (see [3] for a review) and that several additional factors such as assumptions about caloric content and nutritive qualities [4, 5], portion size, sight, and smell of food [3, 6] influence food consumption. Notably though, not all children are equally susceptible to the "obesogenic" environment and recent evidence suggests that personality and cognitive factors could play a crucial role in the regulation of hedonic food intake [7, 8].

Incentive-sensitization theory provides an important framework for understanding the hedonic and motivational processes involved in the consumption of food [9, 10]. This theory posits that individual differences in mesolimbic dopaminergic functioning influence the experience of reward from food and thus its perceived hedonic value. The repeated experience of reward from the consumption of food sensitizes the individual to stimuli associated with food, thereby increasing the incentive salience of food cues. This heightened food cue reactivity then triggers attentional biases and food cravings and, consequently, increased food intake.

Predictions of this model have since been confirmed in adult populations. Functional magnetic resonance imaging (fMRI) studies investigated hypotheses regarding the hedonic and motivational value of food and found increased reward-related brain activation to high-calorie food cues in obese participants [11, 12]. While it is uncertain if these differences are cause or consequence of obesity, another study found that they moreover correlated with less successful weight loss [13]. Furthermore, reward-related functional connectivity was associated with food cravings, both in resting state and when viewing high-calorie stimuli [14, 15], and these cravings were more effortful to regulate with increasing weight [16].

Methodologies with higher temporal resolution also confirmed the predictions of the incentive salience theory. As such, eye tracking studies demonstrated that relative to normal-weight individuals, overweight/obese participants displayed a tendency for larger attentional biases [17] and greater initial attention allocation [18] to high-calorie food. Electroencephalographic (EEG) studies focused on two event-related potentials (ERPs) to examine attentional biases to food cues: The P300, a positive deflection roughly 300 ms post stimulus onset which is thought to be amplified by increased attention allocation to certain stimulus classes or motivationally salient stimuli [19, 20], and the Late Positive Potential (LPP), a slow positive wave with a centro-parietal topography starting roughly 400 ms post stimulus onset [21]. LPP amplitude has been linked to deliberate processing and strategic attention allocation and is known to be increased for emotionally salient stimuli [22–24].

In adults, both P300 and LPP amplitudes were found to be sensitive to the motivational salience of food stimuli, with higher amplitudes for food than for control pictures [25]. In line with incentive-sensitization theory, amplitudes were also increased in hungry as opposed to satiated participants [25, 26], and when high-calorie food was available versus unavailable [27]. On the trait-level, amplitudes were higher in participants who reported increased food intake in response to appetizing food stimuli (external eaters) or in response to negative emotional states (emotional eaters) [28, 29]. Several studies also investigated food craving as well as food intake as observable consequences of the attentional bias posited by incentive-sensitization theory, and P300 but not LPP amplitudes were found to correlate positively with self-reported craving [30] and subjective hunger levels in response to pictures of high-calorie food as well as with subsequent food intake [26].

In contrast, empirical evidence for the incentive salience theory in children and adolescents is less clear: fMRI studies found heightened food cue reactivity in satiated obese compared to normal-weight children [31], but also increased activation in inhibitory brain areas [31, 32]. However, when instructed to regulate food cravings, these areas showed decreased activation in heavier children [33]. Comparable to EEG findings in adults, both P300 and LPP amplitudes were found to be higher for high-calorie food cues, with higher LPP amplitudes in emotional eaters [34]. However, P300 amplitudes for mixed low- and high-calorie food cues were comparable for obese and normal-weight adolescents [35].

A change in time-frequency resolved power, namely event-related desynchronization (ERD) in the EEG alpha band [36–38] is an additional measure of the attentional and semantic processing of stimuli. An alpha band power decrease in response to a stimulus allows for more in-depth processing of the presented information by providing access to the individual's semantic knowledge base [36]. While alpha band power changes have been investigated in some clinical samples (e.g. [39]), this has not been the case for overweight or obese participants. However, given the heightened food cue sensitivity in this population, it could be speculated that alpha band-controlled access to food-related semantic knowledge might be altered in overweight and obese participants when compared to a normal-weight sample.

In summary, there is substantial support for altered food cue responsiveness in overweight/obese participants and several studies with adult samples have investigated the association of food-related attentional biases and body weight. However, few studies also measured subjective food craving or food intake and studies with child or adolescent samples are even scarcer. To our knowledge, no study to date has attempted to connect theory-derived experimental and real life predictions by reporting the assessment of all three constructs – attentional bias, state food craving, and calorie intake – in the same adolescent sample, or to explore food cue-related neural activity with ERPs and ERD. Our study therefore strived to differentiate between low- and high-calorie foods and to replicate the previously reported high-calorie food bias in satiated adolescent participants. We further hypothesized that overweight and obese adolescents would show a stronger attentional bias for high-calorie food than normal-weight controls – as evidenced by higher P300 amplitudes – and that this attentional bias would be associated with higher self-reported state food cravings and higher subsequent snack intake. In addition, overweight/obese participants should show altered ERD in response to food stimuli, representing differences in accessing semantic knowledge upon confrontation with these cues.

Methods

Overweight/obese (OW/OB) adolescents and a matched normal-weight (NW) control group between the ages of 9 and 16 years were recruited via newspaper articles, email announcements, and brochures handed to local paediatric and general practitioner practices. Inclusion criteria were an age- and gender-specific body mass index (BMI) percentile [40] ≥ 90 (OW/OB group) or ≤ 80 (NW group). Exclusion criteria were a history of seizures, compensatory weight control behaviour, psychotic symptoms, suicidality, medical conditions influencing weight and eating behaviour, and food allergies. After a diagnostic screening by phone, potential participants and a parent or guardian were invited for an in-depth diagnostic assessment. Both the adolescent and the parent or guardian gave their informed consent after the study was explained to them. Participants were informed that the exact hypotheses guiding the study could only be revealed afterwards to avoid biasing the results. All study procedures were in accordance with the Declaration of Helsinki [41] and approved by the local Ethics Committee (project number 557/2015B01).

Forty-three adolescents participated in the study. To rule out severe mental health problems, the *Diagnostic Interview for Mental Disorders in Children and Adolescents* (*Kinder-DIPS*) was administered to both the participant and the parent or guardian [42], and eating pathology was assessed by means of the diagnostic items of the *Child Eating Disorder Examination* (ChEDE [43]) as well as the *Child Eating Disorder Examination-Questionnaire (ChEDE-Q* [44]*).* In addition, all participants were measured and weighed in light clothing. EEG appointments were scheduled on a different day, usually within 2 weeks of the diagnostic assessment. To standardize hunger levels, all participants were offered an ad libitum meal before the EEG appointment. Three EEG data sets could not be analysed due to technical difficulties during data collection. Data of 12 participants (six OB/OW) had to be excluded due to excessive noise or movement artefacts, which is comparable to other EEG studies with children and adolescents [45, 46]. The final sample therefore consisted of 28 adolescents, 14 in each group. The two groups were comparable in gender distribution and mean age, but significantly different in BMI percentile standard deviation scores (SDS) and ChEDE-Q global score as well as scores on the ChEDE-Q weight concern and shape concern subscales (see Table 1).

Participants were presented with pictures of food and office supplies in random order. Food pictures were taken from the food-pics database [47], and consisted of 30 high-calorie and 30 low-calorie food items. Food images were chosen to be comparable for contrast, complexity, spatial frequency, and available palatability rating data. Neutral images consisted of 30 pictures of office supplies that were similar in form, colour, and complexity [30]. Luminance for all food and office pictures was adjusted using a modified script from the SHINE toolbox in Matlab (The MathWorks, Natick, MA) [48]. The size of all pictures was 1024 by 768 pixels. Each picture was shown once, leading to a total of 90 trials.

Participants were seated in a sound-attenuated booth with controlled lighting, 60 cm from the screen. After three practice trials to familiarize participants with the experimental design, the study assistant left the booth and picture presentation was started. In addition to the food and office supplies, participants completed a similar task viewing emotional pictures. Results for these pictures are beyond the scope of this article and are therefore not reported here. None of the emotional pictures contained food.

All pictures were displayed in the center of the screen on neutral grey background in random order for 2000 ms with the interstimulus interval (ISI) jittered to last

Table 1 Descriptive data for the overweight/obese group and the matched normal-weight control group

	Overweight/obese	Normal-weight
n (girls)	14 (*7*)	14 (*5*)
Age	12.6 (*1.5*)	13.5 (*1.7*)
BMI percentile SDS	2.2 (*0.44*)[b]	−0.25 (*0.81*)[b]
ChEDE-Q		
Global	1.6 (*1.1*)[a]	0.5 (*0.8*)[a]
Restraint	1.2 (*1.5*)	0.4 (*1.3*)
Eating Concern	1.0 (*1.3*)	0.4 (*0.6*)
Shape Concern	2.3 (*1.4*)[a]	0.7 (*0.9*)[a]
Weight Concern	2.1 (*1.1*)[b]	0.5 (*0.7*)[b]

Note. Means and SDs (in parentheses) for age, BMI percentile SDS, and eating pathology on the Child Eating Disorder Examination Questionnaire (ChEDE-Q) for the two groups. [a]marks significant differences ≤.01, [b]marks significant differences ≤.001

between 1000 ms and 1400 ms to provide an adequate active viewing and baseline duration for EEG data analysis. After each picture, a rating of current craving was collected on a continuous scale ranging from 1 (lowest rating) to 9 (highest rating) (based on 33). Participants were instructed to look at all pictures attentively and subsequently rate how much they would like to eat something at that very moment (see Fig. 1 for a visualization on the time course). Participants reported the ratings using the right index finger and a trackball mouse. It was stressed that there were no wrong answers and that the objective of the study was to simply collect participants' perception of craving at a given point in time. Short breaks were inserted every 30 trials to avoid fatigue.

After the EEG experiment, the elastic cap holding the electrodes was removed and participants were led to another room with a snack buffet consisting of ten different snack foods with a total caloric value of approximately 14, 600 kcal. Participants were told that the study was looking at which foods they liked best and that they could eat as much as they liked. They were only asked to try every item at least once and fill in a rating of preference for the different snacks. Participants were then left alone with the snack buffet for 20 min. All snacks were weighed before and afterwards to calculate the exact amount of consumed calories and macronutrients.

EEG data were collected from 64 Ag/AgCl active electrodes placed according to the extended 10–20 system using actiCap (Brain Products GmbH, Gilching, Germany). Data were recorded in relation to a midline reference electrode placed at Cz, with a sampling rate of 500 Hz. Four additional passive electrodes were placed above and below the right eye as well as on both outer canthi to monitor eye movement. Data were analysed according to current best practice recommendations for electrophysiological data [49] using FieldTrip in Matlab [50]: Data were segmented into three-second epochs around picture onset. Then, slow drifts in the EEG data were removed by de-trending, and a 50 Hz discrete Fourier transform filter was used to remove power line noise. To examine the unbiased EEG-signal, activity from each electrode was referenced to the average of all recorded electrodes. Subsequently, EEG data were visually inspected for movement and technical artefacts. Data sets in which more than 10% of the electrodes were affected by an excessive amount of artefacts were discarded. Eye movement artefacts were identified using independent component analysis (ICA, fastica algorithm) [51] and respective artefacts removed after visual inspection. Finally, noisy electrodes were replaced by the average of three neighbouring electrodes. For each condition, an average of 20 trials per participant could be analysed (neutral: mean = 20.4, low-calorie: mean = 20.4, high-calorie: mean = 20.1). There were slightly more usable trials for low-calorie stimuli in the OW/OB group (mean = 21.6) than in the NW group (mean = 19.1; $p = .04$), but when included as a covariate, this did not affect the significant interaction effects reported below.

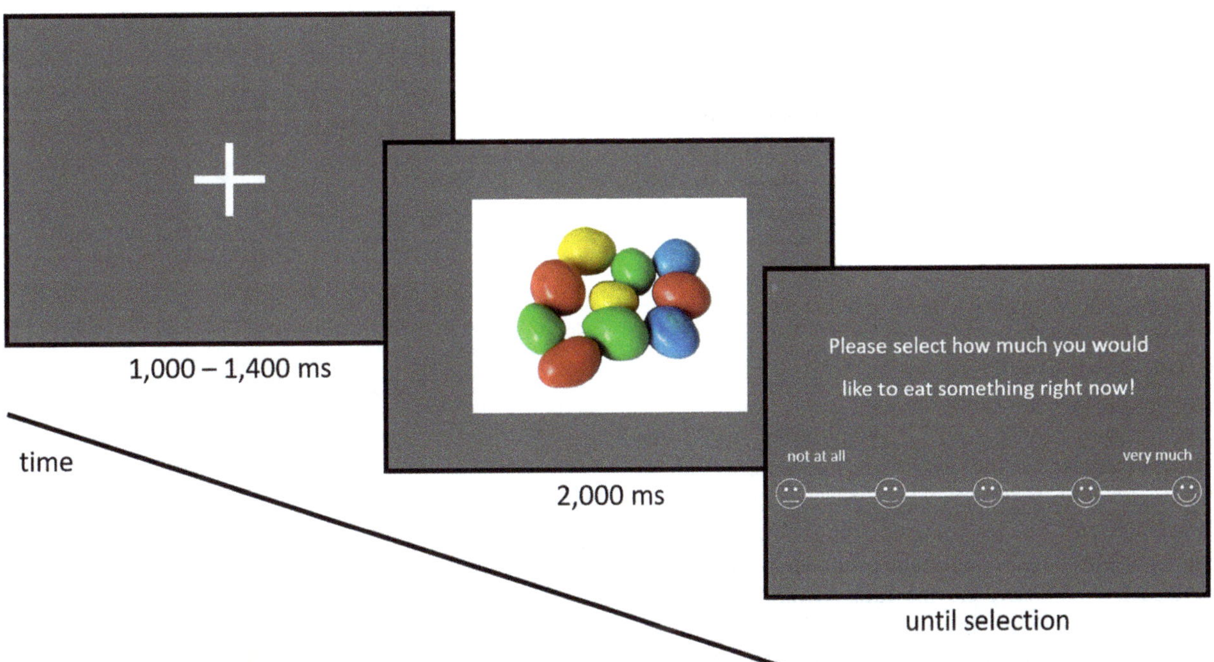

Fig. 1 Time course of one trial, high-calorie condition, with the baseline consisting of 1000–1400 ms presentation of a fixation cross, 2000 ms active picture viewing followed by the participants' response. The next trial started with the ISI after the response

For the analysis of changes in event-related potentials (ERPs), slow fluctuations and high-frequency noise were filtered out of the EEG data using a 0.1 Hz high-pass filter (Butterworth, 2nd order, 2-pass) and a 30 Hz low-pass filter (Butterworth, 4th order, 2-pass) and the average of the baseline interval (– 500 to – 100 ms prior to the stimulus onset) was subtracted from the single trial data. According to our hypothesis, we were interested in late positive ERP deflections (e.g. P300, LPP). To identify these ERP components, the EEG data were pooled across subjects and the electrodes with the largest positive peaks across all participants and conditions were identified (electrodes PO7/PO8) (see "Collapsed Localizers" in [52]). EEG data were subsequently split according to the conditions and averaged to ERPs across these electrodes within each participant. ERPs were then examined for periods of significant interaction of the between-subjects factors Group (OW/OB and NW) and the within-subjects factor Condition (neutral, low-calorie, high-calorie) in the time window from stimulus onset (0 ms) to 1000 ms using a repeated measures analysis of variance (ANOVA) at each timepoint [39, 53–55]. To account for alpha error accumulation due to multiple testing, an effect was only defined as significant if it was below $p < .05$ for at least 10 ms. [56, 57]

To estimate changes in time-frequency -resolved power, single trial EEG data were transformed into the time-frequency domain using a multitaper approach [58]. Time-frequency-resolved power (1–45 Hz, 1 Hz resolution, DPSS tapers) was calculated in steps of 10 ms (window size = 3 cycles per frequency) and the average of the baseline interval (– 500 to – 100 ms prior to the stimulus onset) was removed from the single trial data (so-called relative change). Similar to the analysis of ERPs, time-frequency power was split according to the conditions and averaged for the electrode pair PO7/PO8. It was then examined for periods of significant interaction of the between-subjects factors Group (OW/OB and NW) and the within-subjects factor Condition (neutral, low-calorie, high-calorie) in the time window from stimulus onset (0 ms) to 1000 ms using a repeated measures ANOVA [59]. To account for alpha error accumulation due to multiple testing, 3dClustSim (http://afni.nimh.nih.gov/afni/) [60, 61] was used to estimate the probability of false positives. Accordingly, an effect was only defined as significant if it was below $p < .05$ in at least 34 connected time-frequency windows.

For further analyses, ERP amplitudes and time-frequency power for the significant time windows identified in the ANOVAs were exported, averaged for each participant, and further analysed using IBM® SPSS® Statistics 24. Mean ERP amplitudes, time-frequency power, and also the subjective craving ratings were entered into mixed model analyses of variance (ANOVAs) with the between-subjects factor Group (OW/OB and NW) and the within-subjects factor Condition (neutral, low-calorie, high-calorie). Values of $p < .05$ were considered significant.

Results

Craving data

Craving ratings showed a significant main effect of Condition ($F_{(2, 52)} = 56.91$, $p < .001$, $\eta_p^2 = .69$; see Table 2 for means [*Ms*] and standard deviations [*SDs*]). Post-hoc t-tests conducted separately for Condition showed that across all participants, high-calorie food led to significantly higher mean craving ratings than low-calorie food and neutral items, which had the lowest ratings and were also significantly different from low-calorie food (all *p*-values < .001). There was no main effect of Group ($F_{(1, 26)} = 2.09$, $p = .16$, $\eta_p^2 = .07$) and no interaction of Group and Condition ($F_{(2, 52)} = 0.19$, $p = .73$, $\eta_p^2 = .01$). However, the main effect of Group became marginally significant when all participants were analysed ($F_{(1, 41)} = 4.12$, $p = .049$, $\eta_p^2 = .09$), with the NW group giving slightly higher overall ratings than the OW group.

EEG data

Event-related potentials

The data driven analysis of the event-related potential (ERP) data showed a contiguous significant interaction of Group and Condition for more than 10 ms in the time window of the P300 (276–328 ms).

The subsequent analysis of mean individual amplitudes in this time window showed a significant main effect of Condition ($F_{(2, 52)} = 8.53$, $p = .001$, $\eta_p^2 = .25$; see Table 2 for *Ms* and *SDs*). Post-hoc t-tests conducted separately for Condition showed that across all participants, high-calorie food led to

Table 2 Behavioral and EEG data for the overweight/obese group and the matched normal-weight control group

	Mean subjective craving		
	Neutral	*Low-calorie*	*High-calorie*
Overweight/obese	1.9 (*1.1*)	4.2 (*2.0*)	5.0 (*2.7*)
Normal weight	2.5 (*1.3*)	5.1 (*1.3*)	5.9 (*1.5*)
	P300 amplitude (in μV)		
	Neutral	*Low-calorie*	*High-calorie*
Overweight/obese	16.1 (*7.9*)	19.0 (*8.0*)	19.7 (*8.9*)
Normal weight	22.2 (*9.0*)	21.3 (*9.5*)	23.9 (*9.2*)
	Mean alpha power (relative change)		
	Neutral	*Low-calorie*	*High-calorie*
Overweight/obese	–.0017 (*.0051*)	–.0026 (*.0031*)	–.0011 (*.0040*)
Normal weight	–.0033 (*.0030*)	–.0011 (*.0048*)	–.0016 (*.0035*)
	Mean snack consumption		
	Calories (kcal)	*Fat (g)*	*Carbohydrates (g)*
Overweight/obese	637 (*415*)	29.7 (*19.3*)	80.7 (*54.6*)
Normal weight	558 (*217*)	24.8 (*11.1*)	72.4 (*29.4*)

Note. Means and standard deviations (in parentheses) for subjective craving, P300 amplitude, alpha power, and snack consumption, by group and condition (where applicable)

significantly higher mean amplitudes than low-calorie food ($p = .02$) and neutral items ($p < .001$). Mean amplitudes for low-calorie food and neutral items were not significantly different ($p = .15$). There was no main effect of Group ($F_{(1, 26)} = 1.71$, $p = .20$, $\eta_p^2 = .06$), but the ANOVA confirmed a significant interaction of Group × Condition ($F_{(2, 52)} = 4.56$, $p = .02$, $\eta_p^2 = .15$; see Fig. 2). Post-hoc t-tests conducted separately for Group showed that the OW/OB group displayed significantly higher mean amplitudes for high-calorie food and for low-calorie food than for neutral items ($p = .006$ and $p = .03$, respectively), with the two food categories being not significantly different ($p = .51$). In contrast, the NW group showed significantly higher mean amplitudes for high-calorie food than for low-calorie food ($p = .005$) and for neutral items ($p = .02$), with no significant difference between low-calorie food and neutral items ($p = .17$). Post-hoc t-tests furthermore showed no significant between-group differences for amplitudes regarding the two food-categories and a trend-level difference for amplitudes to neutral stimuli ($p = .07$).

Time-frequency power

Exploratory analyses were carried out to examine changes in time-frequency power. The data driven analysis showed a contiguous significant interaction of Group and Condition lasting from 220 ms to 370 ms in the alpha band (8–12 Hz), indicating differences in condition-specific event-related desynchronization (ERD) between the OW/OB and the NW groups.

The subsequent analysis of mean individual power for this frequency range and time window showed a marginally significant main effect of Condition ($F_{(2, 52)} = 3.20$, $p = .049$, $\eta_p^2 = .11$; see Table 2 for means and standard deviations). Post-hoc t-tests conducted separately for Condition showed that across all participants, high-calorie food led to significantly less mean alpha ERD than neutral stimuli ($p = .01$). Mean alpha ERD for high-calorie and low-calorie food and for low-calorie food and neutral items was not significantly different ($p = .30$ and $p = .18$, respectively). There was no main effect of Group ($F_{(1, 26)} = 0.20$, $p = .90$, $\eta_p^2 = .001$), but the ANOVA confirmed a significant interaction of Group × Condition ($F_{(2, 52)} = 5.63$, $p = .006$, $\eta_p^2 = .18$; see Fig. 3). Post-hoc t-tests conducted separately for Group showed that the OW/OB group had significantly stronger mean alpha ERD for low-calorie food than for high-calorie food ($p = .01$). There was no significant difference for the comparison of high-calorie food and of low-calorie food with neutral items ($p = .29$ and $p = .21$, respectively; see Fig. 3). In contrast, the NW group showed significantly stronger mean alpha ERD for neutral items compared to both high-calorie food and low-calorie food ($p = .02$ and $p = .006$, respectively), with no significant difference between high-calorie food and low-calorie food ($p = .58$). Post-hoc t-tests furthermore showed no significant between-group differences for any of the three categories.

Prediction of snack consumption

There was no significant difference in calorie and macronutrient consumption between the two groups. All participants consumed a substantial amount of the offered high-calorie food with a mean calorie intake of 598 kcal (range: 116 kcal to 1750 kcal). As the Group × Condition interaction for P300 amplitudes a was mainly driven by within-group differences for low-calorie food, mean P300 amplitudes, mean alpha ERD, and mean craving ratings for pictures of low-calorie food were correlated with calorie intake for the two groups. While there were no significant correlations for the NW group, the OW/OB group showed significant correlations for both self-reported craving ($r_{(12)} = 0.56$, $p = .04$) and mean P300 amplitudes ($r_{(12)} = 0.61$, $p = .02$) for pictures of low-calorie food: Participants with higher self-reported craving or higher P300 amplitudes subsequently consumed more snacks than participants with lower values on these two variables. A tendency for a negative association of alpha ERD and subsequent snack intake did not reach significance ($p = .12$).

Discussion

This study intended to examine the association of three supposedly connected concepts in a single sample of adolescents: attentional bias in response to food, self-reported state craving, and increased snack food consumption.

As hypothesized, participants showed increased attention allocation to pictures of food compared to neutral pictures, as evidenced by increased P300 amplitudes for food pictures. Surprisingly, however, a preferential processing for high-calorie food was only present in normal-weight adolescents. These participants had significantly higher P300 amplitudes when viewing high-calorie food than when viewing low-calorie food or neutral items. In contrast, overweight/obese adolescents did not show different P300 amplitudes based on the caloric value of the food pictures: This group also showed a clear distinction between food and non-food pictures, but P300 amplitudes were not different for high- and low-calorie food. This is surprising, as according to incentive-sensitization theory [9, 10] low-calorie food should be associated with weaker sensitization and thus lower cue reactivity than high-calorie food.

While the general attentional bias for food versus non-food items could thus be replicated in an adolescent sample, the most important distinction between overweight/obese and normal-weight participants does not seem to be the processing of high-calorie food, but of low-calorie food. This might help explain the lack of previous findings when investigating ERP correlates of attention allocation in response to food stimuli in obese and normal-weight participants: One study with an adult

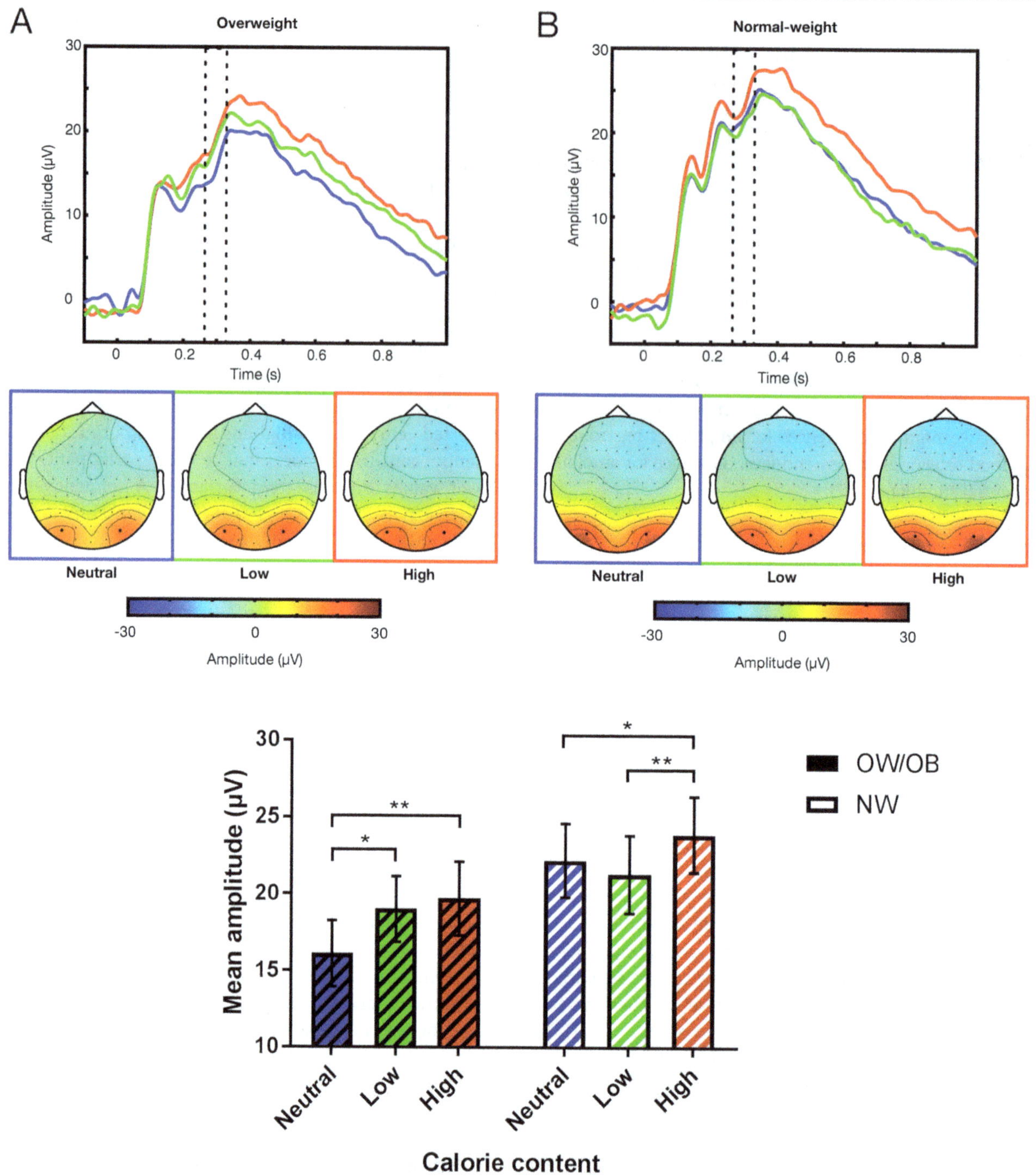

Fig. 2 Grand-average time course for the electrode pair PO7/PO8, topography, and amplitudes by group and condition. The dotted oblong marks the time window of the significant effect; black dots mark electrodes PO7 and PO8, bars denote standard errors; * marks $p < .05$, ** marks $p < .01$

sample compared high-calorie items and neutral items [25], while another study with an adolescent sample compared mixed high-/ low-calorie items and neutral items [35]. No differentiation of high-calorie and low-calorie food was made in these studies. Future studies might thus be well advised to include both high- and low-calorie food and analyse responses to these items separately.

Interestingly, the P300 group difference for low-calorie items in this study was not reflected in self-reported state craving. All adolescents reported highest state craving after viewing high-calorie items and lowest craving

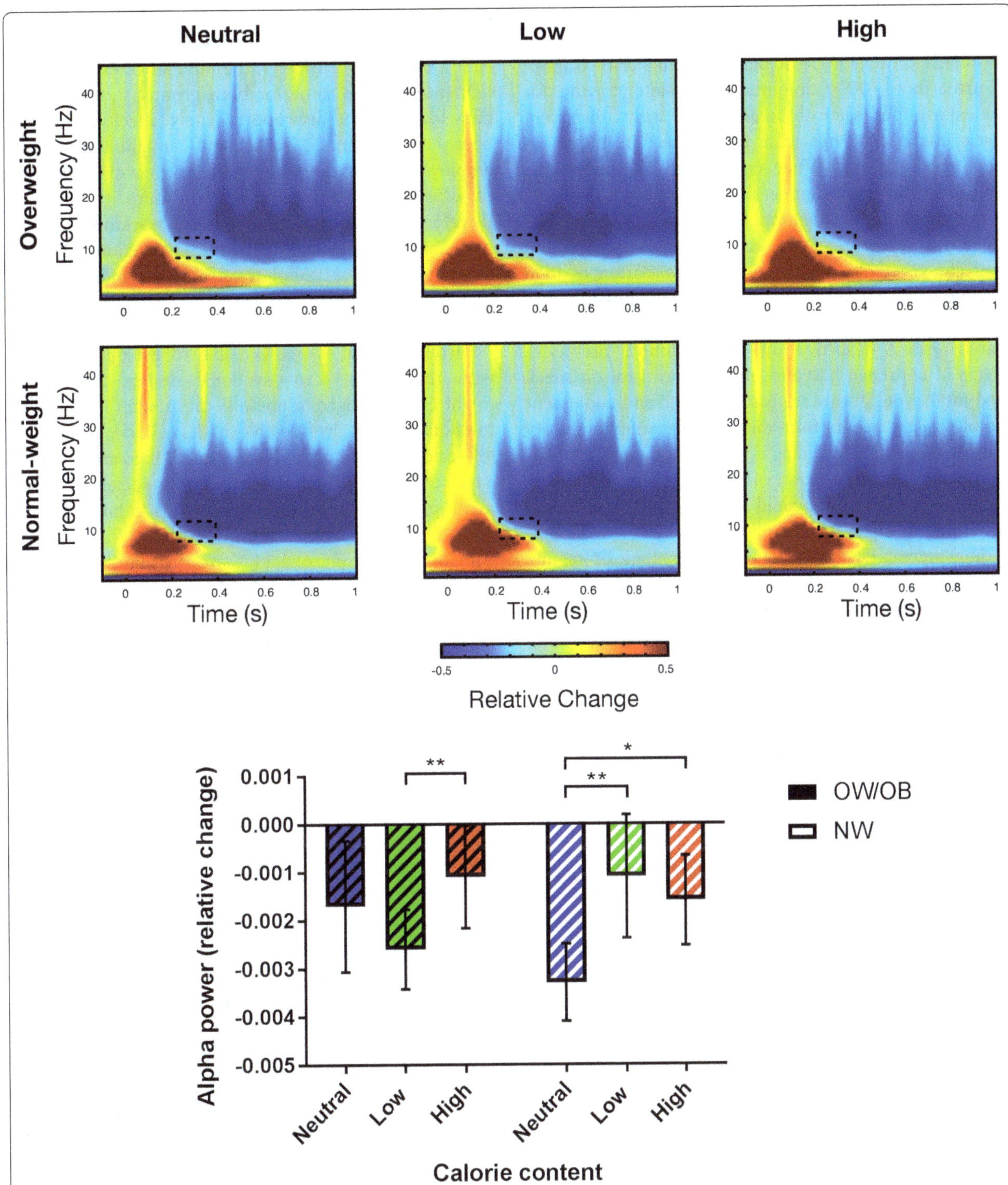

Fig. 3 Mean time-frequency power and mean alpha ERD by group and condition. The dotted oblong marks the time window and frequency range of the significant effect; bars denote standard errors; * marks $p < .05$, ** marks $p < .01$

after viewing neutral items, with craving after viewing low-calorie items in between and no difference between the two groups. Although some studies report a negative association of state craving and BMI [62, 63], these results are in line with previous findings of no association of state craving and BMI in children and adolescents [33] and in adults [14]. In line with state craving ratings, subsequent snack intake was also not significantly different between the two groups. This is surprising given previous findings of correlations between snack intake and BMI in adults [8]. However, studies with children and adolescents also report no difference [64] or even lower snack intake in participants with higher BMI [65].

Furthermore, P300 amplitude and state craving for low-calorie food seem to be associated with subsequent snack intake (but not with each other) in the overweight/obese group. While conclusions are necessarily limited by the small sample size, this association points to the possibility of attentional biases and food cravings being two independent processes triggered by increased food cue reactivity [9, 10] with the association of food cravings and subsequent snack food intake possibly mediated by inhibitory control deficits. As previous research with a healthy adult sample found interactive effects of approach bias and inhibitory control on snack food intake [66], future studies with child and adolescent samples might benefit from directly measuring inhibitory control, while also including a measure of approach bias. In contrast, the association of food cravings and subsequent snack food intake could also be reflective of an external eating style. This would be in line with studies finding increased snack intake after smelling or tasting high-calorie snacks [64] and slower habituation to high-calorie food [67] in overweight children. It might therefore be worthwhile to consider stratifying larger samples of overweight/obese children by their inhibitory control and external eating, and to investigate the possibility of different subtypes of overeating.

The analysis of ERD in the alpha band provides additional information about the processing of food stimuli in the two groups: Neutral stimuli led to strongest ERD in the normal-weight group, which can be explained by their less frequent appearance relative to food stimuli. However, the overweight/obese group showed strongest ERD for low-calorie stimuli. Since ERD was previously hypothesized to indicate access to the individual's semantic knowledge base [36], one could speculate that this might point to a link of greater semantic information and low-calorie food in the overweight/obese group as might be triggered by a social environment emphasizing eating "healthy" food in order to control their weight gain. However, future studies would have to include some measure of semantic memory processing to empirically test for this possibility.

Beyond the small sample size, the present study has several other limitations. Although all participants were demonstrated the EEG's sensitivity with regard to eye and muscle movement, and were instructed to remain as still as possible during data collection, a substantial amount of data had to be discarded due to too many noisy electrodes or movement artefacts. This leaves the possibility of a biased sample with only the less active participants providing usable data. Since there seems to be some concurrence of overeating and attention-deficit/hyperactivity disorder [68], this might have particularly affected overweight/obese adolescents with pathological eating behaviour. However, the number of excluded participants was the same for both groups, indicating that data loss did not disproportionately affect overweight/obese participants. Participants might also have employed different viewing strategies to avoid processing of some of the presented pictures. Future studies might therefore benefit from including eye tracking to ensure participants' compliance with the instructions. Alternatively, it might be useful to include an additional task that is focused on the presented pictures, although this might decrease the observable effects.

Furthermore, it is not possible to establish causality with the current cross-sectional design. Adolescents might be overweight or obese because of an inherited attraction to food irrespective of its calorie content, or low-calorie food might have gained increased importance for these participants because of social and/or familial pressure to consume these foods in an attempt to counteract their overweight or obesity. While the ERP data do not favour one of these possibilities over the other, the analysis of alpha band power actually provides some support for the latter: In the overweight/obese group, ERD was most pronounced in response to low-calorie food, which could indicate a more distinct activation of semantic knowledge [36] in response to these stimuli, as would be caused by previous experiences.

In terms of the clinical applicability of these results, giving recommendations for clinical practice is challenging. While overweight and obesity in adolescence are associated with future morbidity and mortality [69] and thus clearly need to be addressed early on, stressing the importance of consuming low-calorie food might actually lead to paradoxical effects and cause adolescents to eat more. As can be seen on the respective ChEDE-Q subscales, shape and weight concerns were increased in our overweight/obese group, which is characteristic for individuals with eating pathologies (see [70] for a review). It could therefore be speculated that seeing low-calorie food might have intensified these concerns in our overweight/obese participants, which could then have triggered increased craving and attentional bias – a possible mechanism already suggested in Williamson et al.'s influential integrated cognitive-behavioural theory of eating disorders [71]. In clinical practice, it might therefore be worthwhile to move away from the focus on nutrition and also refrain from dividing food into healthy and unhealthy or low-calorie and high-calorie categories to further weight-loss. Instead, it might be worthwhile to attempt interventions that focus on shape- and weight-related issues, e.g. mirror exposure [70], or even more unspecific approaches like mindful eating [72].

Conclusion

To conclude, this is the first study to date to combine data collection for theory-derived cognitive and real life predictions of the incentive sensitization model by assessing attentional bias, state food craving, and snack intake in the same sample while also investigating alpha band power as an informative new measure. Our data indicate that the current research focus in children and adolescents might need to be extended to the investigation of low-calorie food. While all participants showed an attentional bias for high-calorie food, it was the processing of low-calorie food that distinguished the two weight groups on both ERP and ERD measures, and predicted snack food intake in the overweight/obese group. In the future, the assessment of attentional bias to and state craving for low-calorie food in children and adolescents might thus facilitate the creation of more individualized approaches to the early prevention and treatment of overweight and obesity.

Abbreviations

ANOVA: Analysis of variance; BMI: Body mass index; ChEDE (-Q): Child Eating Disorder Examination (–Questionnaire); EEG: Electroencephalogram; ERD: Event-related desynchronization; ERP: Event-related potential; fMRI: Functional magnetic resonance imaging; ICA: Independent component analysis; ISI: Interstimulus interval; LPP: Late Positive Potential; M: Mean; NW: Normal-weight; OW/OB: Overweight/obese; SD: Standard deviation; SDS: Standard deviation score; TFR: Time-frequency response

Acknowledgements

The authors would like to thank all adolescents and their parents for participating in this study, and all students involved in participant recruitment and data collection.

Authors' contributions

SCB and JS designed the study. SCB and EN implemented the design and supervised data collection. SCB and JK analysed the data and wrote the manuscript. All authors read and approved the final manuscript.

Competing interests

The authors declare that they have no competing interests.

Author details

[1]Department of Clinical Psychology and Psychotherapy, University of Tuebingen, Schleichstrasse 4, 72076 Tuebingen, Germany. [2]Department of Clinical Psychology and Psychotherapy, University of Regensburg, Universitaetsstrasse 31, 93053 Regensburg, Germany. [3]Biological Psychology, Christian-Albrechts University, Olshausenstraße 62, 24118 Kiel, Germany.

References

1. Ng M, Fleming T, Robinson M, Thomson B, Graetz N, Margono C, et al. Global, regional, and national prevalence of overweight and obesity in children and adults during 1980-2013: a systematic analysis for the global burden of disease study 2013. Lancet. 2014;384(9945):766–81.
2. Ahluwalia N, Dalmasso P, Rasmussen M, Lipsky L, Currie C, Haug E, et al. Trends in overweight prevalence among 11-, 13-and 15-year-olds in 25 countries in Europe, Canada and USA from 2002 to 2010. Eur J Pub Health. 2015;25:28–32.
3. Wansink B. Environmental factors that increase the food intake and consumption volume of unknowing consumers. Annu Rev Nutr. 2004;24:455–79.
4. Caputo FA, Mattes RD. Human dietary responses to perceived manipulation of fat-content in a midday meal. Int J Obes. 1993;17(4):237–40.
5. Miller DL, Castellanos VH, Shide DJ, Peters JC, Rolls BJ. Effect of fat-free potato chips with and without nutrition labels on fat and energy intakes. Am J Clin Nutr. 1998;68(2):282–90.
6. Rolls BJ, Morris EL, Roe LS. Portion size of food affects energy intake in normal-weight and overweight men and women. Am J Clin Nutr. 2002;76(6):1207–13.
7. Nederkoorn C, Braet C, Van Eijs Y, Tanghe A, Jansen A. Why obese children cannot resist food: the role of impulsivity. Eat Behav. 2006;7(4):315–22.
8. Fay SH, White MJ, Finlayson G, King NA. Psychological predictors of opportunistic snacking in the absence of hunger. Eat Behav. 2015;18:156–9.
9. Berridge KC. 'Liking' and 'wanting' food rewards: brain substrates and roles in eating disorders. Physiol Behav. 2009;97(5):537–50.
10. Robinson TE, Berridge KC. The neural basis of drug craving - an incentive-sensitization theory of addiction. Brain Res Rev. 1993;18(3):247–91.
11. Rothemund Y, Preuschhof C, Bohner G, Bauknecht HC, Klingebiel R, Flor H, et al. Differential activation of the dorsal striatum by high-calorie visual food stimuli in obese individuals. Neuroimage. 2007;37(2):410–21.
12. Stoeckel LE, Weller RE, Cook EW, Twieg DB, Knowlton RC, Cox JE. Widespread reward-system activation in obese women in response to pictures of high-calorie foods. Neuroimage. 2008;41(2):636–47.
13. Murdaugh DL, Cox JE, Cook EW, Weller RE. fMRI reactivity to high-calorie food pictures predicts short- and long-term outcome in a weight-loss program. Neuroimage. 2012;59(3):2709–21.
14. Dietrich A, Hollmann M, Mathar D, Villringer A, Horstmann A. Brain regulation of food craving: relationships with weight status and eating behavior. Int J Obes. 2016;40(6):982–9.
15. Contreras-Rodriguez O, Martin-Perez C, Vilar-Lopez R, Verdejo-Garcia A. Ventral and dorsal striatum networks in obesity: link to food craving and weight gain. Biol Psychiatry. 2017;81(9):789–96.
16. Scharmüller W, Übel S, Ebner F, Schienle A. Appetite regulation during food cue exposure: a comparison of normal-weight and obese women. Neurosci Lett. 2012;518(2):106–10.
17. Castellanos EH, Charboneau E, Dietrich MS, Park S, Bradley BP, Mogg K, et al. Obese adults have visual attention bias for food cue images: evidence for altered reward system function. Int J Obes. 2009;33(9):1063–73.
18. Werthmann J, Roefs A, Nederkoorn C, Mogg K, Bradley BP, Jansen A. Can (not) take my eyes off it: attention bias for food in overweight participants. Health Psychol. 2011;30(5):561–9.
19. Picton TW. The P300 wave of the human event-related potential. J Clin Neurophysiol. 1992;9(4):456–79.
20. Polich J. Updating P300: an integrative theory of P3a and P3b. Clin Neurophysiol. 2007;118(10):2128–48.
21. Schupp HT, Flaisch T, Stockburger J, Junghofer M. Emotion and attention: event-related brain potential studies. In: Anders S, Ende G, Junghoffer M, Kissler J, Wildgruber D, editors. Understanding Emotions. Progress in Brain Research; 2006. p. 31–51.
22. Schupp HT, Junghofer M, Weike AI, Hamm AO. Emotional facilitation of sensory processing in the visual cortex. Psychol Sci. 2003;14(1):7–13.
23. Schupp HT, Cuthbert BN, Bradley MM, Cacioppo JT, Ito T, Lang PJ. Affective picture processing: the late positive potential is modulated by motivational relevance. Psychophysiology. 2000;37(2):257–61.
24. Cuthbert BN, Schupp HT, Bradley MM, Birbaumer N, Lang PJ. Brain potentials in affective picture processing: covariation with autonomic arousal and affective report. Biol Psychol. 2000;52(2):95–111.
25. Nijs IMT, Franken IHA, Muris P. Food cue-elicited brain potentials in obese and healthy-weight individuals. Eat Behav. 2008;9(4):462–70.
26. Nijs IMT, Muris P, Euser AS, Franken IHA. Differences in attention to food and food intake between overweight/obese and normal-weight females under conditions of hunger and satiety. Appetite. 2010;54(2):243–54.
27. Blechert J, Feige B, Hajcak G, Tuschen-Caffier B. To eat or not to eat? Availability of food modulates the electrocortical response to food pictures in restrained eaters. Appetite. 2010;54(2):262–8.
28. Nijs IMT, Franken IHA, Muris P. Enhanced processing of food-related pictures in female external eaters. Appetite. 2009;53(3):376–83.
29. Blechert J, Goltsche JE, Herbert BM, Wilhelm FH. Eat your troubles away: electrocortical and experiential correlates of food image processing are related to emotional eating style and emotional state. Biol Psychol. 2014;96:94–101.
30. Svaldi J, Tuschen-Caffier B, Biehl SC, Gschwendtner KM, Wolz I, Naumann E. Effects of two cognitive regulation strategies on the processing of food cues in high restrained eaters. An event-related potential study. Appetite. 2015;92:269–77.

31. Bruce AS, Holsen LM, Chambers RJ, Martin LE, Brooks WM, Zarcone JR, et al. Obese children show hyperactivation to food pictures in brain networks linked to motivation, reward and cognitive control. Int J Obes. 2010;34(10):1494–500.
32. Davids S, Lauffer H, Thoms K, Jagdhuhn M, Hirschfeld H, Domin M, et al. Increased dorsolateral prefrontal cortex activation in obese children during observation of food stimuli. Int J Obes. 2010;34(1):94–104.
33. Silvers JA, Insel C, Powers A, Franz P, Weber J, Mischel W, et al. Curbing craving: behavioral and brain evidence that children regulate craving when instructed to do so but have higher baseline craving than adults. Psychol Sci. 2014;25(10):1932–42.
34. Wu J, Willner CJ, Hill C, Fearon P, Mayes LC, Crowley MJ. Emotional eating and instructed food-cue processing in adolescents: an ERP study. Biol Psychol. 2018;132:27–36.
35. Hofmann J, Ardelt-Gattinger E, Paulmichl K, Weghuber D, Blechert J. Dietary restraint and impulsivity modulate neural responses to food in adolescents with obesity and healthy adolescents. Obesity. 2015;23(11):2183–9.
36. Klimesch W. Alpha-band oscillations, attention, and controlled access to stored information. Trends Cogn Sci. 2012;16(12):606–17.
37. Klimesch W, Fellinger R, Freunberger R. Alpha oscillations and early stages of visual encoding. Front Psychol. 2011;2:118.
38. Klimesch W. EEG alpha and theta oscillations reflect cognitive and memory performance: a review and analysis. Brain Res Rev. 1999;29(2–3):169–95.
39. Roa Romero Y, Keil J, Balz J, Niedeggen M, Gallinat J, Senkowski D. Alpha-band oscillations reflect altered multisensory processing of the McGurk illusion in schizophrenia. Front Hum Neurosci. 2016;10:Article no. 41.
40. Kromeyer-Hauschild K, Wabitsch M, Kunze D, Geller F, Geiß HC, Hesse V, et al. Perzentile für den Body-mass-Index für das Kindes-und Jugendalter unter Heranziehung verschiedener deutscher Stichproben. Monatsschrift Kinderheilkunde. 2001;149(8):807–18.
41. World Medical Association. World Medical Association Declaration of Helsinki. Ethical principles for medical research involving human subjects. Bull World Health Organ. 2001;79(4):373–4.
42. Schneider S, Unnewehr S, Margraf J, editors. Diagnostisches Interview bei psychischen Störungen im Kindes- und Jugendalter (Kinder-DIPS). 2nd ed. Heidelberg: Springer; 2009.
43. Hilbert A, Buerger A, Hartmann AS, Spenner K, Czaja J, Warschburger P. Psychometric evaluation of the eating disorder examination adapted for children. Eur Eat Disord Rev. 2013;21(4):330–9.
44. Hilbert A, Hartmann AS, Czaja J. Child Eating Disorder Examination-Questionnaire: Psychometrische Eigenschaften der deutschsprachigen Übersetzung. Klinische Diagnostik und Evaluation. 2008;1:447–63.
45. Hill C, Wu J, Crowley MJ, Fearon P. Restrictive feeding practices and adiposity are differentially related to P3b cortical responses to food stimuli in children. Appetite. 2013;63:7–17.
46. Couperus JW, Quirk C. Visual search and the N2pc in children. Atten Percept Psychophysiol. 2015;77(3):768–76.
47. Blechert J, Meule A, Busch NA, Ohla K. Food-pics: an image database for experimental research on eating and appetite. Front Psychol. 2014;5:617.
48. Willenbockel V, Sadr J, Fiset D, Horne GO, Gosselin F, Tanaka JW. Controlling low-level image properties: the SHINE toolbox. Behav Res Methods. 2010; 42(3):671–84.
49. Keil A, Debener S, Gratton G, Junghofer M, Kappenman ES, Luck SJ, et al. Committee report: publication guidelines and recommendations for studies using electroencephalography and magnetoencephalography. Psychophysiology. 2014;51(1):1–21.
50. Oostenveld R, Fries P, Maris E, Schoffelen JM. FieldTrip: open source software for advanced analysis of MEG, EEG, and invasive electrophysiological data. Comput Intell Neurosci. 2011;2011:9. Article ID 156869:9.
51. Hyvarinen A, Oja E. Independent component analysis: algorithms and applications. Neural Netw. 2000;13(4–5):411–30.
52. Luck SJ, Gaspelin N. How to get statistically significant effects in any ERP experiment (and why you shouldn't). Psychophysiology. 2017;54(1):146–57.
53. Kissler J, Herbert C. Emotion, Etmnooi, or Emitoon? - faster lexical access to emotional than to neutral words during reading. Biol Psychol. 2013;92(3):464–79.
54. Kissler J, Koessler S. Emotionally positive stimuli facilitate lexical decisions-an ERP study. Biol Psychol. 2011;86(3):254–64.
55. Schurger A, Cowey A, Cohen JD, Treisman A, Tallon-Baudry C. Distinct and independent correlates of attention and awareness in a hemianopic patient. Neuropsychologia. 2008;46(8):2189–97.
56. Picton TW, Bentin S, Berg P, Donchin E, Hillyard SA, Johnson R, et al. Guidelines for using human event-related potentials to study cognition: recording standards and publication criteria. Psychophysiology. 2000;37(2):127–52.
57. Guthrie D, Buchwald JS. Significance testing of difference potentials. Psychophysiology. 1991;28(2):240–4.
58. Mitra PP, Pesaran B. Analysis of dynamic brain imaging data. Biophys J. 1999;76(2):691–708.
59. Roa Romero Y, Keil J, Balz J, Gallinat J, Senkowski D. Reduced frontal theta oscillations indicate altered crossmodal prediction error processing in schizophrenia. J Neurophysiol. 2016;116(3):1396–407.
60. Cox RW. AFNI: software for analysis and visualization of functional magnetic resonance neuroimages. Comput Biomed Res. 1996;29:162–73.
61. Keil J, Pomper U, Feuerbach N, Senkowski D. Temporal orienting precedes intersensory attention and has opposing effects on early evoked brain activity. Neuroimage. 2017;148:230–9.
62. Ferrer-Garcia M, Pla-Sanjuanelo J, Dakanalis A, Vilalta-Abella F, Riva G, Fernandez-Aranda F, et al. Eating behavior style predicts craving and anxiety experienced in food-related virtual environments by patients with eating disorders and healthy controls. Appetite. 2017;117:284–93.
63. Gearhardt AN, Rizk MT, Treat TA. The association of food characteristics and individual differences with ratings of craving and liking. Appetite. 2014;79:166–73.
64. Jansen A, Theunissen N, Slechten K, Nederkoorn C, Boon B, Mulkens S, et al. Overweight children overeat after exposure to food cues. Eat Behav. 2003; 4(2):197–209.
65. Hofmann J, Meule A, Reichenberger J, Weghuber D, Ardelt-Gattinger E, Blechert J. Crave, like, eat: determinants of food intake in a sample of children and adolescents with a wide range in body mass. Front Psychol. 2016;7:1389.
66. Kakoschke N, Kemps E, Tiggemann M. Combined effects of cognitive bias for food cues and poor inhibitory control on unhealthy food intake. Appetite. 2015;87:358–64.
67. Epstein LH, Robinson JL, Temple JL, Roemmich JN, Marusewski A, Nadbrzuch R. Sensitization and habituation of motivated behavior in overweight and non-overweight children. Learn Motiv. 2008;39(3):243–55.
68. Egbert AH, Wilfley DE, Eddy KT, Boutelle KN, Zucker N, Peterson CB, et al. Attention-deficit/hyperactivity disorder symptoms are associated with overeating with and without loss of control in youth with overweight/obesity. Child Obes. 2018;14(1):50–7.
69. Park MH, Falconer C, Viner RM, Kinra S. The impact of childhood obesity on morbidity and mortality in adulthood: a systematic review. Obes Rev. 2012;13(11):985–1000.
70. Ahrberg M, Trojca D, Nasrawi N, Vocks S. Body image disturbance in binge eating disorder: a review. Eur Eat Disord Rev. 2011;19(5):375–81.
71. Williamson DA, White MA, York-Crowe E, Stewart TM. Cognitive-behavioral theories of eating disorders. Behav Modif. 2004;28(6):711–38.
72. Kumar S, Croghan IT, Biggs BK, Croghan K, Prissel R, Fuehrer D, et al. Family-based mindful eating intervention in adolescents with obesity: a pilot randomized clinical trial. Children-Basel. 2018;5:7.

Body mass index and self-reported body image in German adolescents

Lea Sarrar[1,2*], Marie Vilalta[1], Nora Schneider[3] and Christoph U. Correll[3,4,5]

Abstract

Background: Despite knowledge about eating disorder symptoms in children and adolescents in the general population, relatively little is known about self-reported and sex-specific eating-disorder-related psychopathology, as well as its specific correlates.

Methods: 880 German school-attending adolescents (15.4 ± 2.2 years) and 30 female patients with AN (16.2 ± 1.6 years) were studied. All participants completed the Eating Disorder Inventory-2 and a Body Image Questionnaire.

Results: There were more overweight males than females (15.2% vs 10.1%, $p < 0.001$), but more females with underweight than males (6.2% vs. 2.5%, $p < .001$). Negative body evaluations ($p < .001$) and dissatisfaction (p < .001) were significantly more frequent in females. Compared to underweight female patients with AN, underweight school-attending females had less negative body evaluations ($p < .001$) and lower scores on 5 of the 11 EDI-2 subscales (p < .001; $p < .05$).

Conclusions: Males were more overweight than females, females more underweight. Body image was more important to female than to male youth, yet without reaching pathological values when compared to female patients with AN. Complex emotional and cognitive challenges seem to be a representative factor for eating pathology rather than simply being underweight. These aspects may be relevant for the shift from a thinness-related focus in girls in the general population to the development of an eating disorder.

Keywords: Body mass index, Body image, Adolescents, Underweight, Overweight

Plain English summary

Still too little is known about eating disorder-related psychopathology and its correlates in non-clinical samples, especially with regard to self-report and sex-related differences. Therefore, 880 German school-attending adolescents and 30 female patients with anorexia nervosa (AN) were observed. Males were more overweight than females, females more underweight. Body image was more important to female than to male youth, yet without reaching pathological values. Personality characteristics seem to be maintenance factors in eating disorder pathology, rather than solely being underweight. These aspects may be relevant for the shift from a thinness-related focus in girls in the general population to the development of an eating disorder.

Background

Disturbed eating behaviours have become a serious concern among adolescents [1]. Severe weight concerns, disordered eating symptoms, and body shape perception disturbances have been reported across cultures [2, 3]. During the last decades a drive for thinness [4] as well as an increasing prevalence of obesity [5] and metabolic syndrome [6] have been observed. Clinically relevant eating disorders are among the most frequent chronic illnesses in adolescents [7]. For the German population,

* Correspondence: lea.sarrar@medicalschool-berlin.de
[1]Department of Psychology, Medical School Berlin, Germany, Rüdesheimer Straße 50, 14197 Berlin, Germany
[2]Department of Audiology and Phoniatrics, Charité University Medicine Berlin, Augustenburger Platz 1, 13353 Berlin, Germany
Full list of author information is available at the end of the article

prevalence estimates differ for any threshold eating disorder between 2.9% among females and 0.1% among males, for any subthreshold eating disorder between 2.2% for females and 0.7% for males, and for eating disorder symptoms between 11.5% among females and 1.8% among males [8]. These figures are consistent with those reported in other Western countries [9].

Previous research has demonstrated a high occurrence of disordered eating behaviours in adolescents and suggested the importance of examining preclinical symptoms [10]. Important indicators for eating-disorder-related disturbances are body mass index (BMI; body weight/ body height^2), body image, eating disorder and related psychopathology, such as clinically relevant perfectionism. In this context, body image refers to the perception of oneself and combines perceptual and cognitive-affective components [11]. A distorted body image is part of the diagnostic criteria of AN [12, 13] and body image dissatisfaction and distortion as well as excessive weight concerns are causally or consequently associated with eating disorders. However, whether body dissatisfaction plays a causal role may vary depending on age and sex [14, 15]. Current findings suggest that body image dissatisfaction is becoming more normative and that sex differences, which implicated females as being more underweight and concerned about body shape and fatness, may be decreasing [2]. Importantly, disordered eating behaviours are associated with an increased risk of further health-compromising behaviours, such as suicide and substance use [16–18]. Thus, the evaluation of non-clinical samples provides an opportunity to observe trends in prevalence and severity of unhealthy BMI status, eating disorders as well as weight and shape concerns, which is important for prevention and treatment programming.

Thus, we aimed to examine BMI, body image, eating-disorder-related psychopathology in a school-attending sample of adolescents and to further compare a subset of the school-attending females who were underweight with a clinical sample of patients with AN. Furthermore, we also aimed to replicate previous results with regard to underweight and overweight among adolescents in Germany. At the same time, we aimed to extend prior findings by applying a multidimensional, including self-reported, assessment battery to males and females, including measurements of body image, eating-disorder-related psychopathology. According to prior findings, we hypothesized a higher occurrence of underweight in females. Furthermore, we assumed less eating-disorder-related psychopathology in the underweight school-attending females compared to female patients with AN.

Method

Study population

The study population (Table 1) consisted of 880 school-attending adolescents, of whom 30 school-attending females and 10 school-attending males were underweight ($\leq 10^{th}$ BMI percentile; see 3.4 below). Therefore, a small and comparable size of sex-matched female patients with AN ($n = 30$) was used for further comparisons with the underweight school-attending females.

Adolescents were recruited through German schools. After having received permission to conduct the study, students were asked to complete the questionnaires during class. The order of assessment administration was varied to avoid sequence effects.

Inclusion criteria for the female patients were meeting the diagnostic criteria of an AN (307.1) according to the Diagnostic and Statistical Manual-V (DSM-V [12]). Exclusion criteria were the presence of another eating disorder according to the DSM-V [12]. The AN diagnosis was confirmed by a structured interview based on DSM (SIAB-EX [19];). Female patients were recruited from the Department for Child and Adolescent Psychiatry, Psychosomatics and Psychotherapy, Charité University Medicine, Berlin.

Measures

Body height (in meters) and body weight (in kg) were measured with participants wearing lightweight clothing and no shoes by a digital balance scale (manufacturer 'Korona', max. 150 kg), and a conventional stadiometer. Subsequently, the BMI (body weight/ body height^2) and BMI percentiles were calculated as described by Kromeyer-Hauschild et al. [20]. We defined extreme underweight as being $\leq 3^{rd}$ BMI percentile, underweight as between the $> 3^{rd}$ and $\leq 10^{th}$ BMI percentile (≤ 17.5 kg/m^2 for adolescents ≥ 18 years), overweight $> 90^{th}$ to $\leq 97^{th}$ BMI percentile, and obesity $> 97^{th}$ BMI percentile (more than ≥ 25 to 29.9 kg/m^2 and ≥ 30 kg/m^2 for adolescents ≥ 18 years, respectively).

The Body Image Questionnaire [21] is a self-report device assessing clinically relevant body image distortions as well as non-clinical impairments of body image with a two-factor structure [21]. One scale contains items on the negative evaluation of one's body, the other scale items on the positive perception of one's body. For this study and the associated research questions, we only included the sum and the mean score of the scale "*Negative Evaluations of the Body*" as a measure of body image. The internal consistency of the FKB-20 is good (Cronbach's $\alpha = .84$) indicating its reliability [21].

The Eating Disorder Inventory-2 [22] is a self-report questionnaire assessing eating-disorder-related psychopathology. It contains 11 scales: *Drive for Thinness* (DT), *Bulimia* (B), *Body Dissatisfaction* (BD), *Ineffectiveness* (I), *Perfectionism* (P), *Interpersonal Distrust* (ID), *Interoceptive Awareness* (IA), *Maturity Fears* (MF), *Asceticism* (A), *Impulse Regulation* (IR), *Social Insecurity* (SI). Internal consistency of the scales is satisfactory (Cronbach's $\alpha = .61\text{-}.89$, for eating disorder samples, $\alpha = .73\text{-}.93$ [22]).

Statistical analyses

BMI was calculated for all subjects and categorized into under-, normal- and overweight according to BMI percentiles outlined by Kromeyer-Hauschild et al. [20]. General characteristics of the sample were compared by unpaired t-tests. For the FKB-20, we considered sum scores for the analyses, with regard to EDI-2 age- and sex-adjusted percentiles. FKB-20 and EDI-2 values were divided into quartiles and the groups within these quartiles were compared. Furthermore, for the comparison of underweight girls and patients with AN the subdivision into percentiles was performed. Comparisons of FKB-20 and EDI-2 scores were conducted using Mann-Whitney-U-tests. Additionally, differences between FKB-20 and EDI-2 scores in sex-specific body weight groups were analysed using Kruskal-Wallis-Test. The level of significance was $\alpha = 0.05$ for all statistical tests that were conducted in SPSS 25. In order to avoid the Type I error, post-hoc Bonferroni corrections (adjusted significance level $\alpha = .004$) were applied.

Results

BMI percentiles and groups

Altogether, in the school-attending sample, 0.8% were extremely underweight, 3.8% were underweight, 83.0% were normal weight, 8.6% were overweight and 3.8% were obese (Fig. 1). Significantly more females than males (6.2% vs. 2.5%, $p < .001$) were extremely underweight or underweight (≤ 10th BMI percentile), whereas more school-attending males than females (15.2% vs 10.1%, $p < .001$) were overweight or obese (≥ 90th BMI percentile). All female patients with AN were below the 10th BMI percentile.

Sex-specific findings on body image and eating-disorder-related psychopathology

Based on Mann-Whitney-U tests, we found significantly higher values among school-attending females for the FKB-20 and on the EDI-2 scales DT, BD and I than in school-attending males. Conversely, school-attending males scored significantly higher on the EDI subscale P (Table 2).

Sex-specific findings on body image and eating-disorder-related psychopathology within individual weight percentile groups

Dividing each group according to weight percentiles (extreme underweight/underweight, normal weight and overweight/obese), Kruskal-Wallis-analyses revealed differences between weight percentile groups in school-attending males and in school-attending females for the FKB-20 as well as for the EDI scales, and BD (Table 3).

Comparison of underweight school-attending males and females and school-attending females with female patients with AN

Based on the weight percentile groups, we compared the school-attending males ($n = 10$) and females ($n = 30$) who were underweight (≤ 10th percentile) as well as female patients with AN ($n = 30$). Pairwise comparisons for males vs. females who were underweight (Mann-Whitney-U) revealed no significant group differences. Comparing female patients with AN to school-attending females with underweight (Table 4), we found significantly higher scores for the AN group regarding the

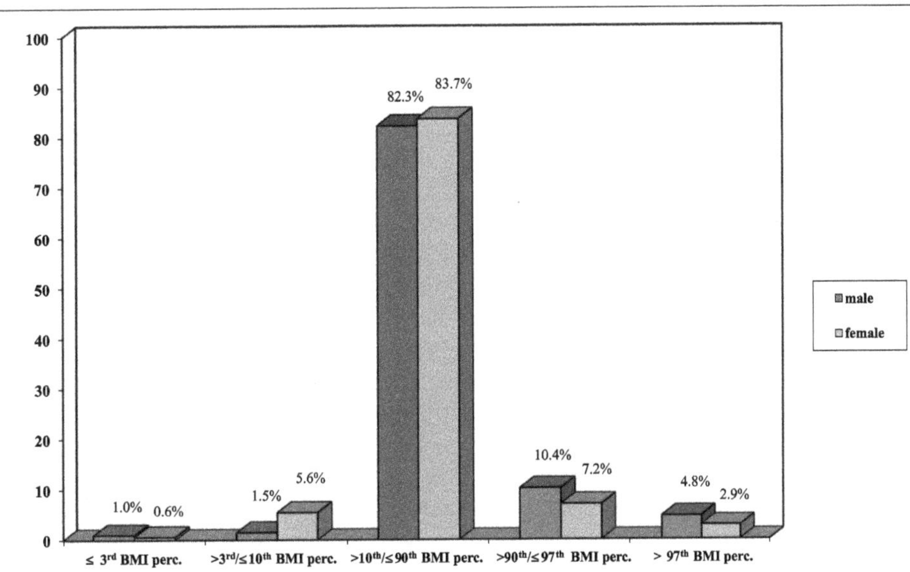

Fig. 1 (Extreme) underweight, normal weight, overweight and obesity in adolescents (school-attending sample, $n = 880$)

Table 1 General characteristics of the school-attending and anorexia nervosa sample

Variable	Total school-attending Sample	School-attending females (M ± SD)	School-attending males (M ± SD)	Female patients with AN (M ± SD)	School-attending males vs. School-attending females *p*-Value°	School-attending females vs. female patients with AN
	$n = 880$	$n = 486$	$n = 394$	$n = 30$		
Age		15.4 ± 2.2	15.3 ± 2.2	16.2 ± 1.6	.835	.008**
Height		1.67 ± 0.7	1.76 ± 0.1	1.67 ± 0.1	.665	< .001***
Weight		58.5 ± 10.6	67.9 ± 14.2	42.5 ± 5.9	< .001***	< .001***
BMI		20.9 ± 3.0	21.7 ± 3.2	15.3 ± 1.4	< .001***	< .001***
BMI percent.		54.5 ± 26.6	63.6 ± 24.2	1.3 ± 2.1	< .001***	< .001***

Notes: *n* = number, *M* mean, *SD* standard deviation, *m* meters, *kg* kilogram, °unpaired t-Tests; ** $p < .01$; *** $p < .001$

FKB-20 as well as on the following EDI-2 subscales: DT, BD, IA, A, and ID.

Discussion

BMI, body image and eating-disorder-related psychopathology

Our findings revealed that 15.2% of male and 10.1% of female adolescents in our school-attending study population were *overweight or obese*. These data are comparable with data by a recent German study as well as European and international studies [5, 23–25]. Although there is some evidence that the rise in the prevalence of overweight and obesity is plateauing [5, 26, 27], prevalence rates are still high and general shifts in the BMI-distribution were found during the last decades [27]. The National Health and Nutrition Examination Survey reported a significantly increasing linear trend in obesity between 1999 and 2000 and 2015-2016, in both adults and youth in the US [28].

Underweight status was more prevalent among school-attending females (6.2%) than school-attending males (2.5%) and occurred less often than overweight/obesity in our study. Accordingly, Schienkiewitz et al. [29] observed comparable rates of underweight in children and adolescents, although no sex differences were found. Nevertheless, other studies have shown sex differences with more underweight in females than males (for example Grajda et al. [30]). Sex differences regarding over- and underweight may result from underlying sociocultural and psychological differences. For instance, males and females differ in calorie consumption, eating styles [31] and body fat distribution [32]. Additionally, females experience more body weight and thinness-oriented body dissatisfaction than males [2, 33].

Our finding regarding more prevalent negative *body evaluations and body dissatisfaction* in school-attending females than school-attending males contrasts with other studies that reported an equal distribution of body dissatisfaction among both boys and girls [2, 34, 35]. However, these studies also report a significantly more thinness-oriented dissatisfaction among females, but also a more muscle-oriented dissatisfaction among males [2, 34, 35].

Regarding *eating-disorder-related psychopathology* we found more ineffectiveness in school-attending females compared with school-attending males which is in line with other findings [36] and could be related to negative body evaluations and body dissatisfaction in the school-attending females in the present study. Surprisingly there was more perfectionism in the school-attending males. It is possible that this finding may also be associated with body-related dissatisfaction in males, but as reported, this finding seems to be more related to a (male-specific) kind of body ideal and dissatisfaction in terms of drive for muscularity than thinness [2, 34, 35]. However, these specific aspects cannot be operationalised with the commonly utilized measures that were used in this study.

Results regarding *body image and eating-disorder-related psychopathology within* the groups of males and females and *individual weight percentile groups* demonstrated that significant differences were found only on body image-related scales. Both sexes showed more body image dissatisfaction in the presence of underweight than in the presence of normal or overweight. This finding is consistent with other studies [37] and underlines that body image dissatisfaction and eating disorder psychopathology are strongly linked, even in school-attending samples.

A *comparison of the underweight school-attending females and female patients with AN* showed greater body image dissatisfaction for the latter. In addition, female patients with AN showed significantly higher scores on the EDI-2 scales of interpersonal distrust, interoceptive awareness and asceticism, pointing out complex emotional and cognitive challenges. The increased values on the eating-disorder-related scales could indicate that these aspects are specific to the eating disorder psychopathology, rather than the underweight status itself. In order to assess eating-disorder-related psychopathology among young people in the general population, the underlying factors mentioned above should be focused on in addition to exclusively screening for drive for thinness [38, 39].

Table 2 Sex-specific findings on body image and eating-disorder-related psychopathology

Variable	Quartile	School-attending males	School-attending females	p-Value°
FKB-20 *Negative Evaluations of the Body*		n = 394	n = 486	< .001*
	1.	13.0	15.0	
	2.	16.0	20.0	
	3.	20.0	26.0	
EDI-D		n = 223[1]	n = 338[1]	< .001*
	1.	0	0	
	2.	0	0	
	3.	0	0.4	
EDI-B	1.	0	0	.414
	2.	0	0	
	3.	0	0	
EDI-BD	1.	0	0	< .001*
	2.	0.1	0.4	
	3.	0. 3	1.1	
EDI-I	1.	0	0	< .001*
	2.	0.1	0.1	
	3.	0.2	0.3	
EDI-P	1.	0.3	0.0	< .001*
	2.	0.5	0.3	
	3.	1.0	0.7	
EDI-ID	1.	0	0	.009
	2.	0.1	0	
	3.	0.4	0.4	
EDI-IA	1.	0	0	.251
	2.	0	0.1	
	3.	0.2	0.2	
EDI-MF	1.	0.3	0.4	.351
	2.	0.5	0.5	
	3.	0.9	0.9	
EDI-A	1.	0	0	.256
	2.	0	0.1	
	3.0	0.3	0.3	
EDI-IR	1.	0	0	.549
	2.	0	0.1	
	3.	0.3	0.3	
EDI-SI	1.	0	0	.440
	2.	0.3	0.3	
	3.	0.5	0.5	

Notes: *n* number, [1]reduced n due to missing data, *FKB-20* Body Image Questionnaire, *EDI* Eating Disorder Inventory-2, °Mann-Whitney-U-test; *$p < .004$ (significant group difference after Bonferroni correction)

Strengths and limitations

When interpreting the results of this study, certain limitations have to be taken into account. First, we used self-report questionnaires. Methodologically, the additional use of a structured interview in our school-attending sample would have been advantageous. Nevertheless, the fact of testing during school days and the related lack of time did not allow for time-consuming individual interviews in such a large sample. For the same reason, we were not able to diagnose any serious

Table 3 Sex-specific findings body image and eating-disorder-related psychopathology within individual weight percentile groups

School-attending males						**School-attending females**			
Variable		**≤ 10th BMI percentile**	**> 10th to ≤ 90th BMI percentile**	**> 90th BMI percentile**	**p-Value°**	**≤ 10th BMI percentile**	**> 10th to ≤ 90th BMI percentile**	**> 90th BMI percentile**	**p-Value°**
	Quartile	*n* = 10	*n* = 324	*n* = 60		*n* = 30	*n* = 407	*n* = 49	
FKB-20 *Negative Evaluations of the Body*	1.	13.3	13.0	15.0	< .001*	14.0	15.0	19.5	< .001*
	2.	15.0	15.0	19.0		18.0	19.0	23.0	
	3.	18.0	19.0	24.0		22.5	26.0	32.0	
EDI-DT		*n* = 5[1]	*n* = 187[1]	*n* = 31[1]	*n* = 223[1]	*n* = 22[1]	*n* = 276[1]	*n* = 40[1]	*n* = 338[1]
	1.	0	0	0	< .001*	0	0	0	< .001*
	2.	0	0	0.1		0	0	0.3	
	3.	0	0	0.4		0	0.4	0.9	
EDI-B	1.	0	0	0	.648	0	0	0	.601
	2.	0	0	0		0	0	0	
	3.	0.1	0	0		0	0	0	
EDI-BD	1.	0	0	0.3	< .001*	0	0	0.4	< .001*
	2.	0	0	0. 8		0.2	0.4	1.1	
	3.	0. 6	0.3	1.3		0.6	1.0	2.0	
EDI-I	1.	0	0	0	.264	0	0	0	.414
	2.	0.2	0	0.1		0.2	0.1	0.2	
	3.	0.5	0.2	0.3		0.3	0.3	0.4	
EDI-P	1.	0.5	0.3	0.2	.828	0	0	0	.661
	2.	0.5	0.7	0.3		0.3	0.3	0.3	
	3.	1.7	1.0	0.5		0.6	0.7	0.7	
EDI-ID	1.	0.1	0.3	0.2	.373	0	0	0	.330
	2.	0.4	0.7	0.3		0	0	0	
	3.	0.8	1.0	0.5		0.1	0.3	0.3	
EDI-IA	1.	0	0	0	.102	0	0	0	.410
	2.	0	0	0.1		0	0.1	0.1	
	3.	0.1	0.2	0.3		0.2	0.2	0.3	
EDI-MF	1.	0.3	0.3	0.4	.380	0.2	0.4	0.3	.218
	2.	0.6	0.5	0.5		0.4	0.5	0.5	
	3.	1.6	0.8	1.0		0.8	0.9	0.8	
EDI-A	1.	0	0	0	.112	0	0	0	.010
	2.	0	0	0.1		0	0.1	0.3	
	3.	0.3	0.3	0.4		0.1	0.3	0.5	
EDI-IR	1.	0	0	0	.818	0	0	0	.546
	2.	0	0	0.1		0.1	0	0.1	
	3.	0.6	0.3	0.2		0.3	0.3	0.3	
EDI-SI	1.	0.1	0	0.1	.621	0	0	0	.578
	2.	0.3	0.3	0.3		0.4	0.3	0.3	
	3.	0.9	0.5	0.5		0.5	0.5	0.7	

Notes: *n* number, [1]reduced n due to missing data, *FKB-20* Body Image Questionnaire, *EDI* Eating Disorder Inventory-2, °Kruskal-Wallis; *$p < .004$ (significant group difference after Bonferroni correction)

Table 4 Differences between school-attending females with underweight and female patients with AN

Variable	Percentile	School-attending females ≤ 10th BMI percentile	Female patients with AN ≤ 10th BMI percentile	p-Value°
		$n = 30$	$n = 29$[1]	< .001*
FKB-20 *Negative Evaluations of the Body*	25.	14.0	24.5	
	50.	18.0	34.0	
	75.	22.5	40.5	
		$n = 22$[1]	$n = 30$	< .001*
EDI-DT	25.	0	0.4	
	50.	0	1.1	
	75.	0	2.1	
EDI-B	25.	0	0	.151
	50.	0	0	
	75.	0	0.3	
EDI-BD	25.	0	0.8	< .001*
	50.	0.2	1.2	
	75.	0.6	1.6	
EDI-I	25.	0	0.1	.005
	50.	0.2	0.7	
	75.	0.3	1.1	
EDI-P	25.	0	0.3	.030
	50.	0.3	0.7	
	75.	0.6	1.0	
EDI-ID	25.	0	0	.004*
	50.	0	0.1	
	75.	0.1	0.6	
EDI-IA	25.	0	0.1	< .001*
	50.	0	0.4	
	75.	0.2	0.6	
EDI-MF	25.	0.2	0.4	.202
	50.	0.4	0.5	
	75.	0.8	0.9	
EDI-A	25.	0	0.3	< .001*
	50.	0	0.4	
	75.	0.1	0.6	
EDI-IR	25.	0	0	.698
	50.	0.1	0.1	
	75.	0.3	0.3	
EDI-SI	25.	0	0.1	.035
	50.	0.4	0.6	
	75.	0.5	1.1	

Notes: *n* number, [1]reduced n due to missing data, *FKB-20* Body Image Questionnaire, *EDI* Eating Disorder Inventory-2, *AN* anorexia nervosa, °Mann-Whitney-U-test; *$p < .004$ (significant group difference after Bonferroni correction)

eating disorders according to the DSM-V [12] in our school-attending sample. Therefore, we cannot eliminate the possibility of clinically relevant eating disorders in the underweight subgroup and it could be false negatives in the school-attending sample. In addition, underweight school-attending females and males in this study may have eating disorder psychopathology with a different severity or duration than those of patients with AN. Due to different and partly small age subgroup sizes in the school-attending survey sample, we have not carried out analyses within these groups, so that the results regarding under- and overweight as well as obesity only apply to the entire sample. As we only screened for underweight and overweight/obesity and the only disease control group was represented by female patients with AN, we cannot generalize our data to other forms of disordered eating behaviour, such as bulimic or binge eating symptoms. Furthermore, we did not collect information about the subtype of AN (restrictive/binge-purge). Moreover, as we did not collect information about the sociodemographic information of all attendees of the schools from which our school-attending sample was drawn, the degree of representativeness of the sample is unclear. Nevertheless, the sex distribution and body measures in our school-attending sample did match well with the previously reported epidemiological data in Germany [40, 41]. In addition, the small size of the patients with AN as well as underweight school-attending females and males limits the representativeness of these samples and generalization of the related findings. Moreover, no control group with AN was available for the underweight school-attending males of our sample. Due to the sample size compared to studies with an epidemiological approach, findings of the present study regarding over- and underweight as well as obese have to be interpreted very carefully. In addition, our data must be treated with caution, as the BMI percentile calculations are based on a reference group from data sets from between 1985 and 1999 [20]. A shift in these percentiles seems possible. Besides, because of the cross-sectional nature of our study we are not able to evaluate if underweight, body image dissatisfaction or other factors could be predictors of eating disorder symptoms.

Despite these limitations, strengths of this study include its relatively large sample size of the school-attending cohort, the multidimensional assessment of body image, eating-disorder-related psychopathology, body height and body weight, and the control group of female patients with AN.

Conclusion

We observed sex differences in the prevalence of (extreme) underweight and overweight/obese in a German school-attending sample. Body image concerns were more prevalent among school-attending females than males. Underweight by itself does not seem to be a representative factor for eating pathology, as female patients with AN differed significantly from school-attending females with underweight in psychopathological factors. These findings underline the importance of a multidimensional assessment of body image and eating-disorder-related psychopathology including self-reports when characterizing an underweight as well as potentially eating disordered sample. Therefore, the evaluation of these aspects in non-clinical samples is important to detect current prevalence rates, and trends in behaviours and attitudes. Further studies should focus on these issues instead of exclusively screening for BMI in non-clinical samples as well as patients with AN. Preventive and treatment programmes should be based on knowledge of underweight and dissatisfaction with body image, but should also focus on emotional, cognitive and personal temperament factors who may be involved in the development of eating disorders. Psychotherapeutic approaches in the treatment of AN and measurement of psychotherapy success should urgently focus these factors in addition to focusing in the key outcome of weight gain and weight restoration. For all, preventive and treatment programmes as well as psychotherapeutic approaches it could be helpful to take personality functions into account as they are described by the Operationalized Psychodynamic Diagnostic System [42] and associated with a lot of psychological disorders in childhood and adolescence including eating disorders [43, 44]. Regarding body dissatisfaction there are indications for a significantly more muscularity-related body ideal in boys [2, 34, 35], which should be deepening investigated in future studies. Existing test instruments should be adapted to these findings.

Abbreviations

A: Asceticism; AN: Anorexia nervosa; B: Bulimia; BD: Body Dissatisfaction; BMI: Body Mass Index; DSM: Diagnostic and Statistical Manual; DT: Drive for Thinness; EDI-2: Eating Disorder Inventory-2; FKB-20: Body image questionnaire; I: Ineffectiveness; IA: Interoceptive Awareness; ID: Interpersonal Distrust; IR: Impulse Regulation; MF: Maturity Fears; P: Perfectionism; SI: Social Insecurity

Authors' contributions

All authors (LS, MV, NS, CC) have participated in the research, have reviewed and agreed with the content of the article. Conceived and designed the experiments: LS NS. Performed the experiments: LS NS. Analysed the data: LS NS. Wrote the paper: LS MV NS CC.

Competing interests

Prof. Dr. Correll has been a consultant and/or advisor to or has received honoraria from: Alkermes, Allergan, Angelini, Boehringer-Ingelheim, Gedeon Richter, Gerson Lehrman Group, Indivior, IntraCellular Therapies, Janssen/J&J, LB Pharma, Lundbeck, MedAvante-ProPhase, Medscape, Merck, Neurocrine, Noven, Otsuka, Pfizer, Recordati, Rovi, Servier, Sumitomo Dainippon, Sunovion, Supernus, Takeda, and Teva. He has provided expert testimony for Bristol-Myers Squibb, Janssen, and Otsuka. He served on a Data Safety Monitoring Board for Boehringer-Ingelheim, Lundbeck, Rovi, Supernus, and Teva. He received royalties from UpToDate and grant support from Janssen and Takeda. He is also a shareholder of LB Pharma.

All other authors have declared that they have no competing or potential conflicts of interest.

Author details
[1]Department of Psychology, Medical School Berlin, Germany, Rüdesheimer Straße 50, 14197 Berlin, Germany. [2]Department of Audiology and Phoniatrics, Charité University Medicine Berlin, Augustenburger Platz 1, 13353 Berlin, Germany. [3]Department of Child and Adolescent Psychiatry, Psychosomatics and Psychotherapy, Charité University Medicine Berlin, Augustenburger Platz 1, 13353 Berlin, Germany. [4]Department of Psychiatry, The Zucker Hillside Hospital, Northwell Health, 75-59 263rd St, Glen Oaks, NY 11004, USA. [5]Department of Psychiatry and Molecular Medicine, Donald and Barbara Zucker School of Medicine at Hofstra/Northwell, 500 Hofstra Blvd, Hempstead, NY 11549, USA.

References

1. Dawson R. Eating disorders in children and adolescents. Pediatr Ann. 2018. https://doi.org/10.3928/19382359-20180523-01.
2. Karazsia BT, Murnen SK, Tylka TL. Is body dissatisfaction changing across time? A cross-temporal meta-analysis. Psychol Bull. 2017. https://doi.org/10.1037/bul0000081.
3. Latzer Y, Azaiza F, Tzischinsky O. Not just a western girls' problem: eating attitudes among Israeli-Arab adolescent boys and girls. Int J Adolesc Youth. 2014. https://doi.org/10.1080/02673843.2012.747973.
4. Keel PK, Forney KJ. Psychosocial risk factors for eating disorders. Int J Eat Disord. 2013. https://doi.org/10.1002/eat.22094.
5. Schienkiewitz A, Brettschneider AK, Damerow S, Rosario AS. Übergewicht und Adipositas im Kindes-und Jugendalter in Deutschland - Querschnittergebnisse aus KiGGS Welle 2 und Trends. Journal of Health Monitoring. 2018a. https://doi.org/10.17886/RKI-GBE-2018-005.
6. Moore JX, Chaudhary N, Akinyemiju T. Metabolic syndrome prevalence by race/ethnicity and sex in the United States, National Health and nutrition examination survey, 1988-2012. Prev Chronic Dis. 2017. https://doi.org/10.5888/pcd14.160287.
7. Herpertz-Dahlmann B. Adolescent eating disorders: update on definitions, symptomatology, epidemiology, and comorbidity. Child Adoles Psychiatr Clin N Am. 2015. https://doi.org/10.1016/j.chc.2014.08.003.
8. Nagl M, Jacobi C, Paul M, Beesdo-Baum K, Höfler M, Lieb R, Wittchen HU. Prevalence, incidence, and natural course of anorexia and bulimia nervosa among adolescents and young adults. Eur Child Adolesc Psychiatry. 2016. https://doi.org/10.1007/s00787-015-0808-z.
9. Swanson SA, Crow SJ, Le Grange D, Swendsen J, Merikangas KR. Prevalence and correlates of eating disorders in adolescents. Results from the national comorbidity survey replication adolescent supplement. Arch Gen Psychiatry. 2011. https://doi.org/10.1001/archgenpsychiatry.2011.22.
10. Herpertz-Dahlmann B, Dempfle A, Konrad K, Klasen F, Ravens-Sieberer U. Eating disorder symptoms do not just disappear: the implications of adolescent eating-disordered behaviour for body weight and mental health in young adulthood. Eur Child Adolesc Psychiatry. 2015. https://doi.org/10.1007/s00787-014-0610-3.
11. Legenbauer T, Thiemann P, Vocks S. Body image disturbance in children and adolescents with eating disorders Current evidence and future directions. Z Kinder Jugendpsychiatr Psychother. 2014. https://doi.org/10.1024/1422-4917/a000269.
12. American Psychiatric Association. Diagnostic and statistical manual of mental disorders. 5th ed. Washington: American Psychiatric Association; 2013.
13. World Health Organization. International classification of diseases. 10th ed. Geneva: Huber; 1997.
14. Culbert KM, Racine SE, Klump KL. Research review: what we have learned about the causes of eating disorders - a synthesis of sociocultural, psychological, and biological research. J Child Psychol Psychiatry. 2015. https://doi.org/10.1111/jcpp.12441.
15. Evans EH, Adamson AJ, Basterfield L, Le Couteur A, Reilly JK, Reilly JJ, Parkinson KN. Risk factors for eating disorder symptoms at 12 years of age: a 6-year longitudinal cohort study. Appetite. 2017. https://doi.org/10.1016/j.appet.2016.09.005.
16. Mandelli L, Arminio A, Atti A, De Ronchi D. Suicide attempts in eating disorder subtypes: a meta-analysis of the literature employing DSM-IV, DSM-5, or ICD-10 diagnostic criteria. Psychol Med. 2018. https://doi.org/10.1017/S0033291718003549.
17. Micali N, Solmi F, Horton NJ, Crosby RD, Eddy KT, Calzo JP, Sonneville KR, Swanson SA, Field AE. Adolescent eating disorders predict psychiatric, high-risk behaviors and weight outcomes in young adulthood. J Am Acad Child Adolesc Psychiatry. 2015. https://doi.org/10.1016/j.jaac.2015.05.009.
18. Smith AR, Zuromski KL, Dodd DR. Eating disorders and suicidality: what we know, what we don't know, and suggestions for future research. Curr Opin Psychol. 2018. https://doi.org/10.1016/j.copsyc.2017.08.023.
19. Fichter M, Quadflieg N. Strukturiertes Inventar für Anorektische und Bulimische Eßstörungen nach DSM-IV und ICD-10 (SIAB). Göttingen: Hogrefe; 1999.
20. Kromeyer-Hauschild K, Wabitsch M, Kunze D, Geller D, Heiß HC, Hesse V, von Hippel A, Jaeger U, Johnsen D, Korte W, Menner K, Müller G, Müller JM, Niemann-Pilatus A, Remer T, Schaefer F, Wittchen H-U, Zabransky S, Zellner K, Ziegler A, Hebebrand J. Percentiles of body mass index in children and adolescents evaluated from different regional German studies. Monatsschr Kinderheilkd. 2001. https://doi.org/10.1007/s001120170107.
21. Löwe B, Clement U. Der Fragebogen zum Körperbild (FKB-20). Literaturüberblick, Beschreibung und Prüfung eines Meßinstrumentes. Diagnostica. 1996;42:352–76.
22. Paul T, Thiel A. Eating Disorder Inventory-2: Deutsche Version. Göttingen: Hogrefe; 2004.
23. Galfo M, D'Addezio L, Censi L, Roccaldo R, Martone D. Overweight and Obesity in Italian Adolescents: Examined Prevalence and Socio-demographic Factors. Eur J Pers Cent Healthc. 2016. https://doi.org/10.21101/cejph.a4367.
24. Marques A, de Matos MG. Trends in prevalence of overweight and obesity: are Portuguese adolescents still increasing weight? Int J Public Health. 2016. https://doi.org/10.1007/s00038-015-0758-8.
25. Toftemo I, Jenum AK, Lagerløv P, Júlíusson PB, Falk RS, Sletner L. Contrasting patterns of overweight and thinness among preschool children of different ethnic groups in Norway, and relations with maternal and early life factors. BMC Public Health. 2018. https://doi.org/10.1186/s12889-018-5952-1.
26. Franssen SJ, Jansen P. Thinness and overweight in children from Amsterdam: a trend analysis and forecast. Ned Tijdschr Geneeskd. 2015; 159(43):A8967.
27. Keß A, Spielau U, Beger C, Gausche R, Vogel M, Lipek T, Körner A, Pfäffle R, Kiess W. Further stabilization and even decrease in the prevalence rates of overweight and obesity in German children and adolescents from 2005 to 2015: a cross-sectional and trend analysis. Public Health Nutr. 2017. https://doi.org/10.1017/S1368980017002257.
28. Hales CM, Carroll MD, Fryar CD, Ogden CL. Prevalence of obesity among adults and youth: United States, 2015–2016. NCHS data brief, no 288. Hyattsville: National Center for Health Statistics; 2017.
29. Schienkiewitz A, Brettschneider AK, Damerow S, Rosario AS. Prävalenz von Untergewicht, Übergewicht und Adipositas bei Kindern und Jugendlichen in Deutschland–Einordnung der Ergebnisse aus KiGGS Welle 2 nach internationalen Referenzsystemen. Journal of Health Monitoring. 2018b. https://doi.org/10.17886/RKI-GBE-2018-087.
30. Grajda A, Kułaga Z, Gurzkowska B, Góźdź M, Wojtyło M, Litwin M. The weight status of school-age children and its association with gross domestic product. Dev Period Med. 2017. https://doi.org/10.1007/s00431-017-2912-1.
31. Bundesministerium für Ernährung und Landwirtschaft (BMEL). Deutschland wie es isst. In: Der BMEL-Ernährungsreport 2016. BMEL. 2016. https://www.bmel.de/SharedDocs/Downloads/DE/Broschueren/Ernaehrungsreport2016.pdf?__blob=publicationFile&v=4. Accessed 05/02/2020.
32. Bredella MA. Sex differences in body composition. In: Mauvais-Jarvis F, editor. Sex and gender factors affecting metabolic homeostasis, Diabetes and Obesity: Advances in Experimental Medicine and Biology. Basel: Springer-Nature; 2017. p. 9–27.

33. MacNeill LP, Best LA, Davis LL. The role of personality in body image dissatisfaction and disordered eating: discrepancies between men and women. J Eat Disord. 2017. https://doi.org/10.1186/s40337-017-0177-8.
34. Balluck G, Toorabally BZ, Hosenally M. Association between body image dissatisfaction and body mass index, eating habits and weight control practices among Mauritian adolescents. Malays J Nutr. 2016;22(3):389–401.
35. Tatangelo, Connaughton C, McCabe M, Mellor D. Preadolescent boys' investment in masculine gender norms and their use of body change strategies. Psychol Men Masc. 2018. https://doi.org/10.1037/men0000087.
36. Quatman T, Watson CM. Gender differences in adolescent self-esteem: an exploration of domains. J Genet Psychol. 2001. https://doi.org/10.1080/00221320109597883.
37. Hyun MY, Jung YE, Kim MD, Kwak YS, Hong SC, Bahk WM, Yoon BH, Yoon H, Yoo B. Factors associated with body image distortion in Korean adolescents. Neuropsychiatr Dis and Treat. 2014. https://doi.org/10.2147/NDT.S63143.
38. Munro C, Randell L, Lawrie SM. An integrative bio-psycho-social theory of anorexia nervosa. Clin Psychol Psychother. 2017. https://doi.org/10.1002/cpp.2047.
39. Oldershaw A, Startup H, Lavender T. Anorexia nervosa and a lost emotional self: a psychological formulation of the development, maintenance, and treatment of anorexia nervosa. Front Psychol. 2019. https://doi.org/10.3389/fpsyg.2019.00219.
40. Gesundheitsberichterstattung des Bundes. Durchschnittliche Körpermaße der Bevölkerung. http://www.gbe-bund.de/oowa921-install/servlet/oowa/aw92/dboowasys921.xwdevkit/xwd_init?gbe.isgbetol/xs_start_neu/&p_aid=i&p_aid=89654477&nummer=223&p_sprache=D&p_indsp=-&p_aid=57158363. Accessed 05/08/2020.
41. Statista. Jugendliche in Deutschland nach Geschlecht im Vergleich mit der Bevölkerung im Jahr 2019. https://de.statista.com/statistik/daten/studie/900346/umfrage/umfrage-in-deutschland-zum-geschlecht-der-jugendlichen/. Accessed 05/08/2020.
42. Operationalized Psychodynamic Diagnostic System Task Force. Operationalized psychodynamic diagnosis OPD-2: manual of diagnosis and treatment planning. Cambridge: Hogrefe & Huber; 2008.
43. Huber E, Bock A, Hans M, Wieser E, Steinmayr-Gensluckner M, Seveck K, Benecke C. Experience of Emotions, Emotion Regulation, and Impaired Structural Integration in Adolescents. Psychotherapie Forum. 2017. https://doi.org/10.1007/s00729-016-0070-y.
44. Obbarius A, Sarrar L. The relation between self-reported symptoms of anorectic eating disorder and personality structure in female adolescents and young adults in an online sample. Psychotherapeut. 2020. https://doi.org/10.1007/s00278-020-00442-w.

An ARFID case report combining family-based treatment with the unified protocol for Transdiagnostic treatment of emotional disorders in children

Sarah Eckhardt[1*], Carolyn Martell[1], Kristina Duncombe Lowe[1], Daniel Le Grange[2,3] and Jill Ehrenreich-May[4]

Abstract

Background: This case report discusses the presentation and treatment of a nine-year-old female with a history of significant weight loss and food refusal using a combined approach of Family-Based Treatment (FBT) and the Unified Protocol for Transdiagnostic Treatment of Emotional Disorders in Children (UP-C).

Case presentation: The patient was diagnosed with avoidant/restrictive food intake disorder (ARFID), separation anxiety disorder, and a specific phobia of choking, and subsequently treated with a modified version of FBT, in conjunction with the UP-C. At the end of treatment, improvements were seen in the patient's weight and willingness to eat a full range of foods. Decreases in anxiety regarding eating/choking, fears of food being contaminated with gluten, and fears of eating while being away from parents were also observed.

Conclusions: These findings highlight promising results from this combined treatment approach, referred to as FBT + UP for ARFID. Further research is needed to evaluate the use of this treatment in patients presenting with a variety of ARFID symptoms.

Keywords: Avoidant/restrictive food intake disorder, Emotional disorders, Family-based treatment, Unified protocol, Transdiagnostic

Background

Avoidant/Restrictive Food Intake Disorder (ARFID), a complex and heterogeneous diagnosis, has been hypothesized along a dimensional model with presentations including sensory sensitivity, fear of aversive consequences, and lack of interest in eating [1, 2]. Significant literature exists on the treatment of pediatric feeding disorders supporting the use of behavioral feeding interventions among young children [3]. Recently, individual case reports/series have suggested other promising approaches for older children, adolescents, and adults with ARFID, using as a base either family-based treatment (FBT) [4–7];, cognitive behavioral therapy (CBT) [8–10];, or other novel approaches [11]. Despite these new approaches being studied, no published, randomized controlled trials have yet to evaluate their efficacy for the treatment of ARFID [2]. What appears to be lacking in the current treatment models is the ability to concurrently address the high rates of comorbid mood and anxiety disorders in patients with ARFID [12, 13], while also remaining focused on the medical complications associated with those patients who present underweight or exhibit significant nutritional deficiencies as part of this diagnosis. Consequently, this case presentation proposes a novel treatment approach that attempts to address both the psychological and emotional comorbidities associated in children and adolescents with ARFID, as well as the hallmark food avoidance features that appear across a heterogeneous array of presentations.

This case study describes the treatment of a patient with ARFID, using a combined approach of FBT [14] and the Unified Protocol for Transdiagnostic Treatment of Emotional Disorders in Children (UP-C) [15]. FBT +

* Correspondence: sarah.eckhardt@childrensmn.org
[1]Center for the Treatment of Eating Disorders, Children's Minnesota, Minneapolis, MN, USA
Full list of author information is available at the end of the article

UP for ARFID was developed through a 3 year case consultation process with treatment developers of both FBT and the UP-C. Treatment focuses on a combination of techniques aimed at addressing both weight gain/normalization of eating and additional symptoms including fear, disgust, and worry or obsessive thoughts, as well as varying forms of functionally-related avoidance behavior and potential concomitant reinforcement of avoidance by parents/caregivers. A major advantage of this combined approach is that it allows the clinician to personalize treatment based on the patient's specific presentation using a core set of evidence-based strategies and assessment tools (e.g., Top Problems [16];). The UP-C is transdiagnostic by definition, and contains evidence-based strategies that are flexible enough to address many of the maintaining symptoms that are unique to ARFID. There is also an adolescent version of the UP-C, which when combined with FBT makes this treatment model acceptable for a wide range of patients (named the Unified Protocol for Transdiagnostic Treatment of Emotional Disorders in Adolescents; UP-A). The UP for adults has previously been adapted for use with other eating disorder populations (anorexia nervosa, bulimia nervosa, and binge-eating disorder), with early results indicating improvments in anxiety sensitivity, experiential avoidance, and mindfulness [17].

While flexible, FBT + UP for ARFID always begins with sessions focused on FBT principles, including collaborative weighing, psychoeducation (specific to ARFID patients and their eating problems), family engagement, separating the eating problem from the child, charging parents with taking control of their child's eating (including increasing volume and variety of foods), promoting weight gain as needed, and a family meal. The UP-C or UP-A is then added to build skills that empower the patient to cope with difficult emotions, address avoidance, and increase tolerance of emotions or disgust responses. The Unified Protocol for Transdiagnostic Treatment of Emotional Disorders (UP) [18] is an emotion-focused, evidence-based treatment that targets the core dysfunction of neuroticism in adults [19]. It has subsequently been adapted to address emotional disorders in youth with the development of the Unified Protocols for Transdiagnostic Treatment of Emotional Disorders in Children and Adolescents (UP-C and UP-A respectively [15];). These protocols bring together cognitive-behavioral techniques, such as cognitive reappraisal, problem-solving and opposite action strategies, including a variety of exposure paradigms and behavioral activation, as well as mindfulness techniques into a single treatment. The UP-C and UP-A present the same skills as the UP; however, the skills have been adapted to be developmentally sensitive in their presentation, as well as in their delivery. Furthermore, the UP-C and UP-A also target core emotional parenting behaviors that are common across emotional disorders in youth (i.e. high levels of criticism, over-control/over protection, inconsistency, and modeling of avoidance [15]). Research has provided support for the efficacy and feasibility of the UP, UP-A and UP-C for individuals with mood, anxiety, and other emotional disorders. The UP, in particular, has been shown to lead to significant improvements at post-treatment [20], as well as maintenance of gains at follow-up time points [21] . The UP-C was originally designed as a group version of the UP-A, with concurrent child and parent group content. However, the UP-C may be delivered in an individual therapy model and explicit directions for doing so are presented in the therapist guide. Preliminary evidence suggests the UP-C may be similarly effective to leading CBT approaches for childhood anxiety, with potential benefits for those youth with higher levels of parent-reported sadness, dysregulation or depressive symptoms [22, 23]. The UP-A has also been shown to improve symptoms of emotional disorders in adolescents. Results from multiple baseline, open-trial and initial wait-list controlled trial studies showed that adolescents evidenced significant improvement in their symptoms after receiving 16 sessions of treatment using the UP-A and gains were maintained at follow-up time points [24–26]. While results of initial patient outcomes for this combined FBT + UP for ARFID approach are not yet available (given this treatment is currently being studied as part of a larger, clinic-wide effectiveness study), feedback from individual patients and practitioners who have been trained in the model through a clinical teaching day at the Academy of Eating Disorders International Conference has been positive [27]. Consent to share the following case was provided by the family and patient. Changes in identifying information were made to protect patient privacy.

Case presentation

"Laura" is a nine-year-old female, who presented with 38 lbs. of weight loss, poor oral intake, and medical instability in the context of fears about eating/choking secondary to a recent diagnosis of gluten intolerance. Ten months before she presented for treatment, Laura felt unwell after eating at a restaurant with her family. Following this experience, she became more anxious with eating, reporting frequent stomach aches and headaches. Laura's family tried a variety of elimination diets, including stopping all dairy and gluten. Laura was seen multiple times by her pediatrician, who ultimately recommended allergy and celiac testing. Over the course of this time Laura lost 29% of her overall body weight. Laura's symptoms continued to worsen, and she was eating little due to anxiety and a sensation of choking when eating. Parents noticed that her hair was falling out, her eyes appeared sunken, and she felt tired every day. She became increasingly afraid of separating from her parents, and her mother began getting calls from Laura's school (3–4 times per day) due to frequent stomach aches or requests to see her mother.

Prior to presentation, Laura's medical work-up showed focal chronic-type peptic duodenitis and reflux esophagitis. She was diagnosed with significant gluten sensitivity/intolerance, with a likely diagnosis of celiac disease. Laura had also been participating in weekly, individual play-based therapy for approximately 4 months to address her separation and other anxiety symptoms, without improvement. Her therapist did not have any expertise or experience in treating ARFID, therefore she was not focusing on weight regain or fears about eating. Laura was started on 20 mg of sertraline (liquid concentrate) 3 months prior to presentation at our service, though family had not seen any notable gains. Upon initial presentation to our team, Laura required hospitalization for 12 days for medical stabilization due to: symptomatic orthostasis, bradycardia, and severe malnutrition. During her hospital stay, Laura was diagnosed with ARFID, her sertraline was increased to 50 mg, and she was started on hydroxyzine, 5 mg TID to target pre-meal anxiety, nausea, and fullness. Following medical stabilization, Laura then began weekly outpatient treatment with her family to address the need for continued weight regain, anxiety/fears with eating, and separation anxiety. Given Laura had previously trended at or above the 85th percentile for BMI, the goal was to return her weight back to her personal healthy weight range.

The underlying assumption of FBT + UP for ARFID is that patients diagnosed with ARFID need a combination of treatment techniques that focus on both weight gain and/or normalizing eating while also addressing additional emotional disorder symptoms (i.e. anxiety, depression, obsessive-compulsive symptoms, emotional/situational avoidance). Patients and their parents begin with traditional FBT for several sessions (see Table 1 for content). Once progress with weight gain/regular eating are underway, the UP-C or UP-A modules are introduced. The UP-C has a flexible approach with core evidence-based principles and concurrent parenting content for emotional disorders that can be individualized for specific ARFID presentations [15]. Once the UP-C is added, the session breakdown continues as follows: 5 min weigh-in and update from patient on how eating is progressing, 30–40 min of individual therapy with the patient focused on the UP-C content, and 10–15 min with the patient and family to review session content, discuss how eating/weight gain are progressing, brainstorm challenges related to eating, and review homework/exposure practice. For younger patients, parents may be present for more/all of the session.

As illustrated in Table 2, over the course of treatment Laura's weight increased from 36.7 kg to 44.7 kg (percent goal weight from 81.4 to 91.4%), with family noting significant improvements in energy level and ability to participate in school and other physical activities. During initial FBT sessions, the focus was on weight gain using foods that Laura felt were safe and could allow her to regain weight efficiently. In session two, a family meal was completed, where the therapist worked to separate the illness from Laura and decrease blame (see FBT manual [14]), as well as discuss rewards that could be utilized to encourage Laura to challenge herself with eating. After two sessions of FBT (and with Laura's weight increasing), the UP-C was added to sessions, though the focus of each subsequent session also remained on weight regain and parental support/empowerment. Of note, Laura's family took to the principles of FBT quickly, but continued to benefit from each session's focus on graphing the patient's weight, problem solving any challenges during weeks where weight was stable or down, and empowering parents to work closely together on how to best refeed their daughter.

The patient and family identified three Top Problems (an ideographic assessment tool by Weisz et al. [16] modified for use in the UP-C and UP-A by Ehrenreich-May et al. [15]) they wanted to address in treatment including: 1) decrease fears of choking/eating feared foods, 2) be away from/eat away from mother, and 3) patient sleeping in her own bed again. Additionally, the therapist reinforced an overarching goal of Laura returning to a healthy weight range as crucial for her recovery. All subsequent treatment sessions involved reviewing Laura's weight/eating, teaching content from the UP-C modules, and discussing home learning assignments.

As treatment progressed and the patient learned skills to better manage her emotions, she became more willing to try foods that she was avoiding. With the help of the treating clinician, Laura created an exposure hierarchy with numerous feared foods and situations (e.g. meats, pasta, nuts, eating with adults other than her mother, eating at restaurants, being away from her mother, and sleeping in her own bed). Because Laura's fears of eating most foods were greatly impacting her overall functioning, the therapist chose to move up exposure work after introducing the three parts of the emotional experience, discussing the cycle of avoidance, and describing true/false alarms. During the exposure work, Laura created a ladder to break down the steps of each exposure, beginning with simply describing the food in a non-judgmental way and later touching, licking, taking a tiny bite, and eventually taking larger bites of these foods. Each of these skills were taught to Laura using specific content from the UP-C. Laura and her parents were encouraged by her success and began implementing exposures outside of sessions.

Laura continued to add more new foods at home and was able to attempt other types of foods in session. Once

Table 1 FBT + UP-C for ARFID session content

Session	Content
FBT Session 1	Collaborative weighing, psychoeducation (specific to ARFID patients), separating the eating problem from the child, charging parents with taking control of their child's eating, and beginning the discussion of utilizing rewards.
FBT Session 2	Engage family in family meal to further assess patient's eating, address any mealtime behaviors that are getting in the way of success, and work to empower parents to begin helping their child make changes to their eating.
FBT Sessions 3+	For very underweight patients, additional FBT sessions focus on building the parental alliance and discussing ways to improve the parent's ability to work together on the task of weight gain and related symptoms (food avoidance, anxieties around eating, etc). For patients who are not underweight or are gaining weight appropriately, the UP session content may begin to be added.
FBT + UP-C Module 1: Introduction to the Unified Protocol for the Treatment of Emotional Disorders in Children	Introduces child/parents to the treatment model/structure and describes the CLUES skills (Consider how I feel, Look at my thoughts, Use detective thinking and problem solving, Experience my feelings, Stay healthy and happy), discusses the purpose of emotions and begins to build emotional awareness, and identifies top problems and treatment goals. Top problems may focus on ARFID related goals or be more wide-range to address other emotional avoidance or related diagnoses.
FBT + UP-C Module 2: Getting to Know Your Emotions	Learn to identify and rate intensity of different emotions, normalizes emotional experiences, discusses the three parts of the emotional experience and the cycle of avoidance, explains true/false alarms, and identifies rewards for new behaviors.
FBT + UP-C Module 3: Using Science Experiments to Change our Emotions and Behavior	Learn about the concept of "acting opposite" and using science experiments to help with acting opposite/emotional behaviors, explains the connection between activity and emotion and assigns emotion and activity tracking as an experiment.
FBT + UP-C Module 4: Our Body Clues	Describe the concept of body clues and their relation to strong emotions, learn to identify body clues for different emotions, teach the skill of body scanning to develop awareness of body clues, help child practice experiencing body clues without using avoidance/distraction through interoceptive exposures.
FBT + UP-C Module 5: Look at my Thoughts	Introduce the concept of flexible thinking and teach children to recognize common "thinking traps."
FBT + UP-C Module 6: Use Detective Thinking	Introduce and apply detective thinking.
FBT + UP-C Module 7: Problem Solving and Conflict Management	Introduce and apply problem solving, discuss use of problem solving for interpersonal conflicts or challenges related to eating.
FBT + UP-C Module 8: Awareness of Emotional Experiences	Teach children about present moment awareness, introduce non-judgmental awareness- especially with relation to strong disgust responses.
FBT + UP-C Module 9: Introduction to Emotion Exposure	Review skills learned to date in the UP-C, review the concepts of emotional behaviors and "acting opposite" in preparation for a new type of science experiment called "exposure," complete a demonstration of an exposure using a toy or other object, work together with child and parents to begin developing plans for upcoming exposures.
FBT + UP-C Module 10: Facing Our Feelings – Part 1	Review the concept of using science experiments to face strong emotions, introduce the idea of safety behaviors and subtle avoidance behaviors (e.g., distraction), practice a science experiment to face strong emotions (sample situational emotion exposure), make plans for future science experiments for facing strong emotions (individualized situational emotion exposures).
FBT + UP-C Module 11: Facing Our Feelings – Part 2	Plan and execute initial situational emotion exposure in session, plan and execute additional situational emotion exposure activities in future sessions and at home.
FBT + UP-C Module 12: Wrap Up and Relapse Prevention	Review Emotion Detective skills learned in the UP-C program, plan for facing strong emotions in the future, celebrate progress made in treatment program, create a plan for sustaining and furthering progress after treatment, distinguish lapses from relapses and help family recognize warning signs of relapse.

in-session exposures became easier for Laura, the therapist had her add interoceptive exposures (e.g. running in place), while also eating feared foods to attempt to evoke increased feelings of anxiety and simulate a more naturalistic experience of distress. As therapy progressed, Laura began eating at restaurants again, as well as in more situations away from her mother (e.g., church, school cafeteria). She was able to stop the use of hydroxyzine, but continued on her sertraline. Treatment ended when Laura returned to eating nearly all foods, in numerous settings (school lunchroom, other's homes) away from her mother, and family felt able to manage remaining avoidance (e.g. working on eating at a greater variety of restaurants while away from their hometown). Laura had also regained weight to the

Table 2 Top problems and weight

	Baseline	End of treatment	5 months post treatment
Top Problems (Parent)			
Fear of choking/eating fear foods	8	3	2
Being away from mother/eating away from mother	8	2	2
Sleeping alone	7	2	0–1
Top Problems (Child)			
Fear of choking/eating fear foods	8	3	1
Being away from mother/eating away from mother	8	2	2–3
Sleeping alone	8	0	0
Weight Presentation			
Kilograms	36.7	44.7	50.4
BMI %ile	41.3	70.7	81.2
% Goal Weight	81.4	91.4	97.1

Top Problems were rated 0–8, with 0 being not a problem and 8 being very much a problem. BMI %ile = Body Mass Index Percentile. % Goal Weight = Percentage of treatment goal weight utilizing the 85th percentile for Body Mass Index

71st percentile for BMI (91.4% of her previously healthy weight range), and her parents felt fully equipped in their ability to continue helping her restore weight. Laura completed 29 sessions over the course of 10 months of weekly or biweekly therapy.

Discussion and conclusions

This case study illustrates that the FBT + UP for ARFID therapy model, which combines and modifies previously developed evidence-based treatments, was feasible and helpful in allowing this patient to gain weight, return to eating a diverse range of foods in a variety of settings, and decrease anxiety about eating/being away from her mother. Notably, when this family returned for a follow-up 5 months after completing treatment, the patient's weight had continued to increase (50.4 kg/81st percentile for BMI/97.1% of goal weight), she had started menstruating, and she was able to separate and eat apart from her mother without significant difficulty. The patient and parents also rated her fears of choking and eating previously feared foods as 1 and 2's on an 8-point likert scale (see Table 2).

This patient was a good treatment candidate for FBT + UP for ARFID given she endorsed significant anxiety prior to treatment and also met criteria for several concurrent anxiety disorder diagnoses. Another major benefit of the treatment is the ability to flexibly offer the various modules that may benefit each patient based on their specific needs and ARFID presentations. For example, this patient benefited from exposure work, learning non-judgmental awareness, and improving awareness of physical sensations, while other patients may need more focus on cognitive reappraisal, problem-solving, and other types of opposite action [15]. Additionally, given Laura had lost a significant amount of weight she required a treatment that also focused on weight restoration as one of its core principles. A major advantage of this combined treatment approach is the ability for clinicians to tailor each session to the specific needs of their individual patient, including returning to solely FBT sessions if weight gain or nutritional dificiencies are not progressing appropriately.

While several novel approaches for the treatment of ARFID have been suggested [7, 10, 11], randomized control trials have yet to be presented regarding their efficacy. Even with some intervention research aiming to address the heterogeneous symptoms of ARFID, no treatment to date has proposed a model that addresses both the varied presentations of ARFID, as well as its full range of common comorbid disorders, in one cohesive approach that is flexible and adaptable to the individual. While the development of symptom specific treatment approaches to ARFID is logical, it does not address the heterogeneous nature of this disorder and can impede dissemination [28]. With so many different presentations of ARFID and high rates of comorbid disorders, one clear treatment that can be used flexibly to adapt to the range of ARFID presentations and co-occurring disorders would provide an efficient and cohesive approach to treating youth with ARFID. Further examination of FBT + UP for a wide-range of ARFID presentations among youth continues. A study to establish an ideal combination of FBT and UP strategies for youth with ARFID between the ages of 6–18 years, and the preliminary efficacy of this approach, is a next logical step in this research.

Finally, some limitations with this case study should be noted. First, it was not possible to ascertain whether FBT in isolation would have worked as effectively for this patient as this combined FBT + UP-C approach. While anxiety reduction has been shown in nutritional-based therapies, such as FBT, it is unclear if patients with profound phobic and other concurrent anxiety would benefit as greatly without specific skills and exposure work inherent in the UP-C. Additional limitations of this case study include the absence of objective assessment of psychological outcomes. That said, this young person made significant improvements in terms of weight, both at completion of treatment and at follow-up. Moreover, *Top Problems* rating by both the patient and parents also appear to indicate meaningful improvements in a variety of behavioral domains. However, without objective measures it is difficult to ascertain whether anxiety reduction allowed for behavioral change, or whether behavioral change caused anxiety reduction over the course of the UP-C. Future studies should attempt to parce out when and for whom this combined treatment approach is most effective.

Abbreviations

ARFID: Avoidant/Restrictive Food Intake Disorder; FBT: Family Based Treatment; FBT+UP: Family Based Treatment with the Unified Protocol; Kg: Kilograms; TID: Three times a day; UP: Unified Protocol for Transdiagnostic Treatment of Emotional Disorders; UP-A: Unified Protocol for Transdiagnostic Treatment of Emotional Disorders in Adolescents; UP-C: Unified Protocol for Transdiagnostic Treatment of Emotional Disorders in Children

Acknowledgements

We acknowledge the generous financial support from the Goven Family Foundation. We would also like to thank Dr. Julie Lesser for her contributions in the initial conceptualization of this treatment model.

Authors' contributions

SE took primary responsibility for the manuscript, including reviewing relevant literature and drafting the paper for publication. CM and KDL assisted with literature review and editing of the manuscript. DLG and JEM contributed to treatment protocol development and critical review of the manuscript. All authors read and approved the final manuscript.

Competing interests

Dr. Le Grange receives royalties from Guilford Press as well as Routledge. He is Co-Director of the Training Institute for Child and Adolescent Eating Disorders, LLC. Dr. Jill Ehrenreich-May receives royalties from the sales of the therapist guide and workbooks for the Unified Protocols for Transdiagnostic Treatment of Emotional Disorders in Children and Adolescents (UP-C and UP-A) from Oxford University Press. She also receives payments for UP-C and UP-A clinical trainings, consultation and implementation support services.

Author details

[1]Center for the Treatment of Eating Disorders, Children's Minnesota, Minneapolis, MN, USA. [2]Department of Psychiatry, University of California, San Francisco, CA, USA. [3]Department of Psychiatry and Behavioral Neuroscience, The University of Chicago, Chicago, IL, USA. [4]Department of Psychology, University of Miami, Coral Gables, FL, USA.

References

1. American Psychiatric Association. Diagnostic and statistical manual of mental disorders: DSM-5: American Psychiatric Association. Arlington: DSM; 2013.
2. Thomas JJ, Lawson EA, Micali N, Misra M, Deckersbach T, Eddy KT. Avoidant/restrictive food intake disorder: a three-dimensional model of neurobiology with implications for etiology and treatment. Curr Psychiatry Rep. 2017;19(8):54.
3. Sharp WG, Jaquess DL, Morton JF, Herzinger CV. Pediatric feeding disorders: a quantitative synthesis of treatment outcomes. Clin Child Fam Psychol Rev. 2010;13(4):348–65.
4. Bryant-Waugh R. Avoidant restrictive food intake disorder: an illustrative case example. Int J Eat Disord. 2013;46(5):420–3.
5. Fitzpatrick KK, Forsberg SE, Colborn D. Family-based therapy for avoidant restrictive food intake disorder: families facing food neophobias. In: Loeb K, Le Grange D, Lock J, editors. Family therapy for adolescent eating and weight disorders. New York: Routledge; 2015. p. 276–96.
6. Loeb K, Le Grange D, Lock J. Family therapy for adolescent eating and weight disorders: new applications. New York: Routledge; 2015.
7. Lock J, Robinson A, Sadeh-Sharvit S, Rosania K, Osipov L, Kirz N, Derenne J, Utzinger L. Applying family-based treatment (FBT) to three clinical presentations of avoidant/restrictive food intake disorder: similarities and differences from FBT for anorexia nervosa. Int J Eat Disord. 2019;52(4):439–46.
8. Mammel KA, Ornstein RM. Avoidant/restrictive food intake disorder: a new eating disorder diagnosis in the diagnostic and statistical manual 5. Curr Opin Pediatr. 2017;29(4):407–13.
9. Dumont E, Jansen A, Kroes D, de Haan E, Mulkens S. A new cognitive behavior therapy for adolescents with avoidant/restrictive food intake disorder in a day treatment setting: a clinical case series. Int J Eat Disord. 2019;52(4):447–58.
10. Thomas JJ, Eddy KT. Cognitive-behavioral therapy for avoidant/restrictive food intake disorder: children, adolescents, and adults. Cambridge: Cambridge University Press; 2018.
11. Zucker NL, LaVia MC, Craske MG, Foukal M, Harris AA, Datta N, Savereide E, Maslow GR. Feeling and body investigators (FBI): ARFID division—an acceptance-based interoceptive exposure treatment for children with ARFID. Int J Eat Disord. 2019;52(4):466–72.
12. Nicely TA, Lane-Loney S, Masciulli E, Hollenbeak CS, Ornstein RM. Prevalence and characteristics of avoidant/restrictive food intake disorder in a cohort of young patients in day treatment for eating disorders. J Eat Disord. 2014;2(1):21.
13. Duncombe Lowe K, Barnes TL, Martell C, Keery H, Eckhardt S, Peterson CB, Lesser J, Le Grange D. Youth with avoidant/restrictive food intake disorder: examining differences by age, weight status, and symptom duration. Nutrients. 2019;11(8):1955.
14. Lock J, Le Grange D. Treatment manual for anorexia nervosa: a family-based approach. 2nd ed. New York: Guilford Press; 2012.
15. Ehrenreich-May J, Kennedy SM, Sherman JA, Bilek EL, Buzzella BA, Bennett SM, Barlow DH. Unified protocols for transdiagnostic treatment of emotional disorders in children and adolescents: therapist guide. New York: Oxford University Press; 2018.
16. Weisz JR, Chorpita BF, Frye A, Ng MY, Lau N, Bearman SK, Ugueto AM, Langer DA, Hoagwood KE. Youth top problems: using idiographic, consumer-guided assessment to identify treatment needs and to track change during psychotherapy. J Consult Clin Psychol. 2011;79(3):369.
17. Thompson-Brenner H, Boswell JF, Espel-Huynh H, Brooks G, Lowe MR. Implementation of transdiagnostic treatment for emotional disorders in residential eating disorder programs: a preliminary pre-post evaluation. Psychother Res. 2019;29(8):1045-61.
18. Barlow DH, Ellard KK, Fairholme CP, Farchione TJ, Boisseau CI, Allen LB, Ehrenreich-May JT. Unified protocol for transdiagnostic treatment of emotional disorders: therapist guide. 2nd ed. New York: Oxford University Press; 2018.
19. Marchette LK, Weisz JR. Practitioner review: empirical evolution of youth psychotherapy toward transdiagnostic approaches. J Child Psychol Psychiatry. 2017;58(9):970–84.
20. Farchione TJ, Fairholme CP, Ellard KK, Boisseau CL, Thompson-Hollands J, Carl JR, Gallagher MW, Barlow DH. Unified protocol for transdiagnostic treatment of emotional disorders: a randomized controlled trial. Behav Ther. 2012;43(3):666–78.
21. Bullis JR, Fortune MR, Farchione TJ, Barlow DH. A preliminary investigation of the long-term outcome of the unified protocol for Transdiagnostic treatment of emotional disorders. Compr Psychiatry. 2014;55(8):1920–7.
22. Kennedy SM, Bilek EL, Ehrenreich-May J. A randomized controlled pilot trial of the unified protocol for transdiagnostic treatment of emotional disorders in children. Behav Modif. 2019;43(3):330–60.
23. Kennedy SM, Tonarely NA, Sherman JA, Ehrenreich-May J. Predictors of treatment outcome for the unified protocol for transdiagnostic treatment of emotional disorders in children (UP-C). J Anxiety Disord. 2018;57:66–75.
24. Ehrenreich-May J, Rosenfield D, Queen AH, Kennedy SM, Remmes CS, Barlow DH. An initial waitlist-controlled trial of the unified protocol for the treatment of emotional disorders in adolescents. J Anxiety Disord. 2017;46:46–55.
25. Ehrenreich JT, Goldstein CR, Wright LR, Barlow DH. Development of a unified protocol for the treatment of emotional disorders in youth. Child Family Behav Ther. 2009;31(1):20–37.
26. Queen AH, Barlow DH, Ehrenreich-May J. The trajectories of adolescent anxiety and depressive symptoms over the course of a transdiagnostic treatment. J Anxiety Disord. 2014;28(6):511–21.
27. Lesser JK, Eckhardt S, Le Grange D, Ehrenreich-May J. Integrating family based treatment with the unified protocol for the transdiagnostic treatment of emotional disorders: A novel treatment for avoidant restrictive food intake disorder. Prague: Academy of Eating Disorders International Conference; 2017. [Clinical teaching day]
28. McHugh RK, Barlow DH. The dissemination and implementation of evidence-based psychological treatments: a review of current efforts. Am Psychol. 2010;65(2):73.

Permissions

All chapters in this book were first published by BioMed Central; hereby published with permission under the Creative Commons Attribution License or equivalent. Every chapter published in this book has been scrutinized by our experts. Their significance has been extensively debated. The topics covered herein carry significant findings which will fuel the growth of the discipline. They may even be implemented as practical applications or may be referred to as a beginning point for another development.

The contributors of this book come from diverse backgrounds, making this book a truly international effort. This book will bring forth new frontiers with its revolutionizing research information and detailed analysis of the nascent developments around the world.

We would like to thank all the contributing authors for lending their expertise to make the book truly unique. They have played a crucial role in the development of this book. Without their invaluable contributions this book wouldn't have been possible. They have made vital efforts to compile up to date information on the varied aspects of this subject to make this book a valuable addition to the collection of many professionals and students.

This book was conceptualized with the vision of imparting up-to-date information and advanced data in this field. To ensure the same, a matchless editorial board was set up. Every individual on the board went through rigorous rounds of assessment to prove their worth. After which they invested a large part of their time researching and compiling the most relevant data for our readers.

The editorial board has been involved in producing this book since its inception. They have spent rigorous hours researching and exploring the diverse topics which have resulted in the successful publishing of this book. They have passed on their knowledge of decades through this book. To expedite this challenging task, the publisher supported the team at every step. A small team of assistant editors was also appointed to further simplify the editing procedure and attain best results for the readers.

Apart from the editorial board, the designing team has also invested a significant amount of their time in understanding the subject and creating the most relevant covers. They scrutinized every image to scout for the most suitable representation of the subject and create an appropriate cover for the book.

The publishing team has been an ardent support to the editorial, designing and production team. Their endless efforts to recruit the best for this project, has resulted in the accomplishment of this book. They are a veteran in the field of academics and their pool of knowledge is as vast as their experience in printing. Their expertise and guidance has proved useful at every step. Their uncompromising quality standards have made this book an exceptional effort. Their encouragement from time to time has been an inspiration for everyone.

The publisher and the editorial board hope that this book will prove to be a valuable piece of knowledge for researchers, students, practitioners and scholars across the globe.

List of Contributors

Liv Sand
Regional Centre for Child and Youth Mental Health and Child Welfare, Ove Heradstveit, NORCE Norwegian Research Centre, RKBU, Nygårdsgaten 112, 5008 Bergen, Norway

Ove Heradstveit
Regional Centre for Child and Youth Mental Health and Child Welfare, Ove Heradstveit, NORCE Norwegian Research Centre, RKBU, Nygårdsgaten 112, 5008 Bergen, Norway
Center for Alcohol & Drug Research, Stavanger University Hospital, Stavanger, Norway

Eva Holmelid, Helene Klundby and Birgitte Søreide
Faculty of Psychology, University of Bergen, Bergen, Norway

Børge Sivertsen
Department of Health Promotion, Norwegian Institute of Public Health, Bergen, Norway
Department of Research & Innovation, Helse Fonna HF, Haugesund, Norway
Department of Mental Health, Norwegian University of Science and Technology, Trondheim, Norway

Cheryl Webb, Sheri Findlay, Neera Bhatnagar, Natasha Snelgrove, Amanda Ritsma and Melissa Kimber
McMaster University, Hamilton, Canada

Jennifer Couturier
Department of Psychiatry & Behavioural Neurosciences, McMaster University, Hamilton, ON L8N3Z5, Canada

Mark Norris and Melissa Brouwers
University of Ottawa, Ottawa, Canada

Leanna Isserlin and Wendy Spettigue
Department of Psychiatry, Children's Hospital of Eastern Ontario, University of Ottawa, Ottawa, ON K1H 8L1, Canada
Children's Hospital of Eastern Ontario Research Institute, Ottawa, ON K1H 8L1, Canada

Gail McVey, Ahmed Boachie, Seena Grewal and Cathleen Steinegger
University of Toronto, Toronto, Canada

Wendy Preskow
National Initiative for Eating Disorders, Toronto, Canada

Catherine Miller and Jennifer Scarborough
Canadian Mental Health Association - Waterloo, Wellington, Dufferin, Kitchener, Canada

Jennifer Coelho and Josie Geller
The Univeristy of British Columbia, Vancouver, Canada

Rachel Loewen, Techiya Loewen and Elizabeth Waite
Woodstock, Canada

Catherine Ford
Ontario Ministry of Health and Long-Term Care, Toronto, Canada

Kerry Bourret
St. Joseph's Care Group - Thunder Bay, Thunder Bay, Canada

Joanne Gusella and David Pilon
Dalhousie University, Halifax, Canada

Adele LaFrance
Laurentian University, Sudbury, Canada

Anick LeClerc
McMaster Children's Hospital, Hamilton, Canada

Monique Jericho and Gina Dimitropoulos
University of Calgary, Calgary, Canada

Yi Wu and Amy Harrison
Department of Psychology and Human Development, Institute of Education, University College London, 25 Woburn Square, London WC1H 0AA, UK

Helene Keery, Sarah LeMay-Russell and Julie Lesser
Center for the Treatment of Eating Disorders, Children's Minnesota, Minneapolis, MN, USA

Timothy L. Barnes
Center for the Treatment of Eating Disorders, Children's Minnesota, Minneapolis, MN, USA
Children's Minnesota Research Institute, Children's Minnesota, Minneapolis, MN, USA

Carol B. Peterson
Department of Psychiatry, University of Minnesota, Minneapolis, MN, USA
The Emily Program, St. Paul, MN, USA

Sasha Gorrell
Department of Psychiatry, University of California, San Francisco, CA, USA

Daniel Le Grange
Department of Psychiatry, University of California, San Francisco, CA, USA
Department of Psychiatry and Behavioral Neuroscience, The University of Chicago, Chicago, IL, USA

Simona Calugi and Riccardo Dalle Grave
Department of Eating and Weight Disorders, Villa Garda Hospital, Via Montebaldo 89 1-37016 Garda (VR), Verona, Italy

Jocelyn Lebow
Department of Psychiatry and Psychology, Mayo Clinic, Mayo Clinic School of Medicine, 200 First Street SW, Rochester, MN 55905, USA
Mayo Clinic Robert D. and Patricia E. Kern Center for the Science of Health Care Delivery, Rochester, MN, USA

Julie Hathaway, Kristin Vickers and Leslie Sim
Department of Psychiatry and Psychology, Mayo Clinic, Mayo Clinic School of Medicine, 200 First Street SW, Rochester, MN 55905, USA

Cassandra Narr, Angela Mattke and Marcie Billings
Department of Pediatric and Adolescent Medicine, Mayo Clinic School of Medicine, Rochester, MN, USA

Robert Jacobson
Mayo Clinic Robert D. and Patricia E. Kern Center for the Science of Health Care Delivery, Rochester, MN, USA
Department of Pediatric and Adolescent Medicine, Mayo Clinic School of Medicine, Rochester, MN, USA

Janna R. Gewirtz O'Brien
Department of Pediatrics, University of Minnesota, Minneapolis, MN, USA

Kirrilly M. Pursey
Faculty of Health and Medicine, University of Newcastle, Callaghan 2308, NSW, Australia

Phillipa Hay
Campbelltown and Camden Hospitals, Campbelltown, NSW, Australia
Translational Health Research Institute (THRI), School of Medicine, Western Sydney University, Sydney, Campbelltown, Australia
Campbelltown Hospital, SWSLHD, Sydney, Campbelltown, Australia

Kay Bussey, Nora Trompeter and Alexandra Lonergan
Department of Psychology and Centre for Emotional Health, Macquarie University, Sydney, NSW, Australia

Kathleen M. Pike
Departments of Psychiatry and Epidemiology, Columbia University Irving Medical Center, New York, NY, USA

Jonathon Mond
Centre for Rural Health, University of Tasmania, Launceston, Australia
School of Medicine, Western Sydney University, Campbelltown, Australia

Deborah Mitchison
Translational Health Research Institute (THRI), School of Medicine, Western Sydney University, Sydney, Campbelltown, Australia
Centre for Emotional Health, Department of Psychology, Macquarie University, North Ryde, New South Wales, Australia

Elizabeth Parker
Department of Dietetics & Nutrition, Westmead Hospital, Wentworthville, NSW 2145, Australia
Sydney School of Health Sciences, Faculty of Medicine and Health, The University of Sydney, Sydney 2006, NSW, Australia

Terri Maister and Anita Stefoska-Needham
SMART Foods Centre, School of Medicine, Faculty of Science, Medicine and Health, University of Wollongong, Wollongong, NSW 2522, Australia

Christine Wearne
Department of Medical Psychology, Westmead Hospital, Westmead, NSW 2145, Australia

Gail Anderson and Linette Gomes
Department of Adolescent & Young Adult Medicine, Westmead Hospital, Westmead, NSW 2145, Australia

Simon Clarke and Michael Kohn
Department of Adolescent & Young Adult Medicine, Westmead Hospital, Westmead, NSW 2145, Australia
Sydney School of Medicine, Faculty of Medicine and Health, The University of Sydney, Sydney, NSW 2006, Australia
Centre for Research into AdolescentS' Health (CRASH), Adolescent & Young Adult Medicine, Westmead Hospital, Westmead, NSW 2145, Australia

Mark Norris
Children's Hospital of Eastern Ontario Research Institute, Ottawa, ON K1H 8L1, Canada
Division of Adolescent Health, Department of Pediatrics, Children's Hospital of Eastern Ontario, University of Ottawa, Ottawa, ON K1H 8L1, Canada

Samantha F. Kennedy
Department of Psychiatry, Michigan State University, 909 Wilson Rd, Room B119, East Lansing, MI 48824, USA

Jeffrey Kovan
Department of Sports Medicine, Michigan State University, East Lansing, MI 48824, USA

Emily Werner
Department of Kinesiology, Michigan State University, East Lansing, MI 48824, USA

Ryley Mancine and Donald Gusfa
Michigan State University College of Osteopathic Medicine, Michigan State University, East Lansing, MI 48824, USA

Heather Kleiman
Grand Ledge High School, Grand Ledge, MI 48837, USA

Julian Baudinet, Mima Simic, Helena Griffiths, Cecily Donnelly, Catherine Stewart and Elizabeth Goddard
Maudsley Centre for Child and Adolescent Eating Disorders, Maudsley Hospital, De Crespigny Park, Denmark Hill, London SE8 5AZ, UK

Adam Burt
School of Medicine, Western Sydney University, Sydney, Campbelltown, Australia

Elizabeth Dale
Ngarruwan Ngadju First Peoples Health and Wellbeing Research Centre, Australian Health Services Research Institute and Illawarra Health and Medical Research Institute, School of Psychology, University of Wollongong, Wollongong, New South Wales, Australia

Alicia Parra Carriedo, Antonio Tena-Suck, Gladys María Bilbao y Morcelle, Mary Carmen Díaz Gutiérrez, Isabel Flores Galicia and Alejandra Ruiz-Shuayre
Universidad Iberoamericana CDMX, México, Mexico

Miriam Wendolyn Barajas-Márquez
Universidad Nacional Autónoma de México, Mexico, Mexico

Eva Naumann and Jennifer Svaldi
Department of Clinical Psychology and Psychotherapy, University of Tuebingen, Schleichstrasse 4, 72076 Tuebingen, Germany

Stefanie C. Biehl
Department of Clinical Psychology and Psychotherapy, University of Tuebingen, Schleichstrasse 4, 72076 Tuebingen, Germany
Department of Clinical Psychology and Psychotherapy, University of Regensburg, Universitaetsstrasse 31, 93053 Regensburg, Germany

Julian Keil
Biological Psychology, Christian-Albrechts University, Olshausenstraße 62, 24118 Kiel, Germany

Lea Sarrar
Department of Psychology, Medical School Berlin, Germany, Rüdesheimer Straße 50, 14197 Berlin, Germany
Department of Audiology and Phoniatrics, Charité University Medicine Berlin, Augustenburger Platz 1, 13353 Berlin, Germany

Marie Vilalta
Department of Psychology, Medical School Berlin, Germany, Rüdesheimer Straße 50, 14197 Berlin, Germany

Nora Schneider
Department of Child and Adolescent Psychiatry, Psychosomatics and Psychotherapy, Charité University Medicine Berlin, Augustenburger Platz 1, 13353 Berlin, Germany

Christoph U. Correll
Department of Child and Adolescent Psychiatry, Psychosomatics and Psychotherapy, Charité University Medicine Berlin, Augustenburger Platz 1, 13353 Berlin, Germany
Department of Psychiatry, The Zucker Hillside Hospital, Northwell Health, 75-59 263rd St, Glen Oaks, NY 11004, USA
Department of Psychiatry and Molecular Medicine, Donald and Barbara Zucker School of Medicine at Hofstra/Northwell, 500 Hofstra Blvd, Hempstead, NY 11549, USA

Sarah Eckhardt, Carolyn Martell and Kristina Duncombe Lowe
Center for the Treatment of Eating Disorders, Children's Minnesota, Minneapolis, MN, USA

Jill Ehrenreich-May
Department of Psychology, University of Miami, Coral Gables, FL, USA

Index

Printed in the USA
CPSIA information can be obtained
at www.ICGtesting.com
LVHW080052211023
761596LV00010BA/2030

9 781646 475841